DRUG DESIGN AND DEVELOPMENT

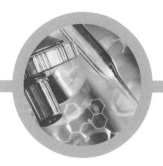

DRUG DESIGN AND DEVELOPMENT

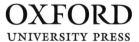

OXFORD
UNIVERSITY PRESS

OXFORD
UNIVERSITY PRESS

Great Clarendon Street, Oxford, OX2 6DP,
United Kingdom

Oxford University Press is a department of the University of Oxford.
It furthers the University's objective of excellence in research, scholarship,
and education by publishing worldwide. Oxford is a registered trade mark of
Oxford University Press in the UK and in certain other countries

© Oxford University Press 2020

The moral rights of the author have been asserted

Impression: 1

Published in the United States of America by Oxford University Press
198 Madison Avenue, New York, NY 10016, United States of America

British Library Cataloguing in Publication Data
Data available

Library of Congress Control Number: 2019957851

ISBN 978–0–19–874931–8

Printed in Great Britain by
Bell & Bain Ltd., Glasgow

TABLE OF CONTENTS

DETAILED TABLE OF CONTENTS

CASE STUDIES

GUIDE TO THE BOOK

Changes to pharmacy education have recently taken place demonstrating an increasing trend towards the integration of pharmaceutical science with the practice elements of pharmacy. One particular area of pharmaceutical science in which students struggle to see the relevance to pharmacy practice is drug design and development i.e. the science involved in bringing a drug to market. This book presents the processes involved in the design and development of new drugs and emphasises the significance of these processes to the practice of pharmacy. Whilst there is general acceptance by students that drug design and development are vital to the pharmaceutical industry, there is a need to demonstrate that an understanding of these subjects is just as important to the pharmacist in hospital or the community.

A novel approach of the book is the consideration of both drug design and development in one volume, which varies from the existing way of presenting these two topics in different texts. This is achieved by presenting the drug journey from discovery to market in an integrated fashion, emphasising the interconnection of all the processes involved. Features are utilised which are designed to help students master the material and encourage them to see the relevance to other aspects of the pharmacy disciplines.

BOX 2.1   HYDROPHOBIC BONDING–DOES IT EXIST AN

There is an amount of uncertainty about how hydrophobic bonds are f
bic bonds were developed as a useful concept to explain the interac
and ligands. It is postulated that thermodynamics can provide an expl
of hydrophobic regions causes a disruption of the ordered structure o
a biological environment. This causes an increase in entropy and thus
ing to an increase in stability. It has also been suggested that lipophil

BOX

Additional material that adds interest or depth to concepts covered in the main text, including how the information is specifically relevant for pharmacists and pharmaceutical scientists.

 DNA and RNA both consist of repeating units of nuc
sugar, and a phosphate group.
The heterocyclic bases in DNA are cytosine, thymine
DNA takes the form of a double helix in which two
bonds. RNA has a single-stranded structure and co

KEY POINT

The important 'take home messages' that you must have a good grasp of are highlighted in these sections. These are designed to help form a basis for your revision.

INTEGRATION BOX 2.3   ACETYLCHOLINE AS A NEURO

Acetylcholine, as a neurotransmitter, acts at two different types
junction and at autonomic ganglia are called nicotinic receptors and
Section 2.2.3). They are so called because they respond to nicoti
target organs within the parasympathetic nervous system are (
Section 2.2.4) and are called muscarinic receptors because they re
of muscarinic receptor. M, receptors are associated with CNS excit
tinal motility. They are excitatory receptors. M, receptors are inhi

INTEGRATION BOX

The material in these boxes explains how the information in the chapter relates to other areas of pharmacy, highlighting the integrated nature of the subject.

**CASE STUDY 2.1   DRUGS INSPIRED BY ENDO
DEVELOPMENT OF β-BLOC**

Adrenergic receptors are all G-protein coupled receptors and one of
into α_1, α_2, β_1, β_2, and β_3. The endogenous agonist for these recepto
tors are present in the heart and stimulation of them increases the f
The development of β-blockers was instituted in the 1950s by Sir Jame
useful in the treatment of angina (and subsequently hypertension, my
For a medicinal chemist looking to develop an antagonist, the best

CASE STUDY

Case studies provide a direct link between the science you are learning across your degree programme and the way in which you will apply this knowledge as a practicing pharmacist or pharmaceutical scientist. Reflection questions and sample answers encourage critical thinking around the points raised in the case study.

There is a small group of drugs which act as enzyme inhib
Irinotecan, a drug derived from the natural product campto
a group of enzymes responsible for the supercoiling, cleavag
(❯ **XR Section 4.1.4**). However the clinical use of irinotecan
toxicity and chemical instability. Drugs used as anti-cance
include doxorubicin and mitoxantrone (❯ **XR Section 4.3.2**
their cardiotoxicity. Also acting in a similar fashion but aga
isomerases, are the fluoroquinolone antibacterial agents.

CROSS REFERENCES

Cross references link related information across the whole textbook, to give you a good idea of how integrated the subject is. These will allow you to understand how one piece of information is applicable across a whole range of subjects.

 Further reading

Copeland, R.A., Harpel, M.R., and Tummino, P.J. (2007) Targeting e
  Therapeutic Targets 11: 967–78.
  A comprehensive review of the role of enzyme inhibitors in drug

Lowe, D. (2010) In the pipeline, *Chemistry World*, September 7: 18.
  An industrial medicinal chemist's perspective on enzyme inhibito

FURTHER READING

At the end of each chapter is a list of additional resources we encourage you to seek out, in your library or online. They will help you gain a deeper understanding of the material presented in the text.

ONLINE RESOURCES

The online materials accompanying *Drug Design and Development* include case studies from the book and 10 multiple-choice questions for each chapter, with answers and feedback.

Go to: www.oup.com/he/rostron1e

LECTURER SUPPORT MATERIALS

For registered adopters of this book, our online resources also feature figures in electronic format, available to download, for use in lecture presentations and other educational resources.

To register as an adopter, visit www.oup.com/he/rostron1e and follow the on-screen instructions.

ABBREVIATIONS

5-FU	5-fluorouracil
5-HT	5-hydroxytryptamine (also known as serotonin)
ACE	angiotensin-converting enzyme
ADME	absorption, distribution, metabolism, and excretion
ADR	adverse drug reaction
ANS	autonomic nervous system
BER	base excision repair
BLA	Biologics License Application
Boc	t-butyloxycarbonyl
cAMP	cyclic adenosine monophosphate
CDM	clinical data management
CHO	Chinese hamster ovary
CJD	Creutzfeldt–Jakob disease
CNS	central nervous system
COMT	catechol-O-methyltransferase
CONH	compound contains a secondary amide
CRF	case report form
CSR	clinical study report
CTD	Common Technical Document
CYP	cytochrome system
DA	dalton
DAG	diacylglycerol
DDT	dichlorodiphenyltrichloroethane
DNA	deoxyribonucleic acid
DSC	differential scanning calorimetry
ED_{50}	the dose of a drug that produces a therapeutic response in 50 percent of the subjects taking it
EDTA	ethylenediamine tetraacetic acid
EFTA	European Free Trade Association
EMA	European Medicines Agency
EPO	erythropoietin
ESTRI	Electronic Standard for Transfer of Regulatory Information
FDA	Food and Drug Administration
fRNA	functional RNA molecule

GABA	gamma-aminobutyric acid
GC	gas chromatography
GCDMP	good clinical data management practice
GCP	good clinical practice
GCSF	granulocyte colony stimulating factor
GDMP	good data management practice
GLP	good laboratory practice
GMCSF	granulocyte-macrophage colony stimulating factor
GMP	good manufacturing practice
GPCR	G-protein coupled receptor
GST	glutathione-S-transferase
HDR	homology-directed repair
HMG-CoA	3-hydroxy-3-methylglutaryl-Co-enzyme A
HMGCoA	hydroxymethylglutaryl coenzyme A
HMGR	hydroxymethylglutaryl-coenzyme A reductase
HPLC-MS	high performance liquid chromatography-mass spectrometry
HTS	high throughput screening
ICH	International Conference on Harmonisation
ICSR	Individual Case Safety Report
IP_3	inositol triphosphate
LD_{50}	the amount of an ingested substance that kills 50 percent of a test population
MAD	multiple ascending dose
MCA	Medicines Control Agency
MDA	Medical Devices Agency
MedDRA	Medical Dictionary for Regulatory Activities
MEPs	molecular electrostatic potentials
MHRA	Medicines and Healthcare products Regulatory Agency
MRC	Medical Research Council
MMR	mismatch repair
mRNA	messenger RNA
MTD	maximum tolerated dose

NADP$^+$	nicotinamide adenine dinucleotide phosphate	SARs	structure-activity relationships
NCEs	new chemical entities	SDS	sodium dodecyl sulphate
ncRNA	non-coding RNA	SMILES	simplified molecular input line-entry specification
NDA	new drug application	SSBs	single strand breaks
NER	nucleoside excision repair	SSRIs	selective serotonin reuptake inhibitors
NSAID	non-steroidal anti-inflammatory drug	TCA	tricarboxylic acid
OTC	over the counter	TCM	traditional Chinese medicine
PAG	polyacrylamide gel	T_g	glass transition temperature
PARP	poly-ADP ribose polymerase	TNF	tumour necrosis factor
PCA	principal component analysis	TPMT	thiopurine-S-methyltransferase
PCR	polymerase chain reaction	tRNA	transfer RNA
QSAR	quantitative structure-activity relationships	UDPGA	uridine diphosphate glucuronic acid
		WHO	World Health Organization
RMM	relative molecular mass	XRD	X-ray diffraction
RNA	ribonucleic acid	XRPD	X-ray powder diffraction
rRNA	ribosomal RNA		
SAD	single ascending dose		

Introduction

The design and development of a new drug involves a wide range of scientific disciplines such as biochemistry, enzymology, medicinal chemistry, proteomics and toxicology. This book will introduce the various aspects of drug design and development, covering both traditional approaches as well as more recent developments. For the sake of simplicity it is usual to divide the entire process of drug design and drug development into what are known as the discovery phase and the development phase. Whilst there has been a tendency to regard these two phases as occurring consecutively, in reality they almost always overlap. This overlap of the two phases is necessary for economic and ergonomic reasons. It could be very wasteful of time and resources to progress one drug candidate through the entire process in a consecutive manner. For example, it would not be appropriate to progress a candidate drug to clinical testing if the pharmacokinetics of that candidate molecule are inappropriate. For the purpose of ease of understanding, this volume will present the necessary topics in the order as shown in Table 1.1. However, it should be borne in mind that the process of drug design and development takes the form shown in Figure 1.1.

Parts 1, 2, and 3 of this book essentially represent the discovery phase and Parts 4 and 5 deal with the development phase. Part 1 covers the targets within the body with which a potential new drug may interact. Usually the identification of a target arises as a result of a detailed investigation of a particular disease state or condition. Most existing targets are endogenous biological molecules such as proteins, nucleic acids, lipids or carbohydrates. Increasingly, however, individual genes are being identified as potential targets and this has led to an increase in the use of gene therapy.

A large number of drugs act upon proteins which are acting as receptors or enzymes. Where proteins act as receptors their role is as part of the body's communication system. An endogenous molecule interacts with the receptor protein resulting in a response (biochemical or physiological). This process is known as signal transduction. Drugs which target these receptors may stimulate or inhibit the receptor's normal response. Chapter 2 deals with a number of the most commonly targeted receptor proteins and their signal transduction processes. Chapter 3 deals with the target protein molecules which act as enzymes. Drugs which target these enzymes usually act as enzyme inhibitors and there is a variety of mechanisms by which this inhibition is brought about. In addition, the differences between human enzymes and those of pathogenic organisms such as bacteria are often exploited.

The drug targets that were initially discovered are those dealt with in Chapters 2 and 3 but, increasingly, nucleic acids are being identified as drug targets (Chapter 4). In particular, drugs with antibacterial, antiviral and anti-cancer activities have nucleic acids as targets. Such drugs may bring about their activity by directly interacting with the structure of nucleic acids but also may target the normal activities of

Table 1.1 Structure of book

Part	Topic
Drug targets	Receptors and signal transduction
	Enzymes as drug targets
	Nucleic acids and protein synthesis as drug targets
	Other drug targets
Drug discovery and design	Sources of lead compounds
	Drug synthesis
	Optimization of lead compounds
	Computer-aided drug design
	Combinatorial chemistry and high throughput screening
	Biotechnology and biopharmaceuticals
Preclinical testing	Drug metabolism
	Pharmacogenetics and pharmacogenomics
	Toxicity testing
Preformulation	Solubility
	Solid state characteristics
	Drug stability
Clinical research	Clinical research and its regulation
	Design and management of clinical trials

Figure 1.1 Drug design and development process

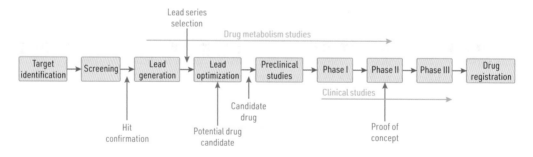

nucleic acids such as transcription, translation and replication. As nucleic acids control the synthesis of proteins, this also can be a drug target, particularly bacterial protein synthesis. Viral nucleic acid synthesis also a drug target.

Less common as drug targets but becoming increasingly important are lipids and, in particular, carbohydrates (Chapter 5). Glycolipids and glycoproteins are important molecules in cell recognition processes and are becoming increasingly important as drug targets.

Having identified a potential target, the next step in drug design is to identify a potential lead compound, i.e. a molecule that is likely to interact with the relevant target in a way which produces a therapeutic effect. The origins of these lead compounds have changed enormously over the years (Chapter 6). The origin of lead compounds was, for many years, natural sources, initially plant sources but, more recently, as better isolation techniques were developed, other sources such as microorganisms, venoms and toxins, marine and animal sources became important (see Table 1.2). As the science of synthetic organic chemistry developed, lead compounds were increasingly synthesized in the laboratory. This process exploited the chemical manipulation of natural products, endogenous ligands and existing drugs (Chapter 7). In parallel to the development of lead compounds it was necessary to develop screening programmes, such as high throughput screening, to provide as much information as possible about the biological activity of the lead compounds.

Once a lead compound has been identified the next step in drug design and development is the optimization of the lead compound (Chapter 8). This optimization may include the following processes: improvement of the interaction with the target, improvement of the pharmacokinetics. Traditional drug design involved making structural changes to the lead compound as well as synthesizing structurally related molecules. These approaches relied upon the skill of the medicinal chemists in predicting what structural changes might lead to improved therapeutic activity. Towards the end of the twentieth century developments in computer technology gave rise to two alternative approaches to drug design. Combinatorial chemistry (Chapter 10) was able to produce large numbers of molecules which were subjected to high throughput screening in order to identify compounds with improved biological activity. Another drug design tool is that of computer-aided drug design (Chapter 9). This technique enables medicinal chemists to model interactions between molecules and a target receptor *in silico*. In this way the optimization of lead compounds can be approached in a much more efficient manner, requiring the synthesis of only those molecules predicted to interact effectively with the target receptor.

For many years drug design was dominated by relatively small organic molecules. However advances in biotechnology have led to the production of so-called biopharmaceuticals (Chapter 11). Initially biotechnology was used simply for the production of existing drug molecules but is now frequently used to produce biologically based drugs such as monoclonal antibodies, antisense oligonucleotides and even gene therapy (see Table 1.3).

Table 1.2 Examples of drugs from natural sources

Source	Drug	Activity
Plants–deadly nightshade	Atropine	Anticholinergic
coca plant	Cocaine	Local anaesthetic
autumn crocus	Colchicine	Anti-tumour
foxglove	Digoxin	Cardiotonic
opium poppy	Morphine	Analgesic
Cinchona	Quinine	Anti-malarial
Microorganisms–Penicillin spp.	Penicillins	Antibiotic
Saccharopolyspora	Erythromycin	Antibiotic
Streptomyces	Vancomycin	Antibiotic
Animal–pig intestines	Heparin	Anticoagulant
pig pancreas	Insulin	Antidiabetic

Table 1.3 Examples of biopharmaceuticals

Biopharmaceutical product	Activity
Interferons	Hepatitis vaccines
Human insulin	Antidiabetic
Erythropoietin	Treatment of anaemia
Herceptin	Treatment of breast cancer
Idarucizumab	Monoclonal antibody for reversal of activity of dabigatran
Fomivirsen	Treatment of cytomegalovirus retinitis
Mipomersen	Treatment of familial hypercholesterolaemia
Specific gene therapy	E.g. treatment of cystic fibrosis

Parts 4 and 5 of the book deal with the development aspects of a new drug. A number of the processes described in Part 4 often take place in parallel with the process in Parts 2 and 3. It is often at this stage that a promising lead compound is rejected, e.g. it if is too insoluble, too easily metabolized, too toxic, etc. If a drug candidate is to be rejected it is more economic for this to be discovered at as early a stage as possible. Hence these development aspects take place at the same time as lead optimization.

Once a drug enters the body it is subject to the body's metabolic processes. Because a drug is almost always a xenobiotic, the principal objective of metabolism is to aid removal of the drug from the body. Drug design and development, therefore, requires a detailed knowledge of drug metabolism (Chapter 12). It is also required to understand that drug metabolism can be affected by numerous factors such as disease, age, gender, diet, and, more recently discovered, genetics. Chapter 13 deals with the influence of genetics on drug activity. Pharmacogenetics, as a science, arose from a study of the factors influencing drug metabolism, but has subsequently developed into the broader study of the influence of genetics on drug activity (see Table 1.4). The sequencing of the human genome has led to the relatively new science of pharmacogenomics, i.e. the influence of the multiple genes of an individual on disease and drug treatment (e.g. individualized drug therapy, non-druggable diseases). Pharmacogenomics presents significant potential but also many challenges to drug design and development.

Toxicity testing is a necessary component of drug development, and is usually carried out at the same time as other aspects of drug design and development, as it makes sense to identify any toxicity problems as early as possible in the process. The types of toxicity tests and the rationale for their usage are described

Table 1.4 Examples of the influence of genetics on drug activity

Genetic polymorphism	Examples of drugs affected
Atypical plasma cholinesterase	Succinylcholine
Fast and slow acetylation	Isoniazid
Cytochrome CYP2C9	Warfarin
Cytochrome CYP 2C19	Diazepam
Cytochrome CYP2D6	Most antidepressants
Thiopurine methyltransferase	Azathioprine
Glucose-6-phosphate dehydrogenase deficiency	Primaquine

in Chapter 14. Also covered are the regulations and guidelines as to which tests are necessary, as well as the additional challenges presented by the newer biopharmaceutical drug candidates.

The ultimate aim for a lead compound is for it to be developed into a new drug suitable for human use. As soon as a potential drug candidate shows sufficient promise in preclinical studies, the pre-formulation aspect of drug development commences. This aspect is also dealt with in Part 4 of the book. Pre-formulation involves investigation of the properties (mainly physicochemical properties) required for the production of a formulation suitable for clinical use. Of particular importance in this regard are the solubility characteristics (Chapter 15), the solid state characteristics (Chapter 16), also known as micromeritics, and the physical and chemical stability of the drug (Chapter 17).

At this stage in the development of a new drug, preclinical research will already have been carried out, involving *in vitro*, *in vivo*, and, increasingly, *in silico* investigations of the pharmacology and toxicology of the new drug candidate. If the results of the preclinical testing are positive, the clinical testing of the drug candidate in human subjects commences and clinical research is the subject of Part 5 of this book. Clinical trials (i.e. clinical testing in humans) are a key part of drug development and, because human subjects are involved, subject to strict regulation. Chapter 18 provides an overview of the regulation and management associated with clinical trials. It should be noted that the regulations related to clinical trials are constantly being updated and the latest versions should always be consulted. In order to produce the most accurate and useful information from clinical trials, the design and management of such trials require careful planning and consideration. Chapter 19 covers important aspects of clinical trial design and management such as target population and selection, nature of the disease, and treatment duration. In order to ensure the validity of any clinical trial there needs to be appropriate test and control groups and processes such as randomization and blinding are key elements. Because of all these requirements of a clinical trial, the outcome of any trial is only as good as the data from the trial, and so clinical data management utilizes good data management practice (GDMP) which is based upon International Conference on Harmonisation (ICH) guidelines.

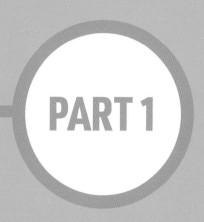

PART 1

Drug Targets

Part 1 will introduce the potential targets with which a drug may interact. In order to design a successful new drug, it is helpful to understand where and how, within the body, the drug is required to bring about its therapeutic activity. It is equally helpful to know where the drug is not intended to act in order to reduce possible side effects and toxicity. Put simply, the specific target for the new drug needs to be understood. At a molecular level, the types of biological molecules likely to be involved as drug targets are lipids, carbohydrates, proteins, and nucleic acids. There are relatively few lipids which act as drug targets and usually the same drug action is involved. This involves disruption of the lipid structure of cell membranes, hence modifying the function of the membrane, for example in the action of general anaesthetics (⟩ **XR Chapter 5**). At present there are even fewer carbohydrates recognized as drug targets, but knowledge in this area is increasing (⟩ **XR Chapter 5**). Most drugs act on proteins or nucleic acids. Enzymes (⟩ **XR Chapter 3**) and nucleic acids (⟩ **XR Chapter 4**) as drug targets will be dealt with in subsequent chapters. Other proteins as drug targets will be dealt with in this chapter and (⟩ **XR Chapter 5**).

Receptors and Signal Transduction

Receptors are proteins or glycoproteins which are very important targets for drug action. Receptors are part of the communication systems within the body. The interaction of the appropriate endogenous ligand with a receptor results in a specific biochemical or physiological response. This response is referred to as signal transduction. Drugs which bind to such receptors can activate or inhibit the normal response associated with that receptor.

2.1 CELLULAR COMMUNICATION

Human cells are often specialized and dedicated to a specific task. In such a complex situation, effective communication is essential. Thus intercellular messaging and response are required for maintenance of control of this effective communication. This communication involves messengers, which may be primary or secondary, interacting with specific recognition sites, known as receptors (❯ XR Section 2.2) to produce the required response.

2.1.1 Primary messengers

These can be classified as endocrine messengers, paracrine messengers or neurotransmitters. **Endocrine messengers**, also called hormones, are produced by specialized endocrine glands and released into the bloodstream to be transported to their target organ. There may be one target organ or many (see Integration Box 2.1 Thyroid hormones).

INTEGRATION BOX 2.1 | **THYROID HORMONES**

Thyroid stimulating hormone (TSH) is secreted by the anterior pituitary gland and has only one target organ–the thyroid gland. Here, it stimulates the release into the bloodstream, of two thyroid hormones, thyroxine (T_4) and triiodothyronine (T_3). These hormones have a large number of targets throughout the body because they are regulators of metabolism in most tissues. T_3 is about three to five times more active than T_4. Additionally, they are also important for growth and development. In this regard they enter cells and T_4 is converted to T_3 which then binds to a nuclear receptor (❯ **XR Section 2.2.6**). A lack of the natural thyroid hormones can be treated by administration of thyroxine in the form of levothyroxine–the (-) isomer of thyroxine. The (+) isomer of thyroxine has little or no physiological activity. Another example of the importance of utilizing a pure enantiomeric form of a stereoisomeric drug can be found in Box 4.2.

Paracrine messengers, sometimes called autocoids, are active locally within the organ in which they are produced, thus having a localized effect (see Integration Box 2.2 Prostaglandins and pregnancy).

INTEGRATION BOX 2.2 | **PROSTAGLANDINS AND PREGNANCY**

The endometrium of the uterus has prostaglandin-synthesizing capacity, in particular for prostaglandins of the E and F series. In a pregnant uterus, release of these prostaglandins causes contractions of the uterus smooth muscle and relaxation of the cervix, aiding delivery of the foetus. Prostaglandins can also have this effect in early and middle pregnancy and can be, therefore, abortifacients. Two prostaglandins are clinically used, these being prostaglandin E_2 (dinoprostone) and 15-methylprostaglandin $F_{2\alpha}$ (carboprost).

Neurotransmitters have an even more localized effect and are chemical messengers between nerve cells or nerve cell and effector organ (see Integration Box 2.3 Acetylcholine as a neurotransmitter).

INTEGRATION BOX 2.3 | **ACETYLCHOLINE AS A NEUROTRANSMITTER**

Acetylcholine, as a neurotransmitter, acts at two different types of receptor. Receptors at the neuromuscular junction and at autonomic ganglia are called nicotinic receptors and are ligand-gated ion channel receptors (❯ **XR Section 2.2.3**). They are so called because they respond to **nicotine**. Acetylcholine receptors associated with target organs within the parasympathetic nervous system are G-protein-coupled receptors (GPCR) (❯ **XR Section 2.2.4**) and are called muscarinic receptors because they respond to **muscarine**. There are five sub-types of muscarinic receptor. M_1 receptors are associated with CNS excitation, gastric acid secretion and gastrointestinal motility. They are excitatory receptors. M_2 receptors are inhibitory and are associated with the heart. M_3 receptors are the most common sub-type and are associated with secretory glands and smooth muscle and are excitatory. M_4 and M_5 receptors are mainly restricted to the CNS but also the salivary gland and nerves of the eye. M_4 receptors are inhibitory and M_5 excitatory.

 Primary messengers are classified as endocrine messengers, paracrine messengers or neurotransmitters.

2.1.2 Secondary messengers

The interaction of a primary messenger with a receptor can, in some cases, lead to the production of another intracellular messenger—a secondary messenger. The role of such messengers will be explained later in this chapter in the sections dealing with the relevant receptor types.

2.2 RECEPTORS

Endogenous molecules and exogenous molecules such as drugs (often referred to as ligands) interact with specific recognition sites known as receptors. The interaction of such molecules with a receptor leads to a specific biological response. Receptors may be intracellular or extracellular. Extracellular receptors are usually found on cell membranes, often possessing an **exofacial** binding site linked to an **endofacial** protein molecule. Intracellular receptor sites can be found in the nucleus (❯ **XR Section 2.2.6**). The nature of receptors is often represented in a very simplistic fashion (see Figure 2.1) but this significantly underestimates the complexity of receptors. Typically a cell may possess multiple receptors and the number of receptors is not fixed. The receptors may be up-regulated or down-regulated, changing the sensitivity of the cell to a particular ligand (see Integration Box 2.4 Development of drug tolerance).

INTEGRATION BOX 2.4	DEVELOPMENT OF DRUG TOLERANCE

The number of receptors per cell and their sensitivity to ligands is not consistent and can vary according to circumstances. Often the pharmacological response to the ongoing administration of a drug decreases with time. In some cases this can be as a result of a reduction in the number of receptors (down-regulation). This feature has been recognized in a number of receptors, including β-adrenoreceptors and hormone receptors. The receptors are taken into the cell by a process known as **endocytosis**. The effect of this down-regulation is often referred to as development of tolerance, but strictly speaking tolerance to a drug can arise due to other processes as well, such as increased metabolic degradation. Conversely, up-regulation leads to an increase in the number of receptors on the cell surface, thus making the cell more sensitive to the ligand. A good example of this is the up-regulation of oxytocin receptors in the uterus during pregnancy (particularly during the third trimester), leading to increased contraction of the uterine smooth muscle.

Figure 2.1 The basic concept of the drug-receptor interaction
(Credit:From Therapeutics and Human Physiology edited by Elsie Gaskell and Chris Rostron (2013). Reproduced with permission of Oxford University Press through PLSclear).

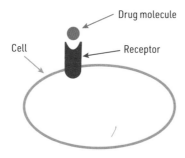

2.2.1 Nature of ligand-receptor interactions

When a ligand binds to a receptor active site, usually a biological response is elicited, which may be either a positive or a negative response. This response is brought about by the interaction of certain structural features of the ligand with specific regions of the receptor site. Such interactions lead to a change in conformation (shape) of the receptor and this change of conformation initiates a cellular response. This is referred to as a signal transduction. It is vital, therefore, when designing a drug to interact with a specific receptor site, to understand the nature of these ligand-receptor interactions.

Ligand-receptor interactions consist of a variety of chemical bonds (see Table 2.1). Usually, it is desirable for most ligands to occupy the receptor site for a relatively short length of time and, as such, ionic or weaker bonds are utilized. Additionally, as most drug-receptor interactions are required to be reversible, relatively weak bonds are involved in drug-receptor binding. Because of the types of functional groups present both in the ligands and the receptor, many of these will be ionized at physiological pH. Consequently, ionic and electrostatic bonds are important in drug-receptor interactions.

Again, because of the nature of the functional groups involved, many possess hydrogen bonding capabilities, either as donors or as acceptors (see Figure 2.2). Add to these electrostatic attractions such as ion-dipole attractions, dipole-dipole attractions and charge transfer complexes (see Figure 2.2) and it becomes apparent the binding forces involved in drug-receptor interactions can be very complex.

Another type of weak force which can be involved in drug-receptor interactions is hydrophobic bonding. The interactions here are between non-polar regions of the ligand and the receptor, although there is some doubt about the exact nature of this type of interaction (see Box 2.1 Hydrophobic bonding—does it exist and, if so, how does it work?).

Another set of attractive forces potentially involved in drug-receptor interactions are Van de Waals forces. Individually these are very weak but may make a contribution if, say, an aromatic ring is involved. Aromatic rings are frequently present in biologically active molecules and their contribution to receptor

Table 2.1 Chemical bonding involved in ligand-receptor interactions

Chemical bond	Approx. bond strength (kcal mol^{-1})	Type of ligand-receptor interaction
Covalent	~ 100	Irreversible bond between ligand and receptor
Ionic bond	~5	Bonding between functional groups ionized at physiological pH
Hydrogen bond	~5	Often a number of these formed Ligand or receptor can be donor or acceptor or both
Ion-dipole Dipole-dipole Charge transfer complex	~5	Arise due to difference in electronegativity resulting in uneven distribution of electrons
Hydrophobic bonds	~1	Interactions between non-polar regions of ligand and receptor
Van der Waals forces	~0.5–1	Induced temporary dipoles caused by ligand and receptor approaching each other
pi-pi interactions	~2–3	Interactions between aromatic rings on the receptor and in the ligand
Cation-pi interactions	~5	Interaction between a cation and an aromatic ring

Figure 2.2 Examples of bonding in drug-receptor interactions

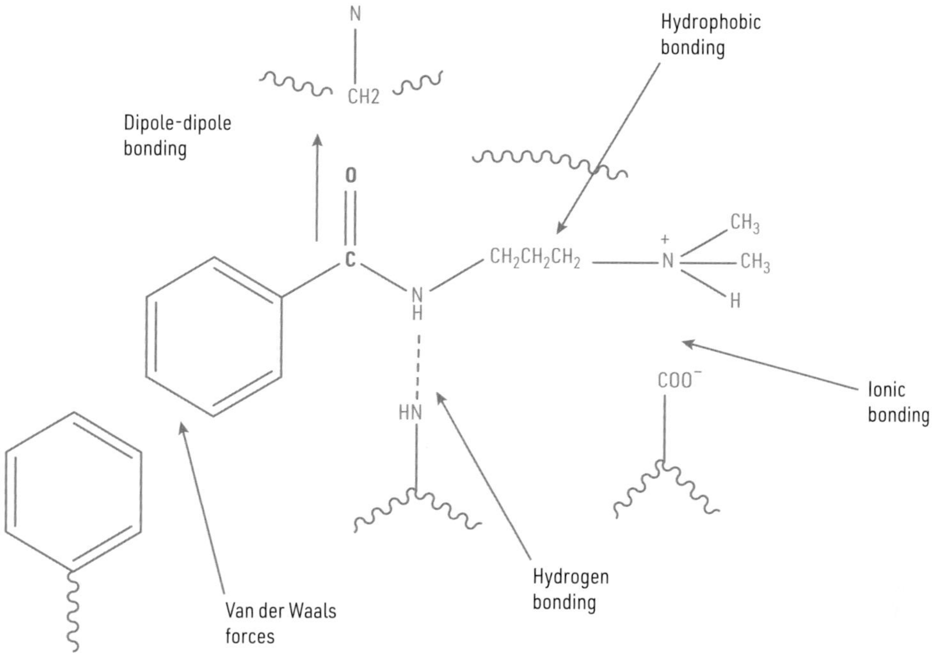

binding may be Van de Waals forces between the flat aromatic ring and an equivalent flat part of the receptor (see Figure 2.2). The presence of aromatic amino acids in receptors and aromatic rings in biologically active molecules could also give rise to interaction between these aromatic rings, called pi-pi interactions or cationic-pi interactions. This type of interaction takes place particularly in G-protein-coupled receptors (❯ **XR Section 2.2.4**). An example of pi-pi interaction is the binding of tryptophan derivatives to the dopamine D_2 receptor, where they bind to aromatic amino acid residues close to the agonist binding site. An example of cationic-pi interaction is between the trimethylammonium ion of acetylcholine and a tryptophan residue at the active site of acetylcholinesterase.

It should be noted that there are instances where an irreversible covalent bond between a drug and a receptor is useful, for example in cancer chemotherapy (❯ **XR Section 4.3.3**) and irreversible enzyme inhibition (❯ **XR Section 3.2.1**).

BOX 2.1   HYDROPHOBIC BONDING—DOES IT EXIST AND, IF SO, HOW DOES IT WORK?

There is an amount of uncertainty about how hydrophobic bonds are formed or, indeed, if they even exist. Hydrophobic bonds were developed as a useful concept to explain the interactions between non-polar regions of receptors and ligands. It is postulated that thermodynamics can provide an explanation of how they work. The coming together of hydrophobic regions causes a disruption of the ordered structure of water molecules which are always present in a biological environment. This causes an increase in entropy and thus a decrease in the energy of the system, leading to an increase in stability. It has also been suggested that lipophilic bonding might be a more appropriate term.

Because most ligand-receptor interactions are required to be reversible, relatively weak bonding forces are involved.

2.2.2 Classification of receptors

Receptors are classified into four main types often known as superfamilies. These are ion channel receptors (❯ **XR Section 2.2.3**) where the endogenous ligands are fast neurotransmitters; G-protein-coupled receptors (❯ **XR Section 2.2.4**) where the endogenous ligands are hormones and slow neurotransmitters; tyrosine kinase receptors (❯ **XR Section 2.2.5**) with insulin and growth factors as endogenous ligands; and nuclear receptors (❯ **XR Section 2.2.6**) with steroid hormones, thyroid hormones, and certain vitamins as endogenous ligands.

2.2.3 Ion channel receptors

Fast neurotransmitters, such as acetylcholine at the neuromuscular junction and gamma-amino butyric acid at the $GABA_A$ receptor in the CNS, interact with ion channel receptors. These ion channel receptors are known as ligand-gated ion channels because they are controlled by chemical messengers (also known as ligands). There is another type of ion channel where a ligand is not directly involved in their control. These ion channels are sensitive to the potential difference in electrical charge which exists across a cell membrane. These are known as voltage-gated ion channels. When the receptor is activated a channel is formed through which ions can enter the cell. These receptors are appropriate for interaction with fast neurotransmitters because the timescale of response is very rapid—of the order of milliseconds.

An ion channel receptor (see Figure 2.3) consists of a collection of (usually) five membrane spanning proteins, forming a pore in the cell membrane. In the resting state the pore is closed, and no ions can cross the membrane. Overall, the receptor consists of an extracellular ligand-binding domain, a

Figure 2.3 The nicotinic acetylcholine receptor (nAChR) is a transmembrane receptor that is an ion channel. (A) shows the ion channel closed, not allowing the entrance of sodium ions (Na^+) into the cell. (B) shows the neurotransmitter acetylcholine activating the receptor, thus opening the ion channel, and Na^+ entering the cell, which leads to the relevant physiological effect

(Credit: From Therapeutics and Human Physiology edited by Elsie Gaskell and Chris Rostron (2013). Reproduced with permission of Oxford University Press through PLSclear).

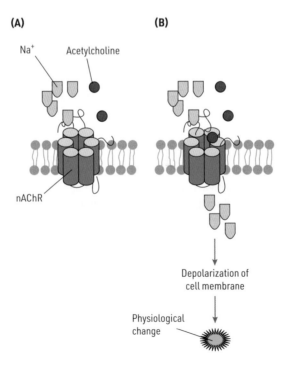

transmembrane domain, and an intracellular anchoring site. The protein molecules consist of five subunits (two α-subunits and one each of β, γ, and δ subunits). The two α subunits are ligand binding sites and both need to be occupied to activate the receptor. Activation causes the channel to open, and ions pass through the membrane causing a potential difference across the membrane, resulting in a biochemical change in the target cell.

The nicotinic acetylcholine receptor is an example of an excitatory ion channel receptor. Stimulation of the receptor allows sodium ions to flow into the cell causing **depolarization**. Depolarization causes the opening of voltage-gated ion channels, allowing even more sodium ions to enter the cell—an amplification of the initial response, leading to muscle contraction. Ion channel receptors can also be inhibitory, for example the GABA$_A$ receptor in the brain. The mode of operation of the receptor is similar but involves the passage of chloride ions. An influx of chloride ions into the cell leads to **hyperpolarization**, causing inhibition of operation of the cell (see Integration Box 2.5 Mode of action of benzodiazepines).

 Ion channel receptors are utilized by fast transmitters. Activation of the receptor opens the channel and allows ions to cross the cell membrane.

INTEGRATION BOX 2.5   MODE OF ACTION OF BENZODIAZEPINES

Benzodiazepines are a group of drugs which possess sedative, hypnotic or anxiolytic properties, depending on their structure. They operate by acting on the GABA$_A$ receptors in the brain. The response of the GABA$_A$ to its natural ligand can be modified by the binding of a separate ligand to a binding site remote from the GABA binding site–this is known as an allosteric binding site. This is the site to which benzodiazepines bind. When they do so they increase the affinity of GABA for its receptor, thus increasing the inhibitory effect. Of course the natural ligand for this allosteric site is not a synthetic drug like a benzodiazepine. Recently some endogenous peptides which bind to this allosteric site have been isolated and named endozepines, potentially useful as new lead compounds for drugs with benzodiazepine-like activities.

2.2.4 G-protein-coupled receptors (GPCRs)

The binding of an endogenous ligand to a G-protein-coupled receptor brings about a change in the concentration of a second messenger, leading to the final cellular response (see Figure 2.4). This is a complex process and involves a regulatory G-protein (G refers to Guanine binding). Because of the complexity of the process, the response time of this type of receptor is of the order of seconds, hence its involvement with slow neurotransmitters such as noradrenaline (see Integration Box 2.6 Adrenoreceptors).

The structure of the receptor consists of a single membrane-spanning polypeptide chain of ~ 400–500 amino acids. The N-terminal of the chain is extracellular and the C-terminus intracellular. The chain consists of seven transmembrane α-helices which surround the ligand binding site, i.e. it is within the cell membrane. The third cytoplasmic loop of the polypeptide chain contains the G-protein binding domain. The G-protein consists of three subunits (α, β and γ) which anchor the G-protein to the cell membrane.

In an unstimulated cell, the G-protein is bound to GDP (guanosine diphosphate). When the receptor is stimulated the GDP is exchanged for GTP (guanosine triphosphate). This causes the α-GTP subunit to break away from the β and γ subunits and associate with a membrane-bound enzyme (such as adenylate cyclase or phospholipase C), thereby activating the enzyme leading to an increase in the concentration of a second messenger (such as cyclic AMP or DAG, and IP$_3$). The G-α subunit has GTPase activity which converts the attached GTP to GDP. The GDP-α subunit has no affinity for the enzyme and re-joins the

Figure 2.4 β_2-adrenoceptors are G-protein-coupled receptors. (A) shows the transmembrane β_2-adrenoceptor associated with the whole G-protein. (B) shows the activation of the adrenoceptor, which stimulates a section of the G-protein (G$_\alpha$) to bind to the membrane-bound enzyme adenylate cyclase, stimulating the production of cAMP, which triggers the physiological changes

(Credit: From Therapeutics and Human Physiology edited by Elsie Gaskell and Chris Rostron (2013). Reproduced with permission of Oxford University Press through PLSclear).

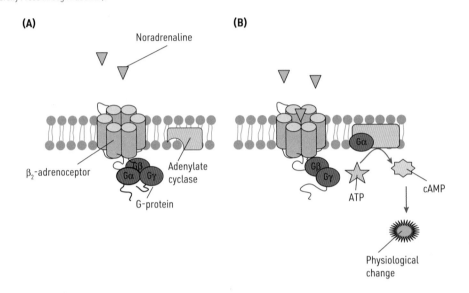

β and γ subunits. The activation of the enzyme produces many second messenger molecules leading to an amplification of the initial receptor stimulation.

Once the purpose of the receptor stimulation has been achieved, the signalling process must be halted. This can be by removal of the ligand from the receptor binding site, by the breakdown of the GTP on the α-subunit or by breakdown of the second messenger (e.g. degradation of cyclic AMP by phosphodiesterases).

GPCRs are probably the most common type of receptor to be utilized as drug targets. It is estimated that 45 per cent of all drugs target GPCRs in some way, although this percentage is gradually falling as new targets are discovered and exploited. Examples of the variety of drugs which interact with GPCRs producing cAMP are salmeterol (a β_2-adrenergic agonist), ranitidine (a histamine H$_2$ antagonist), sumatriptan (a 5 HT agonist), and fentanyl (an opioid μ receptor agonist—which actually inhibits the formation of cAMP). Examples of drugs which interact with GPCRs activating phospholipase C are cetirizine (a peripheral H$_1$ antagonist) and phenylephrine (an α_1-adrenergic agonist).

INTEGRATION BOX 2.6   **ADRENORECEPTORS**

Adrenoreceptors, or adrenergic receptors, are divided into two categories, called α and β receptors. Each of these categories is also divided into sub-types known as α_1, α_2, β_1, β_2, and β_3. All of these are G-protein-coupled receptors and are present in both the CNS and the ANS. α_1-adrenoreceptors are present in smooth muscle and are activated by noradrenaline and adrenaline also activates these receptors. The G-proteins involved are excitatory G-proteins (G$_q$). α_2-adrenoreceptors are inhibitory and are linked to inhibitory G-proteins (G$_i$). β_1-adrenoreceptors are present largely in the heart where they have an excitatory effect (G$_s$) but are also present in the gastrointestinal tract where activation causes the smooth muscle to relax. β_2-adrenoreceptors are found in blood vessels where activation causes vasodilation (G$_s$) and in bronchial smooth muscle where activation causes bronchodilation. The function of β_3-adrenoreceptors is unclear but they are found in smooth muscle in the intestines, the gall bladder, bladder and also in adipose tissue.

G-protein-coupled receptors have been the most common receptors to act as drug targets. Activation of the receptor causes a G-protein to activate a membrane-bound enzyme, leading to the production of a second messenger.

2.2.5 Tyrosine kinase receptors

This type of receptor is involved in the signal transduction of insulin and polypeptide growth factors and, as such, the control of cell growth, cell division, and differentiation. Ligand activation changes cells from the resting state to a cell division cycle. This makes these receptors important targets for anti-cancer drugs (see Integration Box 2.7 Tyrosine kinases as targets for anti-cancer drugs).

The structure of these receptors is much simpler than that of the previous receptor types. They consist of three distinct domains (see Figure 2.5). There is an extracellular domain (N-terminus) which contains the ligand binding site. This is linked by a single helical membrane-spanning domain to a cytoplasmic domain which contains the tyrosine kinase function.

In addition to having a different structure, these receptors have a quite different mode of operation. When a ligand binds to the receptor on the cell surface, this causes the receptors to form dimers. When dimer formation occurs, the tyrosine kinase domains are brought close together causing their activation. Activation results in autophosphorylation, whereby specific tyrosine residues in the cytoplasmic domain of the receptor itself are phosphorylated. These phosphorylated tyrosine residues become high affinity binding sites for target proteins in the cytoplasm, which are themselves phosphorylated at specific tyrosine residues.

Figure 2.5 The insulin receptor is a tyrosine kinase receptor consisting of two identical subunits. (A) shows the insulin receptors not associated with the hormone insulin. (B) shows the association of insulin with its receptors, causing **phosphorylation** of the insulin receptor substrate, autophosphorylation of the receptor, and translocation of the glucose transporter molecules to the cellular membrane, where they transport glucose into the cell

(Credit: From Therapeutics and Human Physiology edited by Elsie Gaskell and Chris Rostron (2013). Reproduced with permission of Oxford University Press through PLSclear).

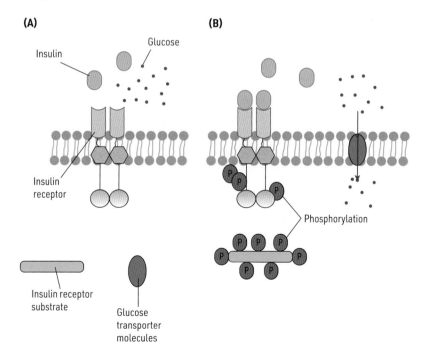

Many cytoplasmic enzymes and proteins have sequence-related regions known as SH2 and SH3 domains. The SH2 domain comprises of approximately one hundred amino acids and this is the site of interaction with the phosphorylated tyrosine kinase domains. The binding of the SH2 domain to the tyrosine kinase induces a conformational change leading to activation of the enzyme or protein. The SH3 domain is approximately fifty amino acids and less is known about its role, although it appears to mediate protein-protein interactions. The response timeframe for this type of receptor varies from minutes to hours.

INTEGRATION BOX 2.7   TYROSINE KINASES AS TARGETS FOR ANTI-CANCER DRUGS

Because of their role in controlling cell division and growth, it is obvious that tyrosine kinases must be involved, in some way, when normal cells become cancerous cells. Indeed, it has been shown that they are found in very high levels in cancer cells. The development of tyrosine kinase inhibitors could be potentially useful in this regard. The problem with this therapeutic approach is that tyrosine kinases are present in normal cells, so selective activity is required. Some progress has been made in this area with approval of the anti-tumour drug imatinib (Glivec®). It is active against the platelet-derived growth factor receptor and is used to treat **leukaemia**. Kinases have become the second most important group of drug targets after G-protein-coupled receptors and are set to become the most important drug targets of the twenty-first century.

Cytokines are peptides which function as regulators of inflammatory and immune responses. Cytokines are the ligands for cytokine receptors which are similar to tyrosine kinase receptors, but they do not have inherent tyrosine kinase activity. In this receptor type dimerization does not cause autophosphorylation but leads to the binding to the intracellular domain of the receptor of a tyrosine kinase enzyme from the cytoplasm. This binding causes the receptor to be phosphorylated. This is then followed by the binding of a SH2 protein and subsequent activation of that protein (see Box 2.2 EPO—an illegal cytokine?). There are two types of cytokine receptors: type 1, for example, the interleukin receptors, and type 2, for example, the interferon receptors.

BOX 2.2   EPO—AN ILLEGAL CYTOKINE?

The role of the cytokine erythropoietin (EPO) in the body is to stimulate red blood cell production. EPO can now be produced by recombinant DNA technology, and can be used to treat anaemia arising from various clinical conditions and usually produces a significant increase in the patient's **haematocrit**. It has long been recognized that an increased haematocrit would be potentially useful in certain endurance sports such as cycling and long-distance running. Once a synthetic version of EPO became available in the 1990s it began to be abused by some competitors in such sports in order to generate an increased blood oxygen-carrying capacity, thereby gaining an unfair advantage over other competitors. As well as being unethical, such a practice is physiologically hazardous. Increasing the red blood cell count beyond normal levels causes increased blood viscosity, leading to reduced blood flow and an increase in the possibility of thrombosis and strokes.

 Tyrosine kinase receptors are involved in cell growth, division, and differentiation. Activation of the receptor results in dimerization, autophosphorylation, and interaction with cytoplasmic proteins.

2.2.6 Nuclear receptors

Nuclear receptors are different from the previous receptor types because, as the name implies, they are found inside the cell and thus their ligands must be able to enter the cell. They were originally thought to be in the cytoplasm because it was from there that they were first isolated, but they are located in the nucleus in live cells.

The structure of the receptor is a large protein of 400–1000 amino acid residues. It has a central section of about sixty residues thought to be the DNA-binding domain (see Figure 2.6). This domain contains two loops, each of about fifteen residues, known as zinc fingers. Each loop consists of four cysteine residues surrounding a zinc atom. Structures such as this are commonly found in proteins that are known to regulate DNA transcription (❯ **XR Section 4.1.2**). The ligand (a hormone) binds to the receptor downstream (towards the C-terminus) of the central section, causing a conformational change, exposing the DNA-binding region and thus allows the binding of DNA. Upstream (towards the N-terminus) from the DNA-binding domain is a domain which controls gene transcription. The DNA-binding domain recognizes specific DNA base sequences, leading to the activation of specific genes. Ultimately, this leads to protein synthesis. Because of this complex sequence of events the response time of this type of receptor is relatively slow, of the order of hours (see Integration Box 2.8 Anti-cancer activity of tamoxifen).

Figure 2.6 Zinc fingers in DNA-binding domain of a nuclear receptor

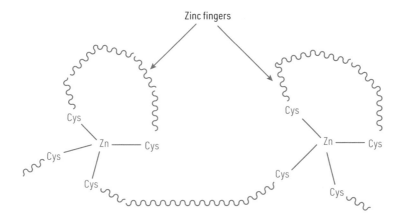

INTEGRATION BOX 2.8   ANTI-CANCER ACTIVITY OF TAMOXIFEN

Tamoxifen is a drug used in the treatment of **oestrogen**-dependent breast cancer. It acts as an antagonist at oestrogen receptors, interfering with the binding of oestradiol. It is a competitive inhibitor at the oestrogen receptors which are overexpressed in about 60 per cent of primary breast cancers. When oestradiol binds to the oestrogen receptors it increases the growth of cancer cells. Tamoxifen prevents this and is often referred to as an anti-oestrogen. However, this is not the whole story. Tamoxifen also can act as a partial agonist of oestrogen receptors in the endometrium, liver, bone, and the cardiovascular system. This could lead to the development of oestrogen-dependent endometrial cancer and the risk of this has to be taken into account when using tamoxifen to treat oestrogen-dependent breast cancer. It is thought that two metabolites of tamoxifen (N-desmethyltamoxifen and 4-hydroxytamoxifen) contribute significantly to the anti-oestrogen effect.

Nuclear receptors interact mainly with hormones and lead, via gene transcription, to protein synthesis.

? Questions

1. Examine the structures of the following endogenous ligands and postulate the types of bonding forces likely to be involved in binding to a receptor site: acetylcholine, noradrenaline, 5-HT.

2. Find an example of a drug which brings about its clinical effect by blocking ion channel receptors.

3. What are the consequences of insulin interacting with a tyrosine kinase receptor?

4. Suggest why the two metabolites of tamoxifen mentioned in Integration Box 2.8 might contribute significantly to its clinical effect.

↺ Chapter summary

- Intercellular communication involves messengers, which may be primary or secondary, interacting with specific targets to produce the required response.

- Ligands bind to receptor sites utilizing a variety of ligand-receptor interactions, including ionic bonds, hydrogen bonds, and electrostatic attractions.

- Receptors are classified into four superfamilies: ion channel receptors, G-protein-coupled receptors, tyrosine kinase receptors, and nuclear receptors.

- Ion channel receptors are mainly involved in fast transmission, operating in the millisecond timeframe.

- Ligand binding at ion channel receptors causes the channel to open, allowing ions to cross the cell membrane into the cell.

- G-protein-coupled receptors operate in the timeframe of seconds and are associated with slow transmission.

- Ligand binding at G-protein-coupled receptors causes activation of a G-protein complex which dissociates and activates a membrane-bound enzyme, releasing a secondary messenger.

- Tyrosine kinase receptors interact with insulin and various growth factors. Signal transduction involves dimerization of the receptors, autophosphorylation of tyrosine residues and interaction with the SH_2 domains of various intracellular proteins. The timeframe of the response can vary from minutes to hours.

- Nuclear receptors are located within the cell and so ligands must be capable of crossing the cell membrane. Ligand binding results in dimerization (but not autophosphorylation) and formation of a gene transcription complex, leading to activation of specific genes. The timeframe of operation of this type of receptor is of the order of hours.

📖 Further reading

Caminero, D.C., Tricarico, D., and Desaphy, J.F. (2007) Ion channel pharmacology, *Neurotherapeutics* 4: 184–98.

Reviews the role of ion channels in a range of diseases and how they can be used as drug targets.

Wigglesworth, M. (2014) *G-Protein-Coupled Receptors in Drug Discovery* in series *Small Molecule Drug Discovery*. The Biomedical & Life Sciences Collection, London: Henry Stewart Talks Ltd. Online at http://hstalks.com. Your university should have a subscription.

An online presentation describing the important role of G-protein-coupled receptors in drug discovery.

Gschwind, A., Fischer, O.M., and Ulrich, A. (2004) The discovery of receptor tyrosine kinases; targets for cancer therapy, *Nature Reviews Cancer* 4: 361–70.

Review of the discovery and role of tyrosine kinase receptors in diseases such as cancer and how this has led to new ways of treating cancer.

Ottow, E. and Weinmann, H. (2008) Nuclear Receptors as Drug Targets: A Historical Perspective of Modern Drug Discovery, in *Nuclear Receptors as Drug Targets*. Weinheim: Wiley-VCH Verlag GmbH & Co. ISBN 978-3-527-31872-8.

A comprehensive review of the role of nuclear receptors in pharmacological research and drug discovery.

(T) CASE STUDY 2.1 DRUGS INSPIRED BY ENDOGENOUS COMPOUNDS— DEVELOPMENT OF β-BLOCKERS

Adrenergic receptors are all G-protein coupled receptors and one of two sub-types—α and β which are sub-divided into α_1, α_2, β_1, β_2, and β_3. The endogenous agonist for these receptors is noradrenaline (Figure CS2.1). The β receptors are present in the heart and stimulation of them increases the force and rate of contraction of cardiac muscle. The development of β-blockers was instituted in the 1950s by Sir James Black. β antagonists, he suggested, would be useful in the treatment of angina (and subsequently hypertension, myocardial infarctions, and cardiac arrhythmias).

For a medicinal chemist looking to develop an antagonist, the best place to start is by examination of the endogenous agonist—noradrenaline (Figure CS2.1). Research determined that the features required for agonist activity were the phenolic OHs, a sidechain OH and an ionizable amine in the sidechain. It was also noted that the stereochemistry of the molecule was important—the R isomer has much greater agonist activity compared with the S isomer. This observation, together with the already identified pharmacophore, was interpreted as a three-point interaction with the receptor site and was known as the Easson–Stedman hypothesis. This interaction has since been confirmed by site-directed mutagenic studies.

Noradrenaline acts as an agonist at both α and β receptors, but what was required was a molecule selective for β receptors. Isoprenaline (Figure CS2.2), as a selective β-agonist, was chosen as the lead compound. One theory regarding the production of an antagonist was to remove one of the necessary points of interaction with the receptor. The phenolic OH groups were chosen and replaced with chlorine atoms to produce dichloroisoprenaline (Figure CS2.3), first synthesized by the Eli Lilly group, which blocks the receptors but still had residual agonist

Figure CS2.1 Noradrenaline

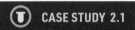

Phenolic groups OH → (HO, 6, 1, 5, 4, 2, 3, HO, 2, 1, OH, NH₂) Ionizable amine

Sidechain OH

Noradrenaline

→

Figure CS2.2 Isoprenaline

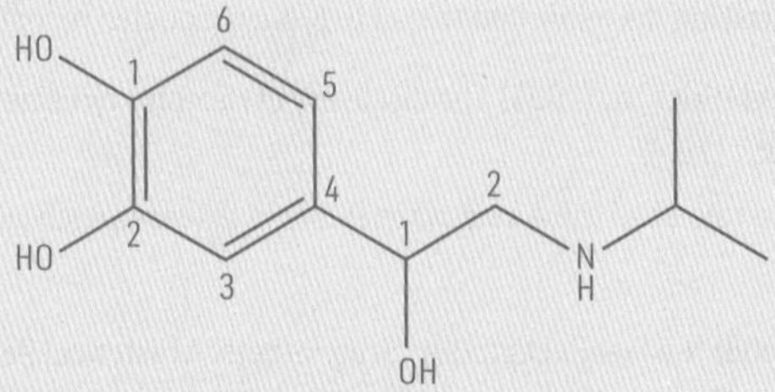

Isoprenaline

Figure CS2.3 Dichloroisoprenaline

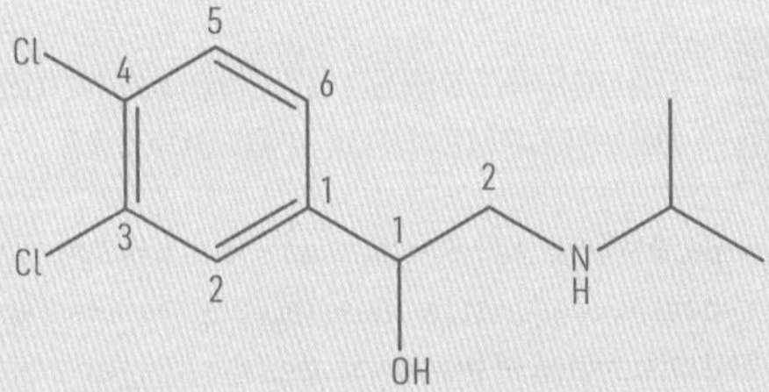

Dichloroisoprenaline

Figure CS2.4 Pronethalol

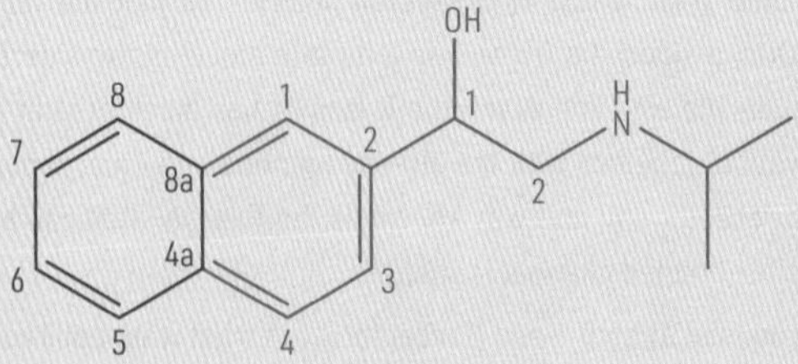

Pronethalol

activity. This finding prompted Sir James Black at ICI to further investigate the possibility of producing a clinically useful β-antagonist. Another common structural change that had been observed to convert an agonist to an antagonist was the addition of an extra aromatic ring. This provides an additional hydrophobic interaction not involved in agonist action. This led to the production of pronethalol (Figure CS2.4–additional aromatic ring in red) which was a much better antagonist but still had some residual agonist activity. Although it did reach clinical trials and was marketed, it was quickly withdrawn due to toxicity.

Research was now carried out on the sidechain, involving the introduction of various linking groups between the naphthalene ring of pronethalol and the ethanolamine sidechain. At this point serendipity was involved. The target compound (Figure CS2.5) required a synthetic starting material of 2-naphthol but only 1-naphthol was available, leading to the synthesis of propranolol (Figure CS2.6) which is regarded as the 'gold standard' of β blockers and was the first of the so-called first-generation antagonists. Detailed structure-activity studies followed (Figure CS2.7) and led to the production of other first-generation antagonists (Figure CS2.8). As can be seen, the structural changes were mainly restricted to the aromatic ring–nadolol where the OH groups were reintroduced,

→

→

Figure CS2.5 Structure of target compound

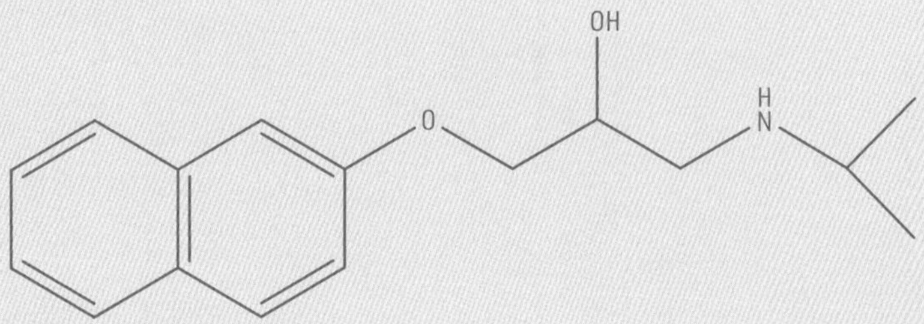

Figure CS2.6 Propranolol

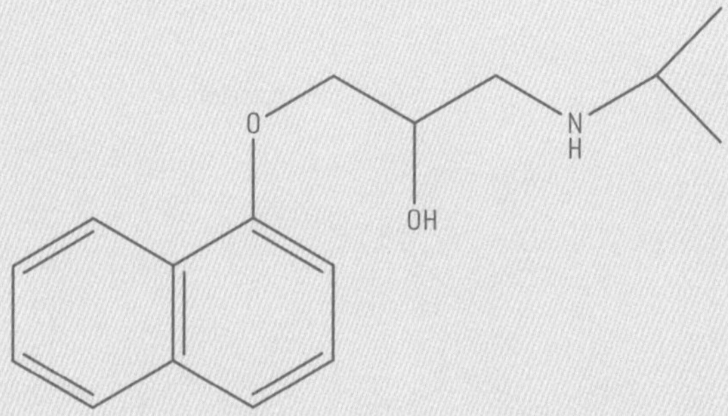

Figure CS2.7 Results of detailed structure-activity studies

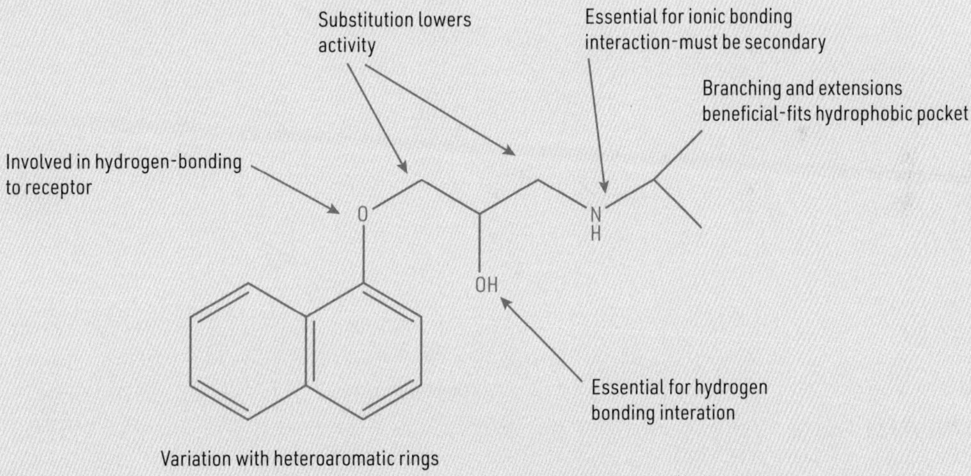

Substitution lowers activity

Essential for ionic bonding interaction-must be secondary

Branching and extensions beneficial-fits hydrophobic pocket

Involved in hydrogen-bonding to receptor

Essential for hydrogen bonding interation

Variation with heteroaromatic rings

pindolol where the aromatic ring was changed to an indole ring, and timolol which has a more complex ring system. The sidechain hydroxyl group and the ionizable amine are retained in all examples.

These molecules (and propranolol) are non-selective antagonists, i.e. they act on both β_1 and β_2 receptors. It would be beneficial to have a selective (cardiac) β_1 antagonist which did not block vascular and bronchial β_2 receptors. Practolol (Figure CS2.9) was the lead compound in this respect and was the first cardioselective β antagonist (the second-generation antagonists) to be marketed but was subsequently withdrawn due to toxic side effects.

→

→

Figure CS2.8 Examples of first-generation β antagonists

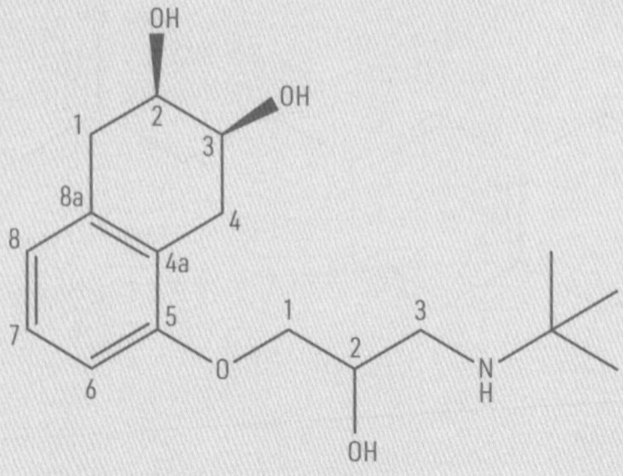

Nadolol

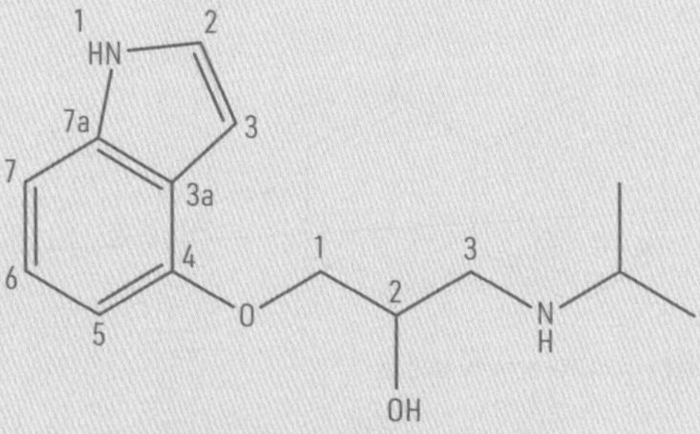

Pindolol

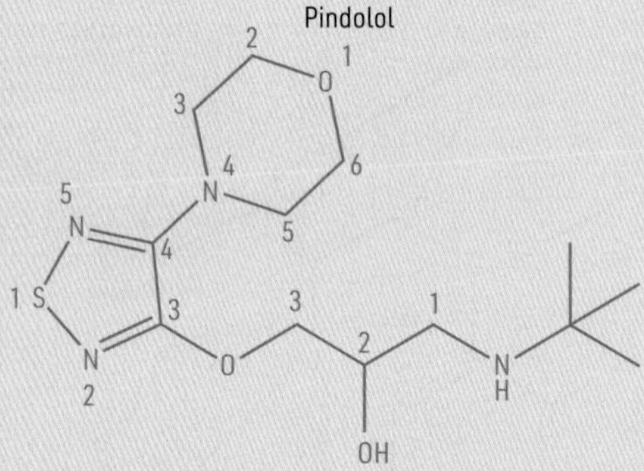

Timolol

Figure CS2.9 Practolol

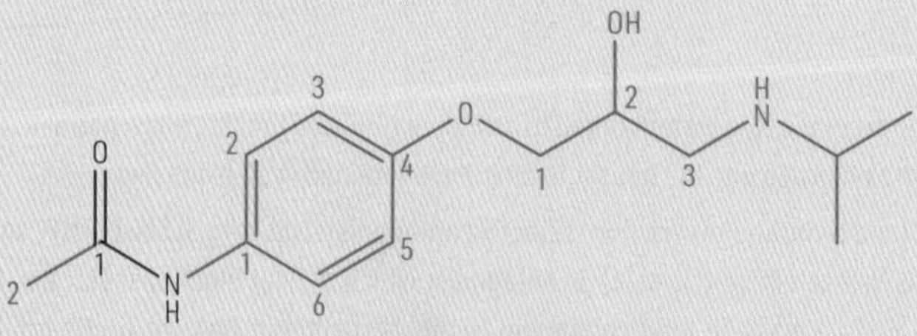

Practolol

→

Figure CS2.10 Examples of second-generation antagonists

(a)

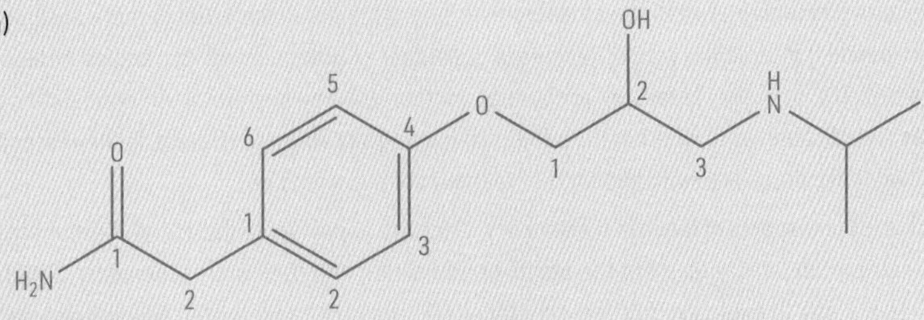

Atenolol

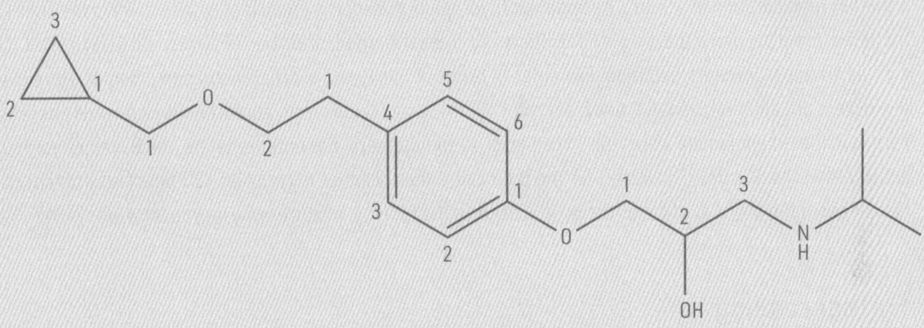

Betaxolol

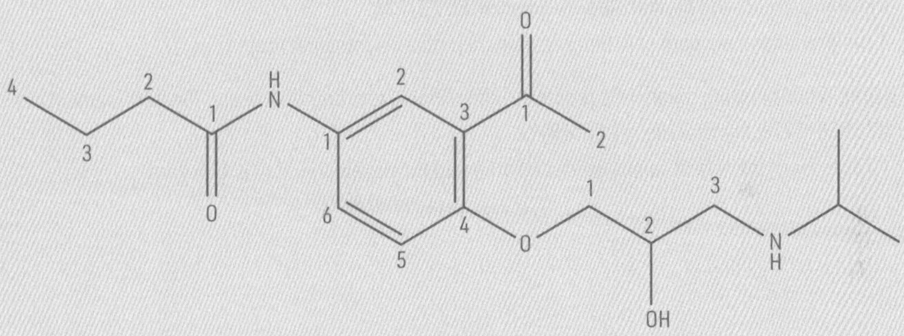

Acebutolol

(b)

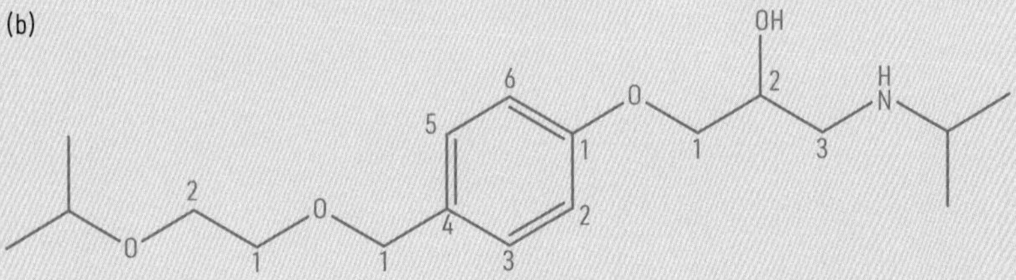

Bisoprolol

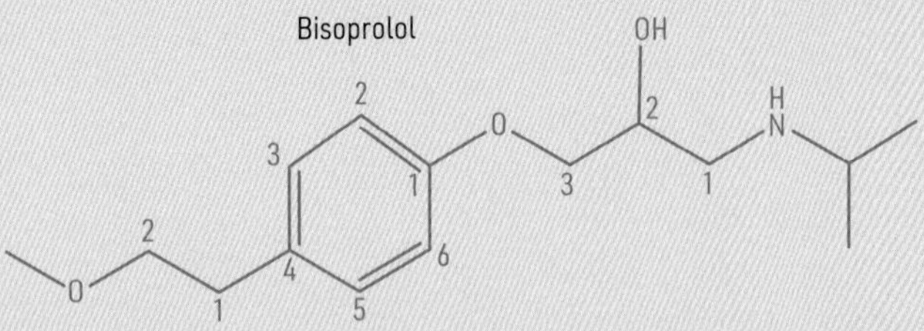

Metoprolol

Structure-activity studies on practolol showed that selectivity was only achieved if the amido functionality (shown in red) was in the para position relative to the ethanolamine sidechain, not in the ortho or meta position. This suggested an extra H-bonding interaction with β_1 receptors. A number of other second-generation antagonists were produced (Figure CS2.10)—atenolol, betaxolol, acebutolol, metoprolol, and bisoprolol. An examination of the para substituents gives an indication as to whether the additional binding site was as a H-bond donor or acceptor. Which do you think it is? All these drugs are indicated for the treatment of hypertension.

There are, of course, other aspects of medicinal chemistry which are important to the use of these antihypertensive agents, namely metabolism, ability to cross the blood-brain barrier, and their stereochemistry. Propranolol has a half-life of 3-4 hours due to extensive first pass metabolism. The other agents (the second-generation antagonists) vary between this value and 14-72 hours—check on their dosing frequency to work out whether a drug has a short or long duration of action. The lipophilic/hydrophilic balance is important with respect to the ability to cross the blood-brain barrier. If the drug is lipophilic it will cross the blood-brain barrier and could give rise to CNS effects such as dizziness, dreams, sedation. Examples of drugs of this type are propranolol and pindolol. More hydrophilic β-blockers are atenolol, nadolol, and bisoprolol. All these molecules from noradrenaline onwards possess a chiral carbon in the ethanolamine sidechain so can exist as enantiomers. For noradrenaline, the R isomer has much more activity than the S isomer. However, for the β blockers the R isomer is typically 100 times less potent than the S isomer but in the majority of cases the drug is used as the racemic mixture—why do you think this is so?

Further reading

J.G. Baker, S.J. Hill, and R.J. Summins (2011) Evolution of β-blockers: From anti-anginal drugs to ligand-directed signalling. *Trends in Pharmacological Science* 32: 227-34.

A comprehensive account of β-blockers and their pharmacological properties.

V. Quirke (2006) Putting theory into practice: James Black, receptor theory and the development of β-blockers at ICI 1958-1978. *Medical History* 50: 69-92.

An account of the role of James Black and others in the development of β-blockers.

Enzymes as Drug Targets

All of the receptors in Chapter 2 are protein molecules. Virtually all enzymes are also proteins and act as catalysts for many of the cell's chemical reactions. Enzymes, both human and non-human, are important drug targets. Many drugs act as enzyme inhibitors, hindering or preventing the catalytic activity of the enzymes. Drugs acting as inhibitors may be reversible or irreversible (**❯ XR Section 3.2.1**). Reversible inhibition may be competitive or non-competitive. A number of useful drugs exploit the biochemical differences between humans and invading organisms such as bacteria (**❯ XR Section 3.2.2**).

3.1 ENZYME SPECIFICITY

The unique tertiary structure of an enzyme usually results in the formation of a specific active site at which the enzyme selectively interacts with its substrate(s). This selectivity is mediated by a range of weak interactions such as hydrogen bonding, and electrostatic, or Van de Waals forces (**❯ XR Section 2.2.1**). In this way an optimal three-dimensional arrangement is achieved between substrate and enzyme.

3.1.1 'Lock and key' model

An attempt to explain enzyme specificity was first put forward by Emil Fischer in the late nineteenth century. This is referred to as the 'lock and key' model. In this model the substrate is the 'key', which fits the 'lock' or active site of the enzyme (see Figure 3.1). Enzyme specificity is explained by this model because, typically, only one key (or substrate) fits a given lock (or enzyme active site).

3.1.2 Induced fit model

The 'lock and key' model, although a useful concept, does not take into account the flexibility of enzymes and their substrates. To accommodate this flexibility, the induced fit model was introduced by Koshland in 1958. In this model it is proposed that the enzyme and the substrate are flexible and can mutually change their conformations, enabling a more effective interaction between the enzyme active site and the substrate, ensuring specificity and enhanced catalytic power and accommodating the change in shape as substrate becomes product (see Figure 3.2).

Figure 3.1 'Lock and Key' model of enzyme-ligand binding

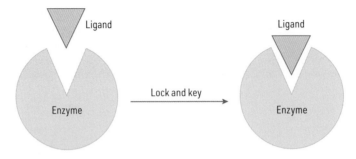

Figure 3.2 'Induced fit' model of enzyme-ligand binding

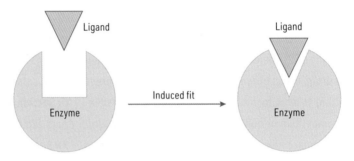

Enzyme specificity is achieved by bringing together substrate and enzyme active site in an optimal three-dimensional arrangement.

3.2 DRUG ACTIONS ON ENZYMES

Many enzymes are targets for drug action. The most common type of drug-enzyme interaction sees the drug acting as an enzyme inhibitor.

3.2.1 Drugs as enzyme inhibitors

In many cases, the drug is a structural analogue of the enzyme's normal substrate, which binds to the enzyme's active site, thus acting as an inhibitor of the normal function of the enzyme. If drugs are to act as enzyme inhibitors, they must be designed such that they are recognized by the active site of the enzyme to which they are targeted. Enzyme inhibition can be irreversible or reversible.

Irreversible inhibitors form covalent bonds with functional groups at or near the enzyme active site. Because covalent bonds are strong bonds and not easily broken the inhibitor becomes permanently attached to the active site, thus permanently modifying the active site. Molecules with this type of inhibitory action are not often used as drugs, however (see Integration Box 3.1 Organophosphates), because they tend to be too toxic, but have been used to map the enzyme's active site because they are permanently bound to the active site. A radio-labelled molecule which is irreversibly bound to the enzyme active site can, on biochemical isolation of the enzyme, allow identification of the amino acid residues to which the radio-labelled molecule is bound, providing useful structural information about the enzyme active site.

INTEGRATION BOX 3.1   **ORGANOPHOSPHATES**

Organophosphates act as irreversible covalent inhibitors of the enzyme acetylcholinesterase. This group of compounds include insecticides such as malathion, herbicides such as glyphosate, and nerve agents such as sarin (see Figure 1). Malathion is used to treat head lice and acts by reacting with a serine residue at the active site of acetylcholinesterase. A phosphorus-oxygen bond is polarized because oxygen is more electronegative than phosphorus thus making the phosphorus susceptible to nucleophilic attack. The result is the formation of a covalent bond between the hydroxyl oxygen of the serine residue and the phosphorus of the insecticide. Malathion, however, has a P = S bond rather than a P = O bond and this is the basis of the selective toxicity towards insects rather than humans. Insects metabolize malathion by replacing the sulphur with oxygen, producing a more powerful inhibitor. Humans, however, hydrolyse the carboxylate ester to produce an inactive molecule which is easily excreted. Nerve gases such as sarin attack acetylcholinesterase by a similar mechanism, but in this case, there is no selective toxicity towards insects.

Figure 1 Organophosphates

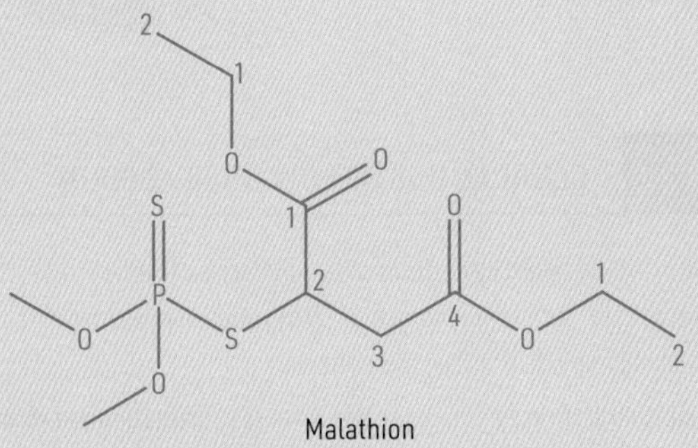

Malathion

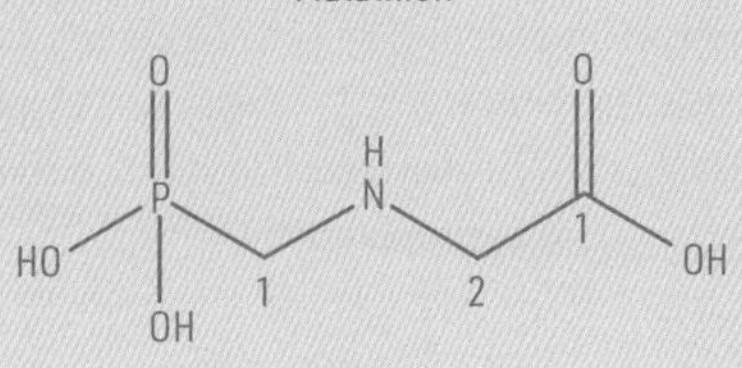

Glyphosate

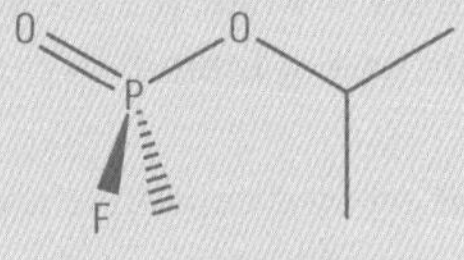

Sarin

One important drug molecule which is known to act by irreversible inhibition, however, is aspirin. Aspirin irreversibly inhibits cyclooxygenase, an enzyme responsible for the production of prostaglandins from unsaturated fatty acids. Aspirin irreversibly inhibits cyclooxygenase by acetylation of serine hydroxyl groups at the active site (see Figure 3.3 and see Integration Box 3.2 Clinical use of low dose aspirin) by a **transesterification** reaction.

Figure 3.3 Aspirin inhibits cyclooxygenase (COX) by acetylating the active site, thus inactivating the enzyme

(Credit: From Therapeutics and Human Physiology edited by Elsie Gaskell and Chris Rostron (2013). Reproduced with permission of Oxford University Press through PLSclear).

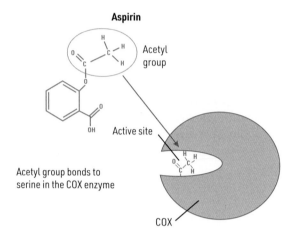

INTEGRATION BOX 3.2   CLINICAL USE OF LOW DOSE ASPIRIN

A small daily dose of aspirin is now taken by millions of people at risk from a stroke, myocardial infarction or follow-ing cardiac surgery to prevent clot formation. A dose of 75 mg aspirin is used in this context, by comparison with the normal dose of at least 300 mg aspirin for other indications.

Aspirin works by irreversibly inhibiting cyclooxygenase. This results in reduced thromboxane A_2 (TXA_2) in platelets and reduced prostacyclin synthesis in the endothelium of blood vessels. Low doses of aspirin, however, are more effective at reducing TXA_2 synthesis than prostacyclin synthesis. As TXA_2 promotes platelet aggregation and pros-tacyclin inhibits platelet aggregation, a preferential reduction in TXA_2 is clinically desirable. A lower dose of aspirin also reduces unwanted side effects such as gastro-intestinal damage.

Most drugs that act as enzyme inhibitors do so by reversible inhibition, which can be competitive or non-competitive. Competitive inhibition is when the inhibitor and the normal substrate compete for binding at the enzyme active site. This type of inhibition can be overcome by increasing the concentra-tion of the normal substrate.

One example of a class of drugs that act by competitive reversible inhibition is the statins. These drugs inhibit the activity of HMG-CoA reductase, a key enzyme involved in the biosynthesis of cholesterol. The drugs have structures that are partially similar to the natural substrate of the enzyme (see Figure 3.4 (a) and Box 3.1 Prodrugs and blockbuster drugs).

Non-competitive inhibition is where the inhibitor does not bind to the enzyme active site and so is not in competition with the normal substrate for the active site. An example of non-competitive inhibition is the action of donepezil. It is an acetylcholinesterase inhibitor given to patients with Alzheimer's disease used to slow down the loss of cognitive abilities. Alzheimer's sufferers have a low level of acetylcholine in the brain and donepezil, as an acetylcholinesterase inhibitor, helps to maintain it at a functional level. X-ray crystallography has shown that donepezil does not actually bind to the acetylcholinesterase active site but to at an allosteric site (▶ **XR Integration Box 2.5**), thus making the inhibition non-competitive. The ability of the enzyme to bind the endogenous substrate is not affected but the enzyme activity is reduced.

 Many drugs bring about their clinical activity by acting as inhibitors of human enzymes.

BOX 3.1   **PRODRUGS AND BLOCKBUSTER DRUGS**

The first statin drug to be introduced was lovastatin, followed rapidly by simvastatin and pravastatin. If the structures of these drugs are examined (see Figure 3.4 (b)), it is not obvious which part of their structures resemble the natural substrate, HMG-CoA. These molecules are, in fact, prodrugs (▶ **XR Section 12.6.4**). The lactone ring which each of them possess is easily hydrolysed by enzymes in the body to produce the acyclic partial structure resembling HMG-CoA.

These molecules contain numerous chiral centres, which make them difficult to synthesize. As a result, second-generation statins—with only two chiral centres (making them much easier to synthesize)—were produced. One example of this class is atorvastatin, which for a number of years has been a 'blockbuster' drug, i.e. a drug which generates over $1 million for its pharmaceutical company each year. In fact, atorvastatin has been in the top ten selling drugs each year since 2001, regularly earning over $10 billion per year for its manufacturer, Pfizer, until the patent expired in 2012.

Figure 3.4 (a) Reaction catalysed by HMG-CoA reductase

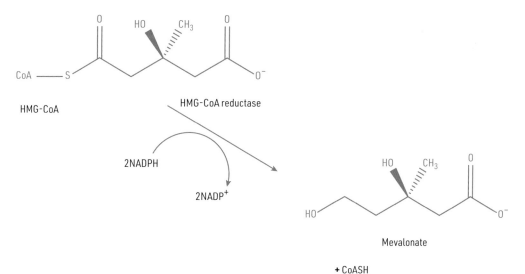

Figure 3.4 (b) Examples of HMG-CoA reductase inhibitors (statins)

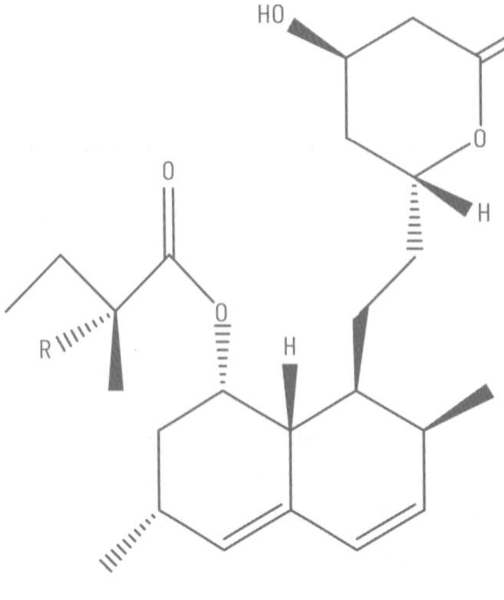

R=H Lovastatin
R=CH$_3$ Simvastatin

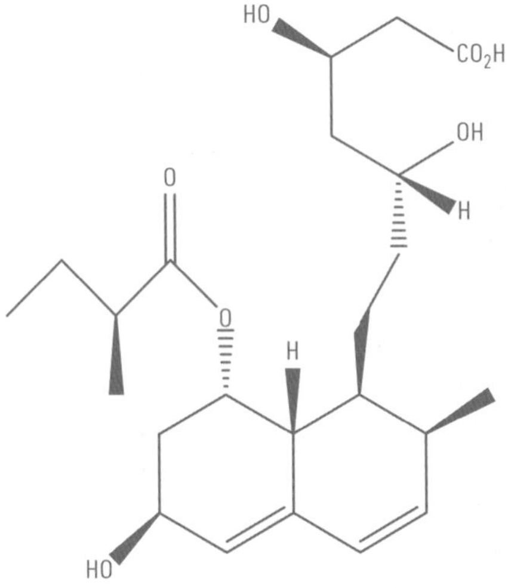

Pravastatin

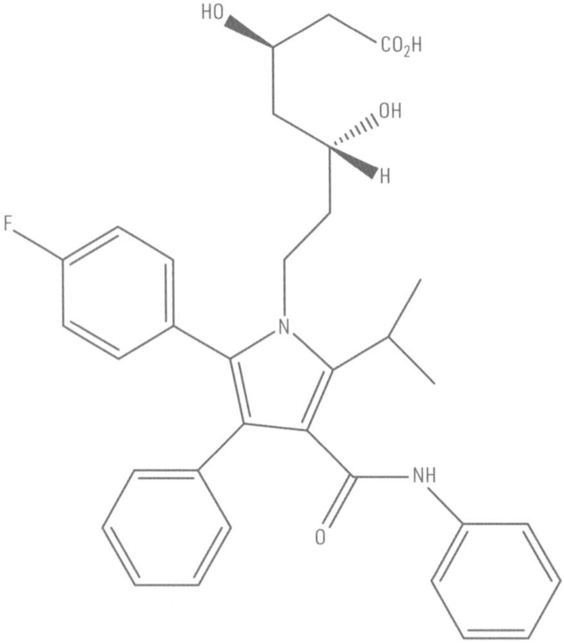

Atorvastatin

3.2.2 Drugs as non-human enzyme inhibitors

The success of a significant number of drugs arises from the way they target the selective activity between an invading organism and the host. This is the molecular basis of chemotherapy. Three classes of biochemical reactions are potential targets for such drugs. Class I reactions are where there is no significant difference between the invading organism and humans (e.g. glycolysis, TCA cycle). Class I reactions are generally not utilized as drug targets as any inhibition caused by a drug would apply equally to the patient and the invading organism.

Pathways in class II reactions exist in invading organism cells but not in human cells and so are more promising as drug targets because they provide an opportunity for drugs to target the invading organism but not the host. A good example of this class is the biosynthesis of folate found in bacterial cells but not in human cells. Humans cannot synthesize folate, so must obtain it from their diet. As such, they have a transport mechanism for its uptake into cells. Bacteria, however, cannot absorb folate and must synthesize it (see Figure 3.6).

PABA (para-aminobenzoic acid) is essential for the biosynthesis of folate, a fact that acts as the basis of the action of the sulfonamide group of drugs. Sulfonamides compete with PABA for the enzyme dihydropteroate synthase, thus inhibiting the synthesis of folate. This inhibition arrests bacterial cell growth and division. Because the nature of the inhibition is competitive, the sulfonamides are bacteriostatic and not bacteriocidal.

The effectiveness of the competitive inhibition of dihydropteroate can be enhanced by the folate antagonist trimethoprim. Folic acid, once biosynthesized, is an essential coenzyme in the bacterial and human biosynthesis of the nucleotide base thymidine (part of DNA). This pathway is essentially identical in both humans and microorganisms. However, one of the enzymes in the pathway, dihydrofolate reductase, is much more sensitive to folate antagonists in bacteria than in humans. Consequently, the combination of a sulfonamide and trimethoprim is more successful than either drug alone (see Figure 3.6).

In class III reactions the pathways for producing certain macromolecules exhibit significant differences between humans and microorganisms. Such reactions are also good targets for selective toxicity towards the invading organism. A good example of drugs which are used in this context is those that interfere with the biosynthesis of peptidoglycans, a constituent of bacterial cell walls but not of human cell walls. Many antibiotic drugs act in this way. Penicillins and cephalosporins inhibit **transpeptidation** which causes cross-linking between the peptide chains. Vancomycin inhibits the release of peptide building units, preventing addition of the peptide building unit to the growing **peptidoglycan** chain (see Integration Box 3.3 Antibiotic resistance).

 Many chemotherapeutic agents exploit the biochemical differences between humans and microorganisms.

INTEGRATION BOX 3.3   **ANTIBIOTIC RESISTANCE**

In a report in 2013, Dame Sally Davies, the Chief Medical Officer for England, stated that 'antibiotic resistance posed a catastrophic threat'. Man's ability to treat life-threatening bacterial infections with antibiotics has been one of the greatest achievements of medical treatment. However, bacteria have been equally as effective at developing resistance to these antibacterial drugs. This situation is, essentially, evolution in action. Bacteria have a very rapid generation time. This means that there is an increased possibility of a mutation occurring which will produce a bacterial strain that is resistant to a particular antibacterial drug. Antibiotic resistance arises via a number of biochemical mechanisms.

→

These include the production of enzymes, such as β-lactamases, that inactivate the drug. These enzymes can be se-lective for specific classes of antibiotic, e.g. penicillinases for penicillins and cephalosporinases for cephalosporins. In some cases, bacteria develop drug-specific efflux mechanisms such as those for tetracyclines and fluoroquinolones. In this situation bacteria develop genes which code for the production of 'resistance' proteins which promote the active removal of antibiotics back out through the bacterial cell membrane, lowering their concentration and effectiveness.

Plasmid-mediated resistance can lead to the formation of an enzyme which has little affinity for the drug, such as a dihydrofolate reductase with very low affinity for trimethoprim. The ease with which bacteria can transfer genetic material via plasmids and **transposons** can rapidly lead to the development of strains of bacteria with mul-tiple resistances to available antibiotics, e.g. multiple resistant *Staphylococcus aureus* (MRSA). (Although, strictly speaking, the M stands for Meticillin, it could equally well represent 'multiple'.) An increased understanding of the genetic code of bacteria and how this controls their mechanism of protein synthesis will, hopefully, lead to the iden-tification of new targets for antibacterial drugs.

Figure 3.5 Effect of drugs on bacterial folate biosynthesis

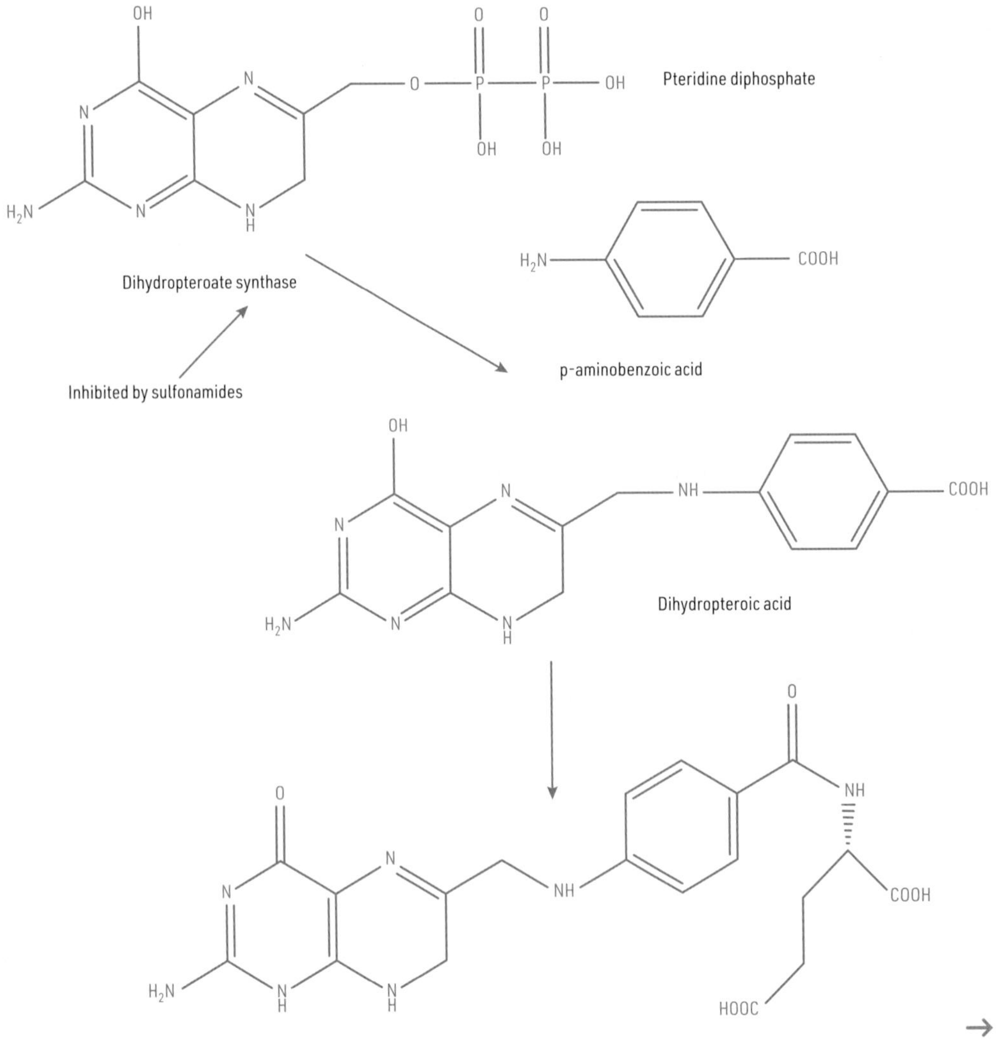

→

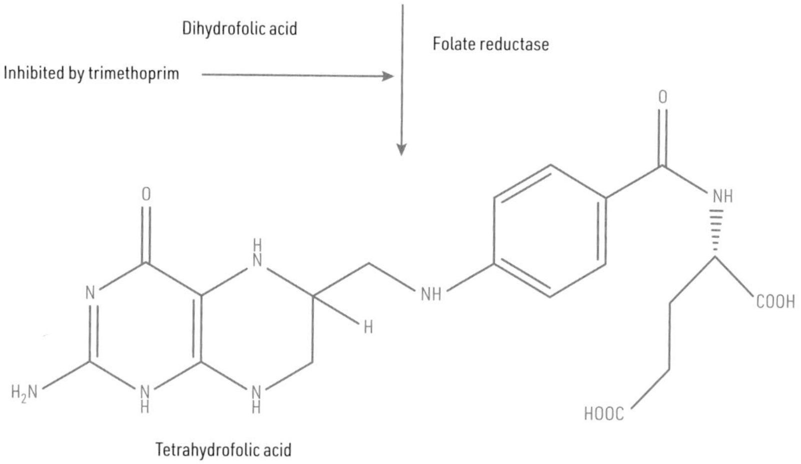

Dihydrofolic acid

Folate reductase

Inhibited by trimethoprim ⟶

Tetrahydrofolic acid

3.2.3 The challenges of enzymes as drug targets

The most significant challenges to the use of enzymes as drug targets are cell permeability, selectivity, and metabolic inactivation. Many enzymes have polar active sites and the types of molecules which would be expected to interact with such sites are usually difficult to get to cross cell membranes. Consequently, it is difficult for such molecules to reach the enzyme active site.

Many enzyme active sites are very similar (e.g. phosphatases) and, therefore, inhibitors are likely to act at similar active sites to the desired one and this may lead to adverse effects. One approach to this problem is to develop allosteric inhibitors which do not bind at the active site itself.

The vast majority of molecules which are targeted towards enzyme active sites will be molecules which are not normally present in the body (i.e. **xenobiotics**). As such the body's normal defences will attempt to remove them from the body as quickly as possible. This process usually involves metabolism to a molecule which is easily excreted, usually via the urine (❯ **XR Chapter 12**). Useful drugs, therefore, need to be sufficiently protected against these processes to allow them to reach the enzyme active site in order to bring about the desired action.

> Cell permeability, selectivity, and metabolic inactivation are the main challenges to the use of enzymes as drug targets.

? Questions

1. How can irreversible inhibitors be used to map enzyme active sites?

2. Sulfonamides compete with PABA for the active site of dihydropteroate synthetase. Show the probable binding sites of both PABA and a sulfonamide with the enzyme active site.

3. In what ways might bacterial resistance to antibiotics be reduced?

Chapter summary

- Enzyme inhibitors can be reversible or irreversible. The former are more commonly used as drugs. The inhibition may be competitive or non-competitive.

- Many drugs exploit the difference between human biochemistry and that of invading organisms such as bacteria.

- Classes II and III categories of biochemical reactions are more useful to exploit as here the differences between humans and microorganisms are greatest.

- Because of their ability to evolve rapidly, bacteria have developed significant resistance to many of the existing antibiotics.

- The main challenges of enzymes as drug targets are cell permeability, selectivity, and avoidance of metabolic inactivation.

Further reading

Copeland, R.A., Harpel, M.R., and Tummino, P.J. (2007) Targeting enzyme inhibitors in drug discovery, *Expert Opinion on Therapeutic Targets* 11: 967–78.

A comprehensive review of the role of enzyme inhibitors in drug discovery.

Lowe, D. (2010) In the pipeline, *Chemistry World*, September 7: 18.

An industrial medicinal chemist's perspective on enzyme inhibitors as drug candidates.

Tackling antimicrobial resistance (2015) *RSC News*, May 12–13.

Views on antimicrobial resistance from the Royal Society of Chemistry.

Broadwith, P. (2013) Re-arming the antibiotic arsenal, *Chemistry World* October 10: 48–51.

An article which describes the approaches being taken to produce new antibiotics.

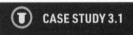 **CASE STUDY 3.1** **DRUGS INSPIRED BY XENOBIOTICS–DEVELOPMENT OF ANGIOTENSIN CONVERTING ENZYME INHIBITORS AND ANGIOTENSIN II RECEPTOR BLOCKERS**

Angiotensin converting enzyme (ACE) in plasma was discovered in 1956. ACE is responsible for converting the inactive decapeptide angiotensin I to form the octapeptide angiotensin II which is a potent vasoconstrictor and causes high blood pressure if present in excessive amounts. ACE also degrades bradykinin and, therefore, increases circulating levels of bradykinin. Inhibition of ACE could find use in the treatment of heart failure and hypertension. In the early 1960s a Brazilian scientist identified a substance, bradykinin potentiating factor (BPF), in the venom of the Brazilian pit viper (*Bothrops jararaca*) (Figure CS3.1) which potentiated

$\rightarrow$

→

the action of bradykinin. Pit viper venom was historically used as an arrow poison and caused death by uncontrolled lowering of blood pressure. How do you think it achieves this? However, an understanding of the mode of action of this poison led to the development of ACE inhibitors being used to combat hypertension. This scientist took his isolated BPF to John Vane's pharmacology research group and, subsequently, the research group was able to isolate peptides with ACE-inhibitory activity because they had developed a specific *in vitro* assay for measuring ACE activity. The original pentapeptide (BPF), as well as potentiating bradykinin activity, also inhibited ACE activity and lowered blood pressure in animal models but it was rapidly degraded. Subsequently, workers at Squibb Laboratories produced a series of larger peptides of which a nonapeptide, teprotide, was extremely stable. It was an effective antihypertensive but lacked oral activity (why do you think this is?). However, the peptide work had also led to the development of key test systems for evaluating ACE inhibitory activity, including a simple guinea-pig ileum test which was highly predictive of antihypertensive activity.

Figure CS3.1 Brazilian pit viper (*Bothrops jararaca*)

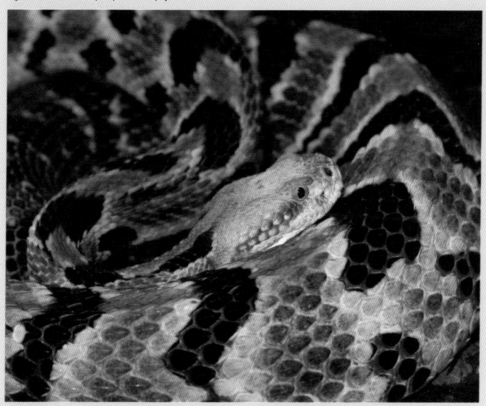

→

→

ACE is a metalloprotease enzyme (i.e. it contains a metal ion) and is responsible for hydrolysis of peptide links. In ACE this metal is zinc and is present as the zinc ion Zn^{++} (Figure CS3.2). It is coordinated to the nitrogen of two histidine residues and the carboxylate group from an acidic amino acid. The fourth ligand is an activated water molecule. ACE is responsible for the hydrolysis of a peptide bond in angiotensin I, resulting in the removal of a dipeptide to produce angiotensin II (Figure CS3.3). The zinc ion activates the bound water molecule so that it attacks the carbonyl group of the peptide bond, essentially catalysing the hydrolysis.

The first ACE inhibitor to be developed was captopril. The rational drug design process was based on the hypothesis that ACE and carboxypeptidase A acted by similar mechanisms. 2-benzylsuccinic acid (Figure CS3.4) was already known to be a potent inhibitor of carboxypeptidase A but it did not inhibit ACE, however it was used as a lead compound. The active site of carboxypeptidase A contains two important binding sites—an arginine residue and a zinc ion. The suggestion was that, for 2-benzylsuccinic acid, one carboxyl group interacted with arginine and the other carboxy group with the zinc ion (Figure CS3.5). It binds strongly to the active site but doesn't undergo hydrolysis because there is no amide (peptide) bond present and it, therefore, blocks the receptor. Carboxypeptidase

Figure CS3.2 In ACE this metal is zinc and is present as the zinc ion Zn^{++}

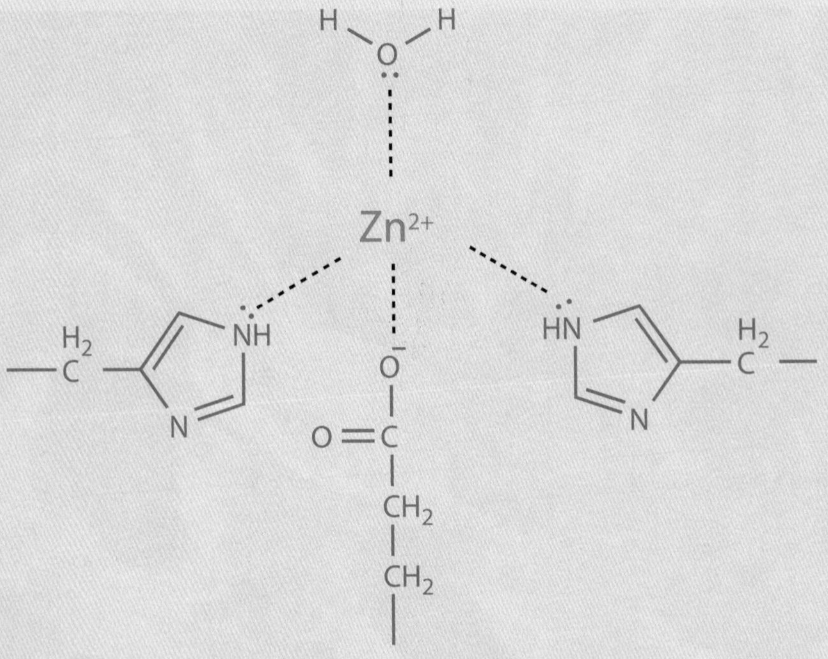

Figure CS3.3 Action of angiotensin converting enzyme (ACE)

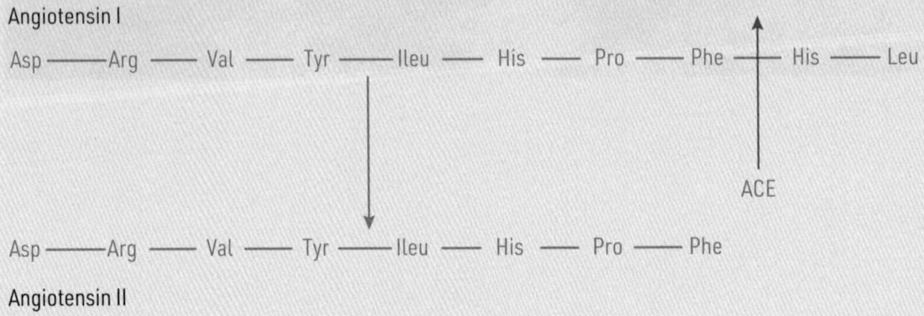

Angiotensin I

Asp —— Arg —— Val —— Tyr —— Ileu —— His —— Pro —— Phe ——|—— His —— Leu

ACE

Asp —— Arg —— Val —— Tyr —— Ileu —— His —— Pro —— Phe

Angiotensin II

→

→

A only removes one amino acid from a peptide chain, but ACE removes two. Thus an assumption was made that the distance between the two binding sites would be greater, so it was decided to produce a molecule similar to 2-benzylsuccinic acid but somewhat bigger. The work with the pit viper venom peptides suggested the dipeptide Ala-Pro. This suggestion led to the synthesis and testing of succinylproline (Figure CS3.6), a molecule which did inhibit ACE. However there was no equivalent of the hydrophobic benzyl group present in benzyl succinic acid so a hydrophobic group (methyl—highlighted in red) was introduced (Figure CS3.7). An attempt to find a group which would interact more effectively with the zinc ion led to the introduction of a thiol group which further increased the inhibitory activity—this was captopril (Figure CS3.8). Why do you think the introduction of an SH group increases the activity? The design process from PBF to captopril is summarized in Figure CS3.9. The equivalent of

Figure CS3.4 2-benzylsuccinic acid

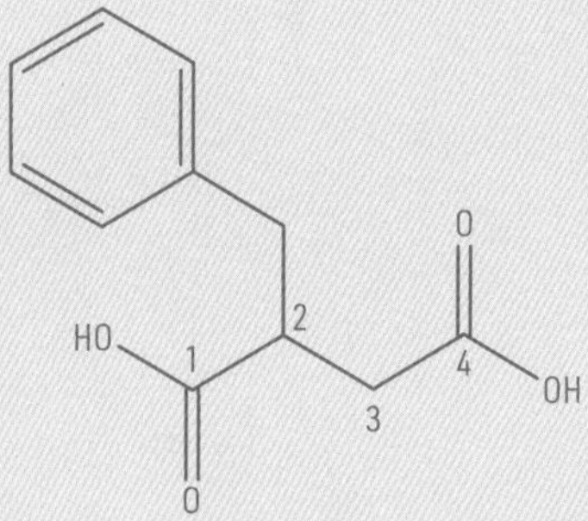

2-benzylsuccinic acid

Figure CS3.5 Proposed interaction of 2-benzylsuccinic acid with enzyme active site

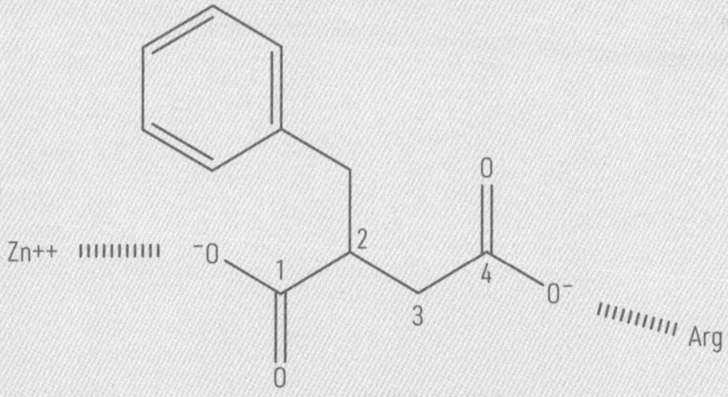

Figure CS3.6 Succinylproline

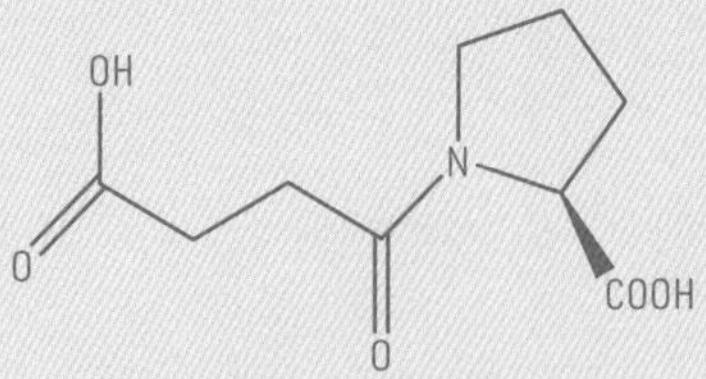

Succinylproline

→

→

Figure CS3.7 Addition of methyl group to increase hydrophobicity

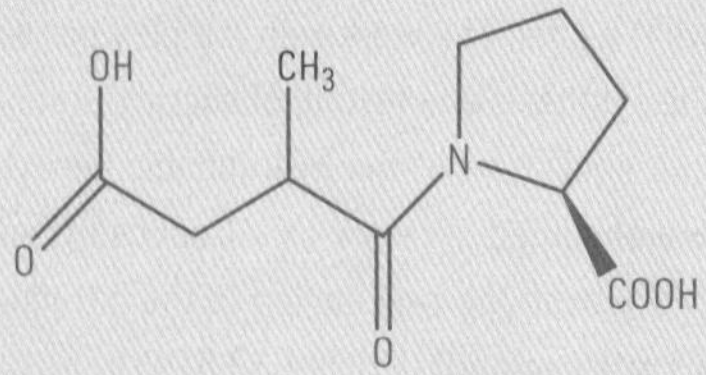

Figure CS3.8 Captopril

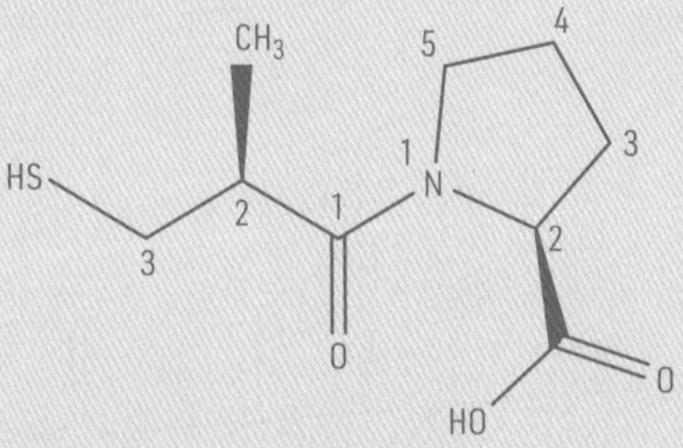

Captopril

Figure CS3.9 Journey from BPF to captopril

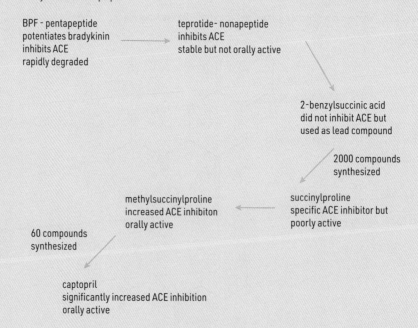

BPF – pentapeptide
potentiates bradykinin
inhibits ACE
rapidly degraded

teprotide– nonapeptide
inhibits ACE
stable but not orally active

2-benzylsuccinic acid
did not inhibit ACE but
used as lead compound

2000 compounds
synthesized

methylsuccinylproline
increased ACE inhibiton
orally active

succinylproline
specific ACE inhibitor but
poorly active

60 compounds
synthesized

captopril
significantly increased ACE inhibition
orally active

→

→

Figure CS3.10 Enalapril

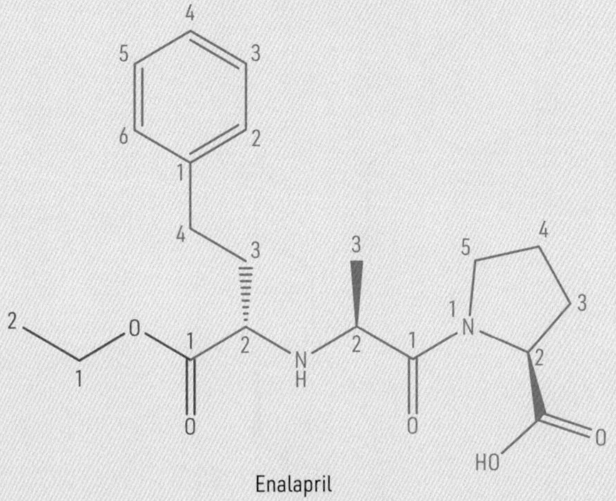

Enalapril

the phenylalanine residue (present in angiotensin I) was introduced to enhance interaction with the enzyme active site to yield enalapril (Figure CS3.10).

However, the original assumption that the binding was the same in ACE and carboxypeptidase A was subsequently shown not to be the case. As a result of a greater knowledge of the ACE receptor, the drug lisinopril (Figure CS3.11) was developed. It should be noted that enalapril is actually an inactive prodrug. For the ACE inhibitor activity to take effect the ethyl ester (highlighted in red in Figure CS3.10) must be hydrolysed back to the carboxylate group (enalaprilat) once the prodrug has been absorbed into the bloodstream Enalaprilat itself is inactive orally and medicinal chemists converted the carboxy group to an ester (enalapril) which is suitable for oral delivery and is metabolized to the active form. Lisinopril possesses the necessary carboxy group (highlighted in red in Figure CS3.11).

One of the significant side effects of ACE inhibitors is an interference with bradykinin levels and this produced, in some patients, a persistent dry cough which becomes debilitating. Inhibition of ACE prevents the breakdown of bradykinin which is a bronchoconstrictor and this can give rise to the persistent dry cough. In order to avoid this, the suggestion was made to antagonize the product of ACE–angiotensin II which is an octapeptide. A number of structural variations of angiotensin II were produced but with only limited success. However this did lead to the development of a series of imidazole-5-acetic acids (Figure CS3.12) which acted as antagonists. Further structural modifications led to the production of losartan (Figure CS3.13). Losartan is metabolized to the carboxylic acid (highlighted in. Figure CS3.14) which is required for binding to the receptor site. Further development led to production of a range of 'sartan' derivatives–candesartan, irbesartan, valsartan etc., known as angiotensin II receptor blockers (ARBs) (Figure CS3.15) which are not inhibiting angiotensin converting enzyme (ACE). Candesartan possesses an ester which is metabolized to the free acid required for binding. Irbesartan does not have an acid group but can hydrogen bond to the receptor via the amide. Valsartan already possesses an acid group.

But what about the rest of the complex structures–what else are structural requirements? Losartan has an imidazole ring and candesartan has a benzimidazole ring but irbesartan and valsartan have no imidazole ring, so maybe

→

→

Figure CS3.11 Lisinopril

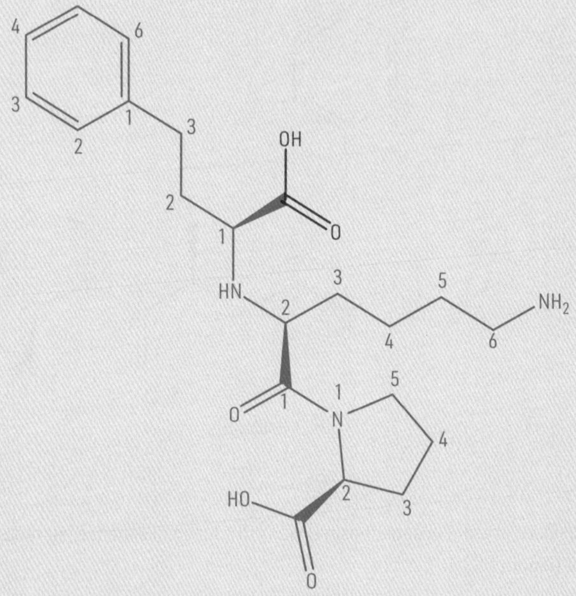

Lisinopril

Figure CS3.12 Imidazole derivatives

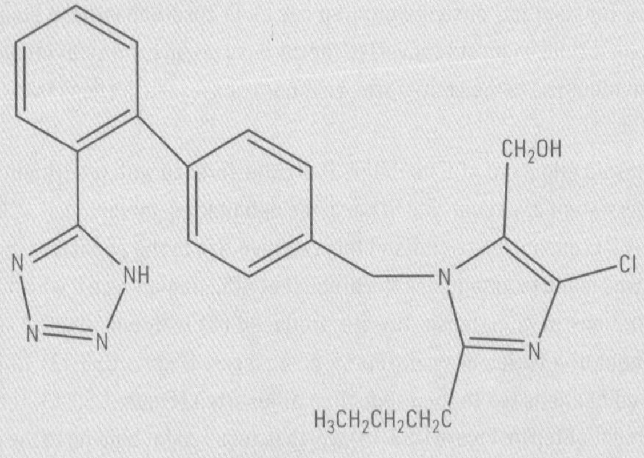

the imidazole ring is not a structural requirement. The tetrazole ring appears to be a structural requirement as it is present in all the structures, as also is the biphenyl system.

Subsequent research on ACE showed that the C-terminus domain is involved in angiotensin hydrolysis and hence blood pressure regulation. However, the N-terminus domain appears to be involved with the bradykinin system and

→

→

Figure CS3.13 Losartan

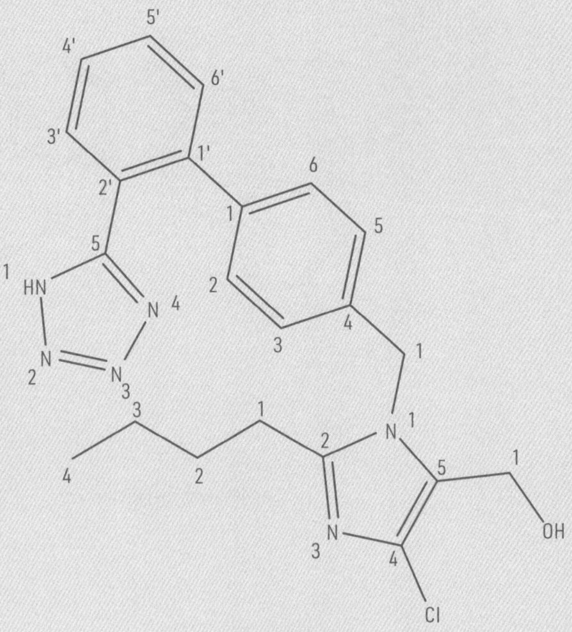

Losartan

Figure CS3.14 Losartan metabolite

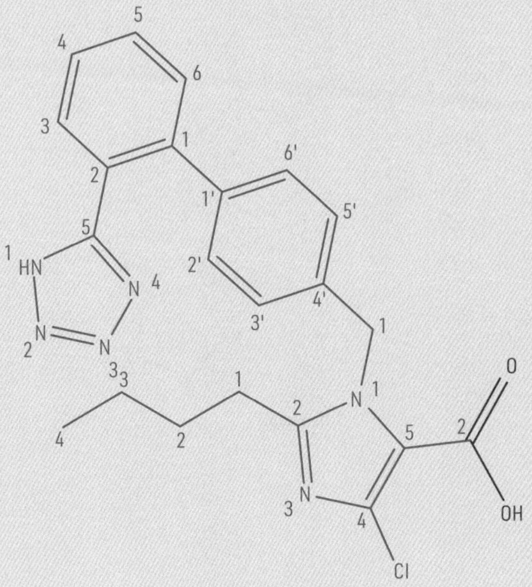

Losartan metabolite

→

→

Figure CS3.15 Examples of other sartans

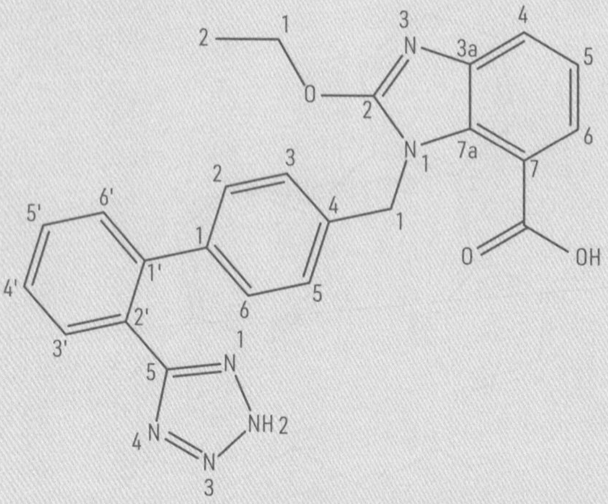

Candesartan metabolite

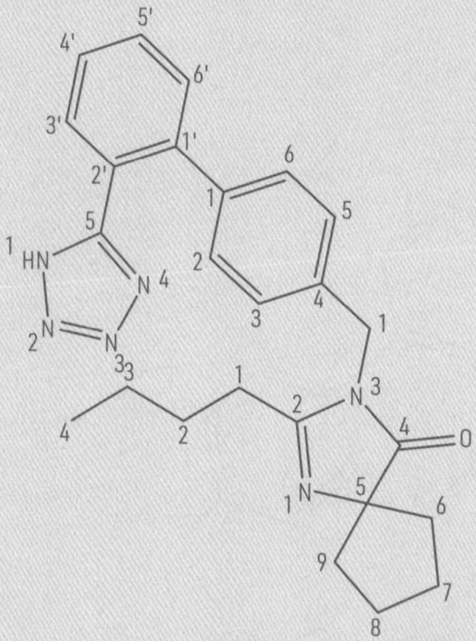

Irbesartan

→

→

Figure CS3.15 (*Cont.*)

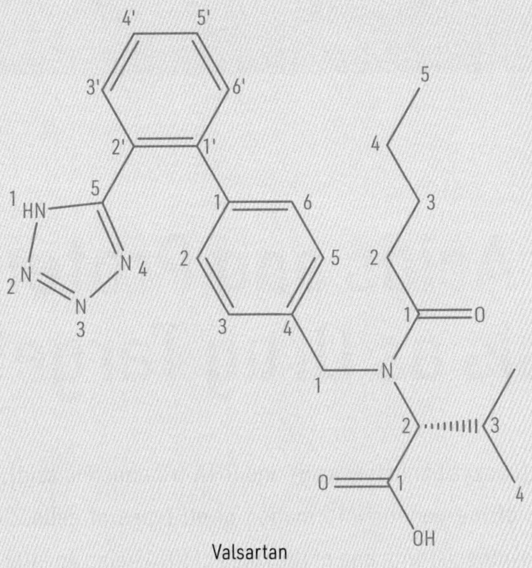

Valsartan

hence the persistent cough and angioedema. Consequently future work will be concentrated of on development of inhibition at the C-terminus.

Further reading

D.W. Cushman and M.A. Ondetti (1991) History of the design of captopril and related inhibitors of angiotensin converting enzyme. *Hypertension* 17: 589–92.
An account of the development of ACE inhibitors by workers who were involved in the project.

J. Bryan (2009) From snake venom to ACE inhibitors—the discovery and rise of captopril. *Pharmaceutical Journal*. 17 April.
An account of the development of and the initial problems of dosage with ACE inhibitors.

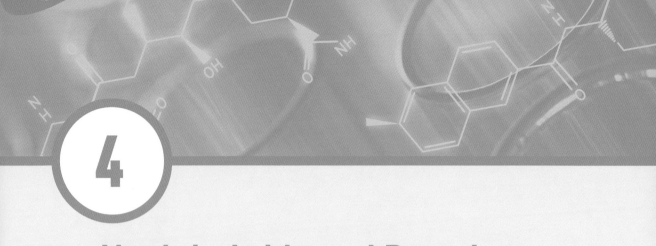

Nucleic Acids and Protein Synthesis as Drug Targets

The nucleic acids, DNA (deoxyribonucleic acid) and RNA (ribonucleic acid), are responsible for the storage and processing of the genetic information of all types of cells. Sequences of DNA carry instructions for protein synthesis, with one of the roles of RNA being an intermediate in this process. Many drugs, such as antibacterial, antiviral, and anti-cancer drugs, target nucleic acids and protein synthesis.

4.1 STRUCTURE AND FUNCTION OF NUCLEIC ACIDS

Some classes of anti-cancer drugs bring about their activity by interfering with the normal structure of nucleic acids. It is important, therefore, to understand the normal structure of nucleic acids (❯ XR Section 4.1.1). Other classes of anti-cancer drugs target the synthesis of nucleic acids. They do so at all stages of nucleic acid synthesis, namely transcription (❯ XR Section 4.1.2), translation (❯ XR Section 4.1.3), and replication (❯ XR Section 4.1.4).

4.1.1 Structure of nucleic acids

DNA and RNA are biopolymers composed of repeating monomeric units known as nucleotides (see Figure 4.1). Each nucleotide consists of three distinct components—a heterocyclic base, a ribose sugar and a phosphate group. The ribose sugar units are covalently bonded to the heterocyclic bases and are known as nucleosides. The sugar is 2'-deoxyribose in DNA and ribose in RNA.

In the nucleic acid polymers the nucleotides are joined together by alternating phosphate and sugar groups to form the nucleic acid backbone. A phosphodiester bond is formed between the 3' position of the sugar in one nucleotide and the 5' position of the next sugar residue. The nucleotides are always joined in the 5' to the 3' direction. The heterocyclic bases are of two types—pyrimidines and purines. The pyrimidine bases are cytosine (C) and thymine (T), and the purine bases are adenine (A) and

Figure 4.1 The nucleotide strand

(Credit: From Therapeutics and Human Physiology edited by Elsie Gaskell and Chris Rostron (2013). Reproduced with permission of Oxford University Press through PLSclear).

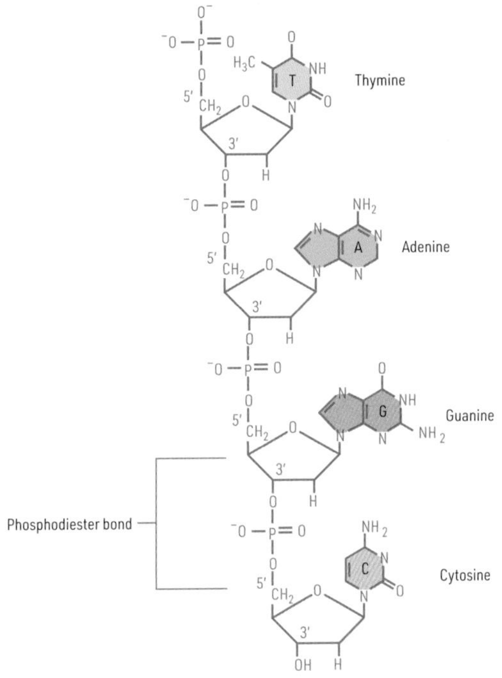

guanine (G). These four bases are present in DNA; in RNA, however, thymine is replaced by uracil (U) (see Figure 4.2).

The sequence of nucleotides within a nucleic acid molecule is represented by single letter abbreviations of the heterocyclic bases; by convention, the sequences are always written in the 5' to the 3' direction. Normally, DNA in cells is in the form of a double helix in which two separate strands of DNA are held together by hydrogen bonds between the heterocyclic bases. The strands are joined together in an antiparallel manner with one strand running in the 5' to the 3' direction and the other strand running in the 3' to the 5' direction.

The hydrogen bonds between the heterocyclic bases are very specific. Adenine and thymine are always joined by two hydrogen bonds, and guanine and cytosine are always joined by three hydrogen bonds. In RNA, thymine is not present so adenine bonds with uracil. Because of this specific hydrogen bonding, the base sequence of each strand of the DNA is matched and so the base sequence is said to be complementary between the strands.

This double helix structure is very stable and protects the sequence of bases on the inside of the double helix, ensuring the integrity of the genetic code. When cells are required to synthesize specific proteins, the relevant parts of the genetic code, known as genes (see Box 4.1 The differences between human and bacterial genomes), are expressed via RNA molecules. Expression of genes means that the coded information within the specific genes is copied into RNA molecules (transcription), followed by decoding and protein synthesis (translation).

RNA is different in structure from DNA. Unlike DNA, RNA usually exists as a single strand and is found in a variety of three-dimensional shapes as opposed to the double helix of DNA. There are three principal

Figure 4.2 Nucleic acid heterocyclic bases

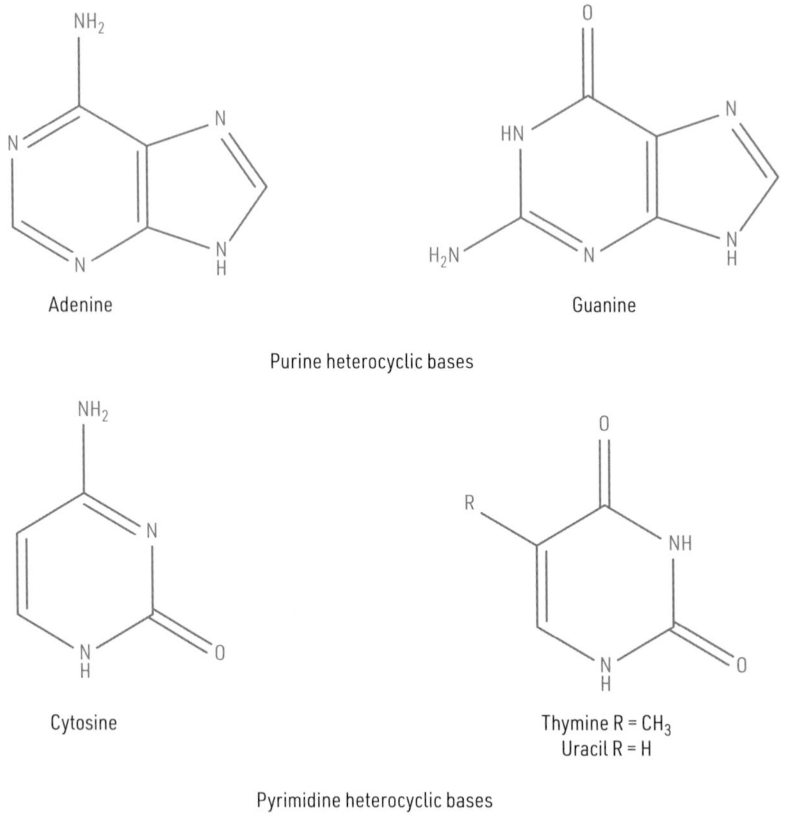

Adenine

Guanine

Purine heterocyclic bases

Cytosine

Thymine R = CH_3
Uracil R = H

Pyrimidine heterocyclic bases

types of RNA: messenger RNA (mRNA), transfer RNA (tRNA), and ribosomal RNA (rRNA). They each have a particular role in the transcription of genes and the synthesis of specific proteins by translation. These are the types of RNA which are currently the targets for drugs. In addition, there are functional RNA molecules (fRNA), often also referred to as non-coding RNA (ncRNA). fRNA molecules are not translated into protein. The roles of fRNA are only just beginning to be investigated and may, in the future, produce yet more drug targets.

BOX 4.1   THE DIFFERENCES BETWEEN HUMAN AND BACTERIAL GENOMES

The human genome consists of twenty-three pairs of linear chromosomes whereas the bacterial genome consists of a single circular chromosome. The amount of DNA in a human cell is ~ 1000X the amount of DNA in a bacterial cell. Human chromosomes are contained in the nucleus whereas the bacterial chromosome is present in the cytoplasm. The bacterial chromosome is haploid whereas human chromosomes are diploid. The large amount of DNA in a human cell is supercoiled and attached to histone proteins. Human DNA has non-coding sequences called introns which are absent in bacteria.

DNA and RNA both consist of repeating units of nucleotides, which are composed of a heterocyclic base, a ribose sugar, and a phosphate group.

The heterocyclic bases in DNA are cytosine, thymine, adenine, and guanine. In RNA thymine is replaced by uracil. DNA takes the form of a double helix in which two separate nucleotide strands are held together by hydrogen bonds. RNA has a single-stranded structure and consists of three principal types—mRNA, tRNA, and rRNA.

4.1.2 Transcription

Transcription is the process by which the genetic code, contained within DNA, is copied in the form of an RNA molecule and then transferred to a ribosome (❭ **XR Section 4.1.3**).

Transcription takes place in three phases—initiation, elongation, and termination. It involves the unwinding of the DNA double helix and the copying of the genetic code in the form of an mRNA molecule. Initiation involves the formation of an RNA polymerase II transcription complex. RNA polymerases are enzyme complexes that are responsible for transcribing the genetic code from DNA to RNA. Eukaryotic cells have three different versions of this enzyme complex—RNA polymerase I, II, and III. RNA polymerase II is responsible for the transcription of genes coding for protein into mRNA. For the elongation phase the RNA polymerase II separates from the initiation complex and moves along the DNA strand which is to be transcribed in a 3' to 5' direction, unwinding the DNA double helix as it moves. The RNA molecule is formed in the 5' to 3' direction, and nucleotides complementary to those on the DNA strand are added to the growing messenger RNA (mRNA) molecule. The mRNA so produced has exactly the same base sequence as the coding strand of DNA except that thymine is replaced by uracil. This molecule is known as pre-mRNA. Termination occurs when RNA polymerase II releases the mRNA transcript (see Figure 4.3).

Genes contain protein-coding sequences known as exons separated by non-coding sequences known as introns. Intron sequences copied within the mRNA are removed and the coding sequences are joined together. This splicing process results in the production of a mature mRNA (see Figure 4.4).

Figure 4.3 The RNA Pol II transcription initiation complex and the arrangement of regulatory sequences. RNA Pol II, RNA polymerase II; URE, upstream regulatory elements; Inr, initiator

(Credit: From Therapeutics and Human Physiology edited by Elsie Gaskell and Chris Rostron (2013). Reproduced with permission of Oxford University Press through PLSclear).

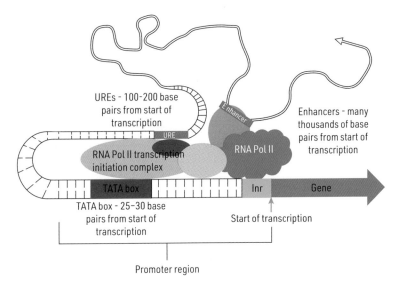

Figure 4.4 Splicing of mRNA

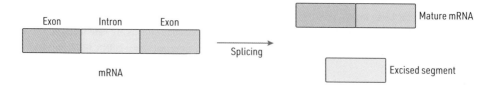

 Transcription involves the unwinding of the DNA double helix and the copying of a specific portion in the form of an mRNA molecule.

4.1.3 Translation

Translation takes place within the ribosomes. Ribosomes are the site of protein synthesis and consist of a mixture of ribosomal RNA (rRNA) and ribosomal protein.

The mature mRNA molecule is transported to a ribosome ready for translation into a protein. The translation process involves transfer RNA (tRNA) which has an interesting structure that is widely referred to as a cloverleaf shape. The tRNA is held in this shape by hydrogen bonds between complementary base pairs (see Figure 4.5). One of the loops of the cloverleaf structure contains an **anticodon** which is a triplet of bases complementary to the **codon** in the mRNA which corresponds to a particular amino acid. Because of the complementarity, the tRNA can only bind to the part of the mRNA that has the correct codon. This ensures that only the correct amino acid can be attached.

Ribosomes consist of a mixture of about 65 per cent ribosomal RNA (rRNA) together with about 35 per cent protein. A ribosome has two parts known as the large subunit (60S) (see Integration Box 4.1

Figure 4.5 Cloverleaf representation of tRNA

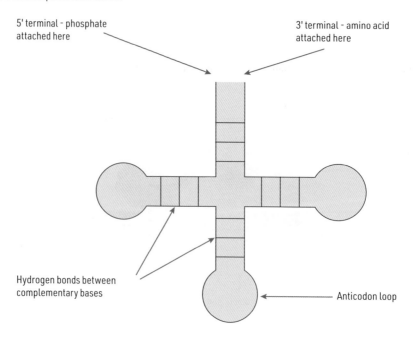

Ribozymes) and the small subunit (40S) which are joined together during translation. An initiation tRNA molecule attaches itself to the small 40S subunit of the ribosome. This initial tRNA molecule always carries the amino acid methionine. The 40S subunit scans the mRNA for the start codon (AUG) and then triggers the 60S subunit to join the 40S subunit thus forming an active ribosome. The ribosome now scans along the mRNA in the 5' to 3' direction. Appropriate tRNA molecules provide the amino acids which are linked together to form the growing polypeptide chain. When the ribosome reaches a stop codon (UAG, UGA, or UAA) the polypeptide chain is released, and the ribosome complex dissociates.

INTEGRATION BOX 4.1   **RIBOZYMES**

As Chapter 3 explained, enzymes, the biological catalysts that can speed up reactions in living systems, are proteins. However, in the 1970s, an RNA molecule was discovered to have enzymatic activity. The scientists who made this discovery coined the name 'ribozyme' for this non-protein catalytic molecule. Ribozymes form part of the large ribosomal subunit, catalysing the linkage of amino acids in protein synthesis. They also take part in a number of RNA processing reactions such as RNA splicing (**❯ XR Section 4.1.2**) and transfer RNA biosynthesis. The first ribozyme to be discovered was named the hammerhead ribozyme because of the resemblance of its shape to a hammerhead shark. There are now several types of ribozyme which have been identified. It has been proposed that ribozymes could have a role in the treatment of disease, particularly gene therapy of viral diseases. However, the problem of the short half-life of ribozymes in the body has yet to be overcome. If you want to know more about ribozymes there is an excellent review to be found in Further reading at the end of the chapter.

 Translation of the mRNA molecule involves transfer to a ribosome where tRNA molecules provide the appropriate amino acids to form the polypeptide chain.

4.1.4 DNA replication

DNA replication takes place during the S phase of the cell cycle (S = DNA Synthesis). The cell cycle is a series of events which occur every time cells divide (see Figure 4.6). Replication commences by the unwinding of a section of the double helix, either at the end of or within the DNA helix. No matter where the origin of the replication, it is initiated by the formation of a protein complex known as the origin recognition complex. This complex then attracts other proteins such as helicases and topoisomerases. Helicases, as the name suggests, are enzymes which unwind the DNA double helix. Topoisomerases work in advance of the helicases cutting, uncoiling and resealing the DNA strand. The separated strands then act as templates for new daughter strands.

As the nucleotide bases of each strand are exposed, they are hydrogen bonded with new complementary nucleotide bases, a process catalysed by enzymes known as DNA polymerases. DNA polymerase, however, is only capable of producing a new DNA strand in the 5' to 3' direction. Consequently the daughter strand which starts at the 3' end of the original DNA strand can be produced in one continuous operation and is called the leading strand. The strand running in the opposite direction, i.e. 5' to 3', cannot proceed in this way. This is known as the lagging strand and the complementary strand has to be produced in a series of small fragments, each of which still grows in the 5' to 3' direction. Thus, the DNA polymerase copies the lagging strand in a series of fragments, known as Okazaki fragments. These fragments are eventually joined together by the enzyme DNA ligase to form a second daughter strand (see Figure 4.7).

Figure 4.6 The cell cycle

(Credit: From Therapeutics and Human Physiology edited by Elsie Gaskell and Chris Rostron (2013). Reproduced with permission of Oxford University Press through PLSclear).

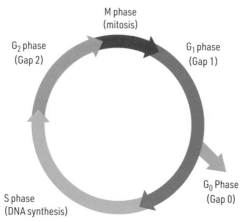

Figure 4.7 Eukaryotic replication

(Credit: From Therapeutics and Human Physiology edited by Elsie Gaskell and Chris Rostron (2013). Reproduced with permission of Oxford University Press through PLSclear).

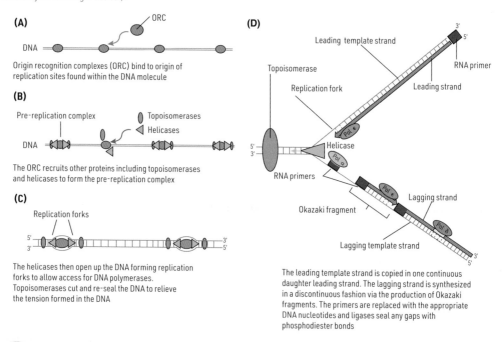

(A) Origin recognition complexes (ORC) bind to origin of replication sites found within the DNA molecule

(B) The ORC recruits other proteins including topoisomerases and helicases to form the pre-replication complex

(C) The helicases then open up the DNA forming replication forks to allow access for DNA polymerases. Topoisomerases cut and re-seal the DNA to relieve the tension formed in the DNA

(D) The leading template strand is copied in one continuous daughter leading strand. The lagging strand is synthesized in a discontinuous fashion via the production of Okazaki fragments. The primers are replaced with the appropriate DNA nucleotides and ligases seal any gaps with phosphodiester bonds

 DNA replication involves the unwinding of the double helix, with each of the two separate strands acting as templates for new daughter strands.

4.2 BACTERIAL PROTEIN SYNTHESIS AS A DRUG TARGET

The synthesis of protein differs between prokaryotic (bacterial) cells and eukaryotic (human) cells. Although the overall process is similar, the difference lies in the structure of the ribosomes involved. As seen previously (➲ **XR Section 4.1.3**) the ribosomes in eukaryotic cells consist of 60S and 40S subunits. The prokaryotic ribosomes consist of 50S and 30S subunits. This difference is the basis for the action of some antibiotics.

Bacterial protein synthesis involves different ribosomal subunits to human protein synthesis.

4.2.1 Macrolide antibiotics

A class of molecules which interfere with bacterial protein synthesis are the macrolides, typically represented by erythromycin (see Figure 4.8). Macrolides inhibit the process of transpeptidation—the transfer of amino acids to the growing peptide chain. They do this by binding to the 50S subunit of the bacterial ribosome. Newer members of the macrolides are clarithromycin and azithromycin (see Figure 4.8).

The macrolides are mainly active against Gram-positive bacteria. The macrolides, in particular erythromycin, possess a very bitter taste. Erythromycin esters are tasteless, but they have no antibacterial activity and so must be hydrolysed in the body to erythromycin—they are prodrugs (❯ **XR Section 12.6.4**). Usually erythromycin, in oral administration, is administered as enteric-coated or delayed release preparations because it is particularly acid labile.

 Macrolide antibiotics interfere with bacterial protein synthesis and are active mainly against Gram-positive bacteria.

4.2.2 Aminoglycoside antibiotics

The **aminoglycosides** (exemplified by streptomycin, tobramycin, gentamicin, and neomycin) (see Figure 4.9) also act by interfering with bacterial protein synthesis. They bind to the 30S subunit of the bacterial ribosomes causing misreading of the codons resulting in the insertion of incorrect amino acids into the growing peptide chain. The aminoglycosides are active mainly against Gram-negative and some Gram-positive organisms. Streptomycin is particularly active against *Mycobacterium tuberculosis*. Gentamicin is the most commonly used member of this class.

As might be expected from their structure, the aminoglycosides are extremely polar and are not absorbed significantly from the gastro-intestinal tract. Indeed neomycin is used to 'sterilize' the gastro-intestinal tract prior to abdominal surgery. Dose-related toxic effects can occur with the aminoglycosides, in particular ototoxicity and nephrotoxicity. Commonly ototoxicity may lead to hearing impairment. Aminoglycoside-resistant bacterial strains can be a problem. Resistance arises via inactivation by microbial enzymes (see Integration Box 4.2 Aminoglycoside resistance).

INTEGRATION BOX 4.2   **AMINOGLYCOSIDE RESISTANCE**

Although active mainly against Gram-negative bacteria, there are now Gram-positive bacteria which are resistant to the aminoglycosides. The resistance arises largely by these bacteria being able to synthesize enzymes which can phosphorylate, adenylate (add an adenine group) or acetylate amino or hydroxyl groups of the aminoglycosides. At present, these inactivating enzymes have been identified, as have their sites of attack. If this site of attack (functional group) is not present, then resistance to that antibiotic does not develop. For example, gentamicin does not possess the 3-hydroxy group acted upon by O-phosphotransferases and so is resistant to those enzymes, unlike streptomycin which possesses the 3-hydroxyl group (shown in red in Figure 4.9). Knowledge and understanding of these inactivation processes can potentially lead to development of aminoglycosides which are not susceptible to bacterial enzyme inactivation.

Figure 4.8 Examples of macrolide antibiotics

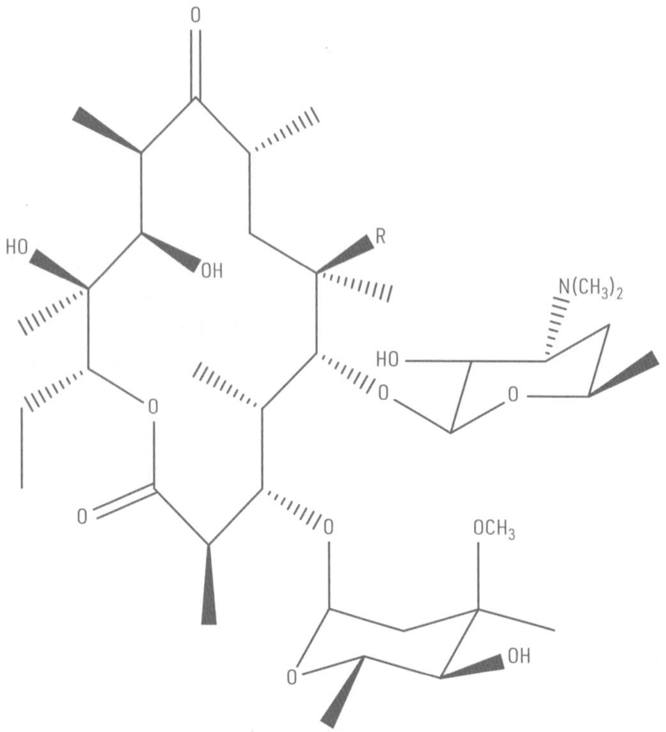

Erythromycin R=OH
Clarithromycin R=OCH$_3$

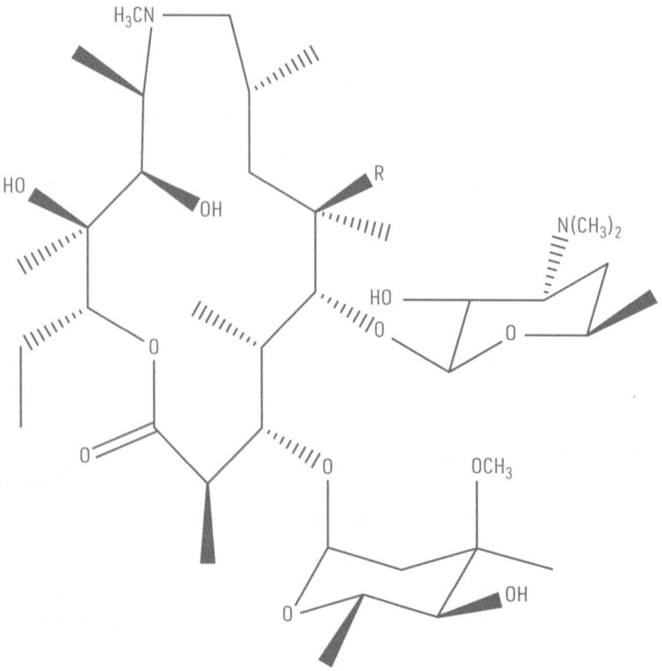

Azithromycin R=OH

Figure 4.9 Examples of aminoglycoside antibiotics

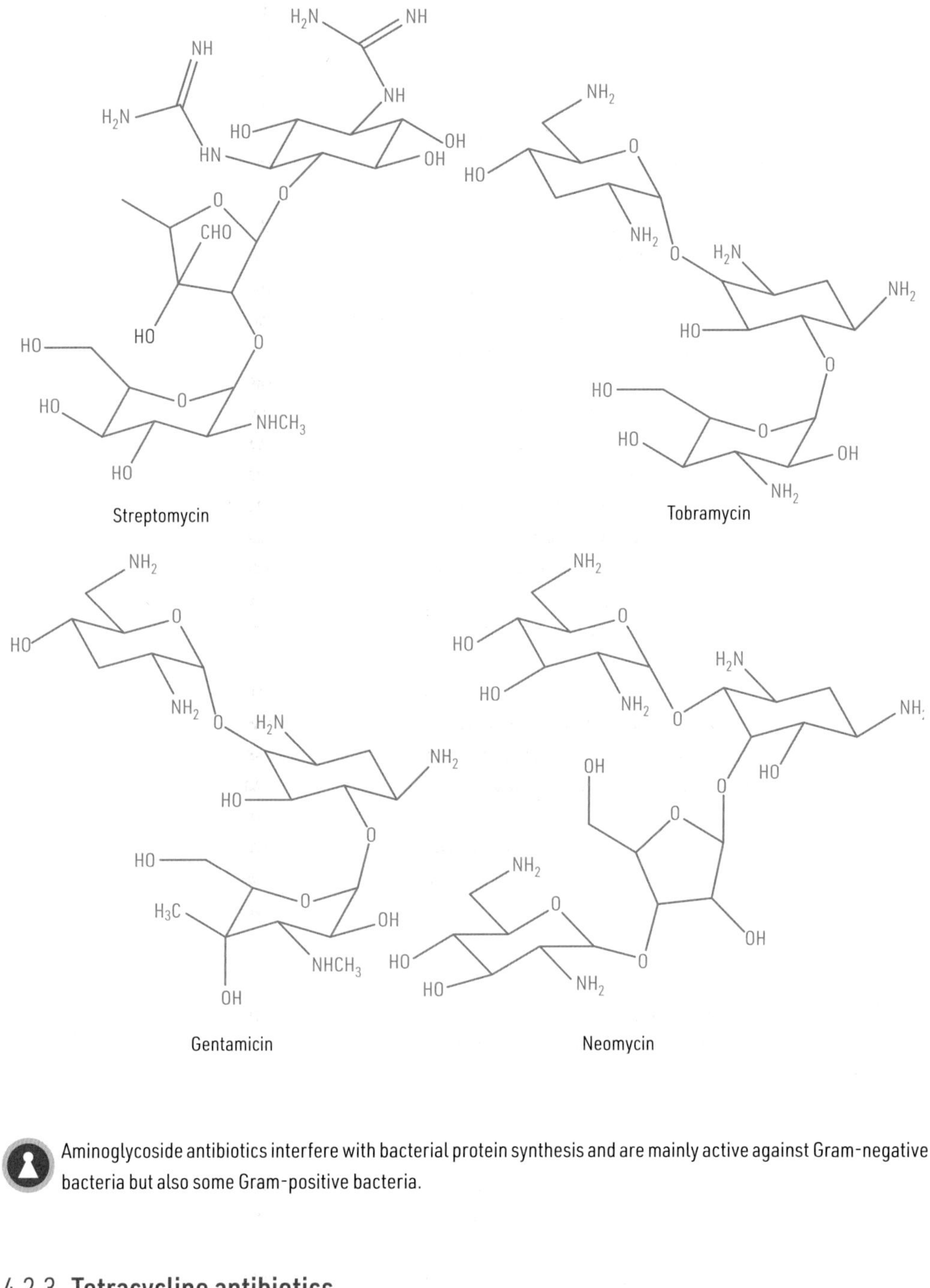

Streptomycin

Tobramycin

Gentamicin

Neomycin

Aminoglycoside antibiotics interfere with bacterial protein synthesis and are mainly active against Gram-negative bacteria but also some Gram-positive bacteria.

4.2.3 Tetracycline antibiotics

The tetracyclines are a very important class of **broad-spectrum** antibacterial agents. Figure 4.10 illustrates the range of tetracyclines in clinical usage today (see Box 4.2 Stereochemistry of the tetracyclines).

Figure 4.10 Structures of some clinically used tetracyclines

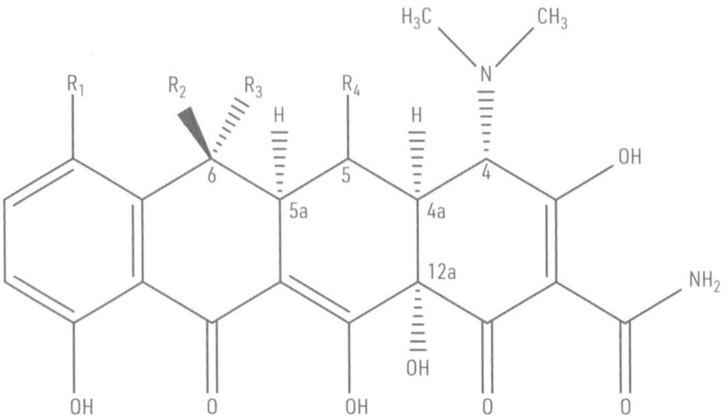

Tetracycline R_1= H R_2=CH_3 R_3=OH R_4=H
Chlortetracycline R_1=Cl R_2=CH_3 R_3=OH R_4=H
Oxytetracycline R_1=H R_2=CH_3 R_3=OH R_4=OH
Demeclocycline R_1=Cl R_2=H R_3=OH R_4=H
Doxycycline R_1=H R_2=H R_3=CH_3 R_4=OH
Minocycline R_1=N$(CH_3)_2$ R_2=h R_3=H R_4=H

BOX 4.2   STEREOCHEMISTRY OF THE TETRACYCLINES

As can be seen from Figure 4.10, the generic structure of the tetracyclines shows five potential chiral centres at carbons 4, 4a, 5, 5a, 6, and 12a depending upon substitution. X-ray crystallography has been used to establish the absolute stereochemistry. A change of stereochemistry solely at the 4 position reduces activity. Such a change is known as epimerization. This process occurs spontaneously under acidic conditions at room temperature to produce a 50:50 equilibrium mixture of the α-epimer (active) and the β-epimer (much less active). This accounts for the reduced clinical activity of old solutions of tetracyclines.

The tetracyclines bind to the smaller subunit of ribosomes of both prokaryotic and eukaryotic cells. However they bind to the ribosomes of mammalian cells with much lower affinity and do not achieve sufficient intracellular concentrations to interfere with mammalian protein synthesis. Binding to the 30S subunit of bacterial ribosomes prevents the binding of aminoacyl-tRNA to the 30S subunit.

The tetracyclines have a very broad spectrum of antibacterial activity, being active against a wide range of Gram-positive and Gram-negative organisms. However, their action tends to be bacteriostatic rather than bacteriocidal. Partly because of this, a great many strains of bacteria have developed resistance to the tetracyclines, reducing their usefulness. There are three separate mechanisms responsible for the development of resistance to tetracyclines—an energy-dependent efflux mechanism, development of ribosomal resistance, and enzymatic oxidation. The first of these is mediated by plasmids and is the most clinically significant resistance mechanism.

Tetracyclines have a strong affinity for metal ions, forming stable **chelates** with calcium, magnesium and iron ions. Hence, absorption of tetracyclines is reduced in the presence of foods and drugs containing such ions, such as milk, some antacids, and iron supplements (see Integration Box 4.3 Tetracyclines and children don't mix).

INTEGRATION BOX 4.3   **TETRACYCLINES AND CHILDREN DON'T MIX**

Tetracyclines are able to form stable chelates with a number of metal ions including calcium. This ability to form complexes with calcium means that they are incorporated into developing bones and teeth, by formation of tetracycline-calcium orthophosphate complexes. If taken during pregnancy, this can lead to bone malformation. If given to children, deposition of these complexes in teeth can lead to permanent discolouration of the teeth due to a photochemical reaction of the complexes.

 Tetracyclines are broad spectrum antibiotics and interfere with bacterial protein synthesis. They form chelates with metal ions, in particular calcium.

4.2.4 Chloramphenicol

Chloramphenicol is a drug which interferes with bacterial protein synthesis (see Figure 4.11). Its mechanism of action is blocking the transfer of amino acids to the growing peptide chain. It has a wide spectrum of antibacterial activity but is mainly bacteriostatic rather than bacteriocidal. It causes bone marrow suppression and, therefore, is limited to treatment of serious infections (see Integration Box 4.4 Grey baby syndrome). Because it is widely distributed in body tissues including the cerebrospinal fluid it is used systemically to treat meningitis. Topically, it can be safely used for the treatment of eye infections and is a POM (pharmacy only medicine) in this context. If administered orally, chloramphenicol is usually administered as the palmitate ester in order to mask its extremely bitter taste.

Figure 4.11 Chloramphenicol

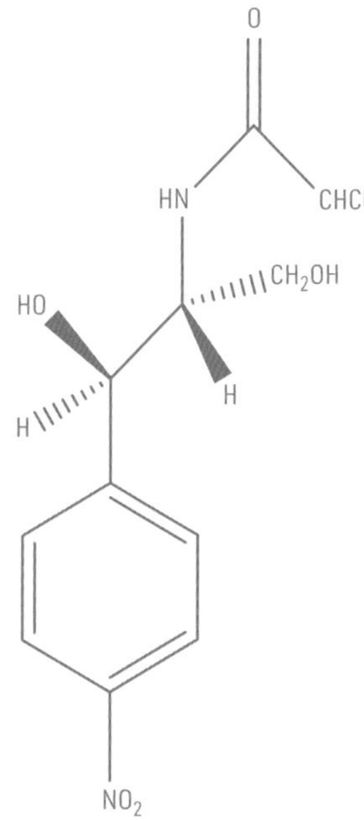

INTEGRATION BOX 4.4   **GREY BABY SYNDROME**

The normal range of metabolic routes is not fully developed in the foetus and the newly-born (❯ **XR Section 12.5.2**). One example of this relates to the metabolism of chloramphenicol. One of the major routes of metabolism of chloramphenicol is glucuronidation of the hydroxyl group by glucuronyl transferase to form a highly water-soluble glucuronide which is readily excreted. In neonates, the levels of glucuronyl transferase are too low and chloramphenicol builds up to a toxic level, leading to a collection of symptoms known as 'grey baby syndrome' which can be fatal. Thirty days after birth the level of glucuronyl transferase increases and the problem disappears.

4.3 NUCLEIC ACIDS AS DRUG TARGETS

Drugs which target nucleic acids can broadly be divided into two types—those which target nucleic acid synthesis and those which target nucleic acid molecules themselves. Drugs that target nucleic acid synthesis are either antimetabolites or enzyme inhibitors. Drugs that target existing nucleic acid molecules are alkylating agents, intercalators and chain-cleaving agents. More recent research has been focused on drugs which interfere with DNA repair mechanisms.

4.3.1 Antimetabolites and enzyme inhibitors

These are molecules which prevent the production of normal cellular metabolites. Clinically speaking, most **antimetabolites** are related to metabolites in the biosynthesis of nucleic acids. They usually have structures which are very similar to the natural metabolites in the cell. Their mode of action is either to replace the endogenous metabolite, leading to incorporation into the biosynthetic pathway, or to inhibit an enzyme in the normal metabolic pathway (see Box 4.3 Difficulty of classification of drug action).

Antifolates have structures which resemble folic acid (see Figure 4.12). In normal cellular metabolism folates are converted into tetrahydrofolates by dihydrofolate reductase. These tetrahydrofolates are necessary for the biosynthesis of purine and thymine nucleotides required for DNA synthesis (see Figure 4.12). The most important antifolate is methotrexate (see Figure 4.13), being one of the most widely used antimetabolites in cancer chemotherapy. Methotrexate inhibits dihydrofolate reductase, and so could be classified as an enzyme inhibitor (❯ **XR Section 3.2.1** and see Box 4.3 Difficulty of classification of drug targets).

BOX 4.3   DIFFICULTY OF CLASSIFICATION OF DRUG TARGETS

Chapter 3 of this volume dealt with drugs which have enzymes as their targets. This chapter deals with drugs that have nucleic acids as targets. You could be forgiven for thinking that this classification of targets is rigid, but it is not. Many drugs act by more than one mechanism and, therefore, have more than one target. Most drugs exhibit side effects and many of these arise because the drug interacts with a target other the one for which it is being used clinically. Additionally there are drugs which are classified in one way, but equally could be placed in a different class. One example of this is methotrexate. It is a drug which targets nucleic acids but inhibits dihydrofolate reductase and thus could be classified as an enzyme inhibitor.

Figure 4.12 Folate metabolism

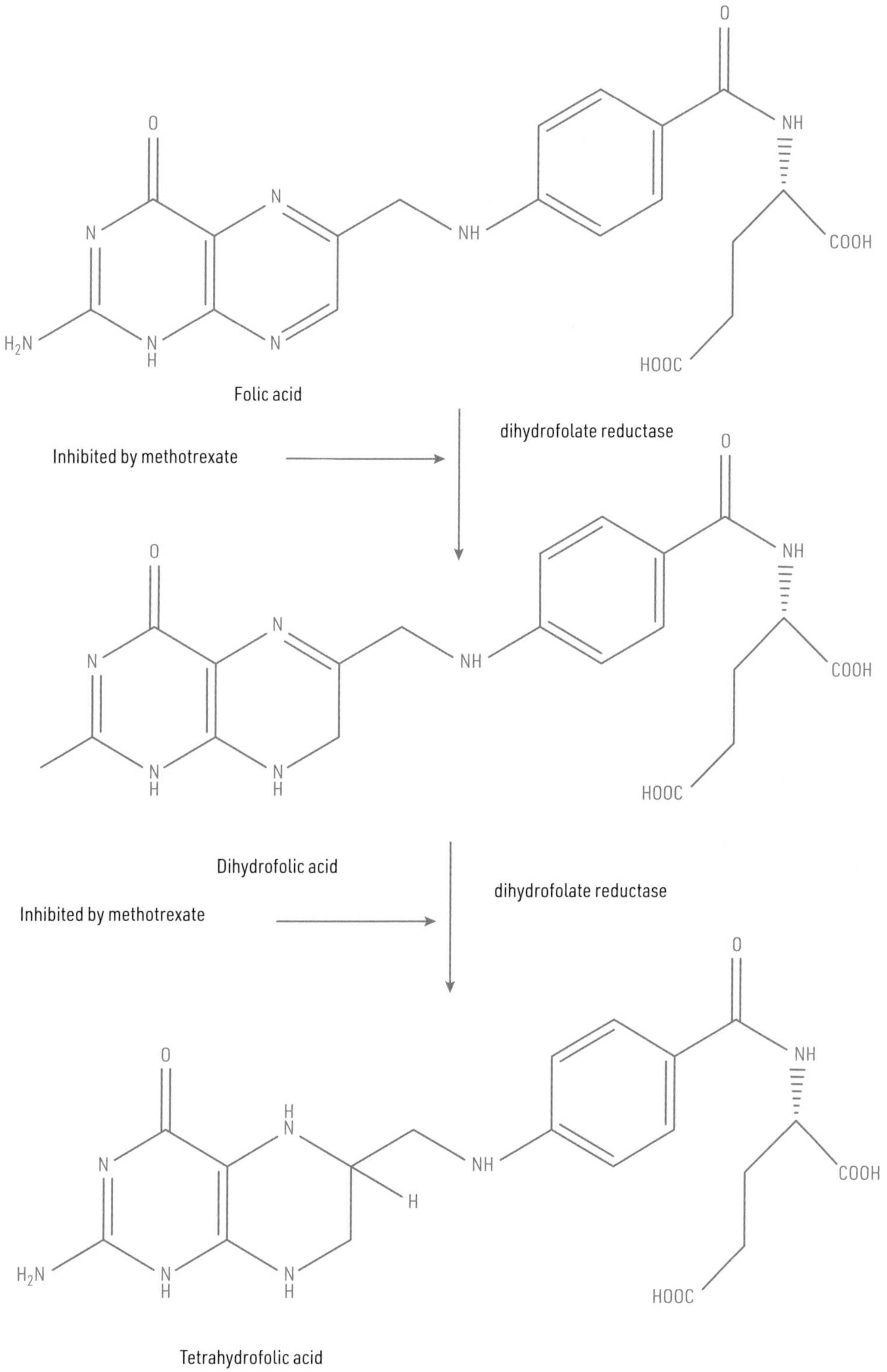

Folic acid

Inhibited by methotrexate   ⟶   dihydrofolate reductase

Dihydrofolic acid

Inhibited by methotrexate   ⟶   dihydrofolate reductase

Tetrahydrofolic acid

Figure 4.13 Methotrexate

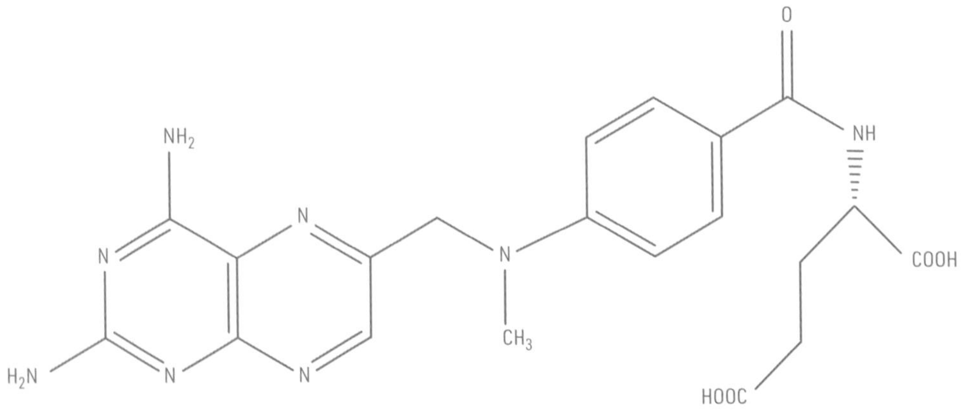

Methotrexate

Methotrexate is a slow-binding reversible inhibitor which resembles an irreversible inhibitor because its affinity for dihydrofolate reductase is so high. Clinically, methotrexate is used to treat various types of cancer, including acute lymphocytic leukaemia and, in combination therapies, breast cancer, lung cancer, and head and neck tumours (see also Integration Box 4.5 Methotrexate and rheumatoid arthritis). Methotrexate possesses a range of unwanted side effects such as gastro-intestinal disturbances, oral and gastric ulceration and bone marrow suppression.

INTEGRATION BOX 4.5 · METHOTREXATE AND RHEUMATOID ARTHRITIS

Rheumatoid arthritis is an auto-immune disease which causes severe inflammation and pain in the joints. Methotrexate can be used, at low doses, to treat such conditions. It does not cure the disease but reduces the symptoms. Methotrexate is known as a disease-modifying anti-rheumatic drug (DMARD). It reduces the activity of the immune system, causing the body to reduce the production of antibodies which affect the joints. This clinical use is, of course, subject to the same range of side effects as when it is used as an anti-cancer drug.

 Antifolates, such as methotrexate, inhibit dihydrofolate reductase, preventing normal folate metabolism.

The main purine antimetabolites are mercaptopurine and thioguanine (see Figure 4.14). They are both 6-thiol analogues of the 6-hydroxypurine bases, hypoxanthine, and guanine respectively. In order to be active they are converted, in the cell, to the respective ribonucleotides. These non-endogenous ribonucleotides bring about their anti-cancer action by a number of different mechanisms, such as inhibition of purine biosynthesis (mercaptopurine) and incorporation into the structure of DNA (thioguanine). Both drugs have the unwanted side effect of bone marrow depression (see Integration Box 4.6 Azathioprine usage).

Figure 4.14 Purine antimetabolites

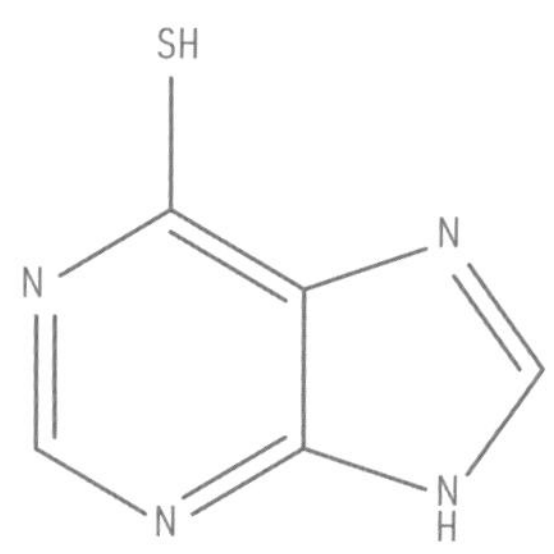

Mercaptopurine

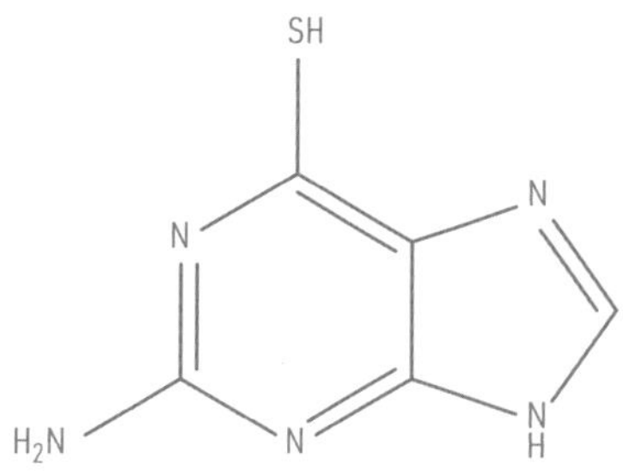

Thioguanine

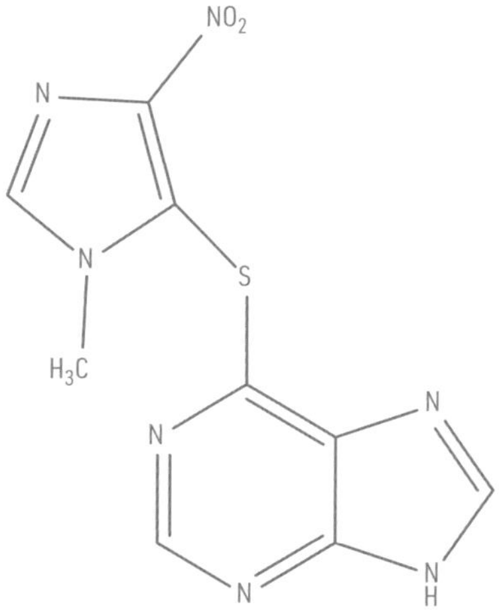

Azathioprine

INTEGRATION BOX 4.6	AZATHIOPRINE USAGE

6-Mercaptopurine is rapidly eliminated from the body. Because of this, a prodrug is used–azathioprine (see Figure 4.14). Azathioprine is easily absorbed when taken orally and is extensively, but slowly, converted to 6-mercaptopurine, thus providing a more sustained action. The conversion is brought about by the action of glutathione which removes the nitroimidazole ring, releasing the free SH group of 6-mercaptopurine.

 Purine antimetabolites have different modes of action. 6-Mercaptopurine inhibits purine biosynthesis whereas thioguanine is incorporated into the structure of DNA.

The most clinically useful pyrimidine antimetabolites are fluorouracil and cytarabine (see Figure 4.15). Fluorouracil acts by interfering with thymidylate synthesis. It is converted into a false nucleotide (5-fluoro-2'-deoxyuridine monophosphate) which inhibits thymidylate synthetase. This inhibition is due

Figure 4.15 Pyrimidine antimetabolites

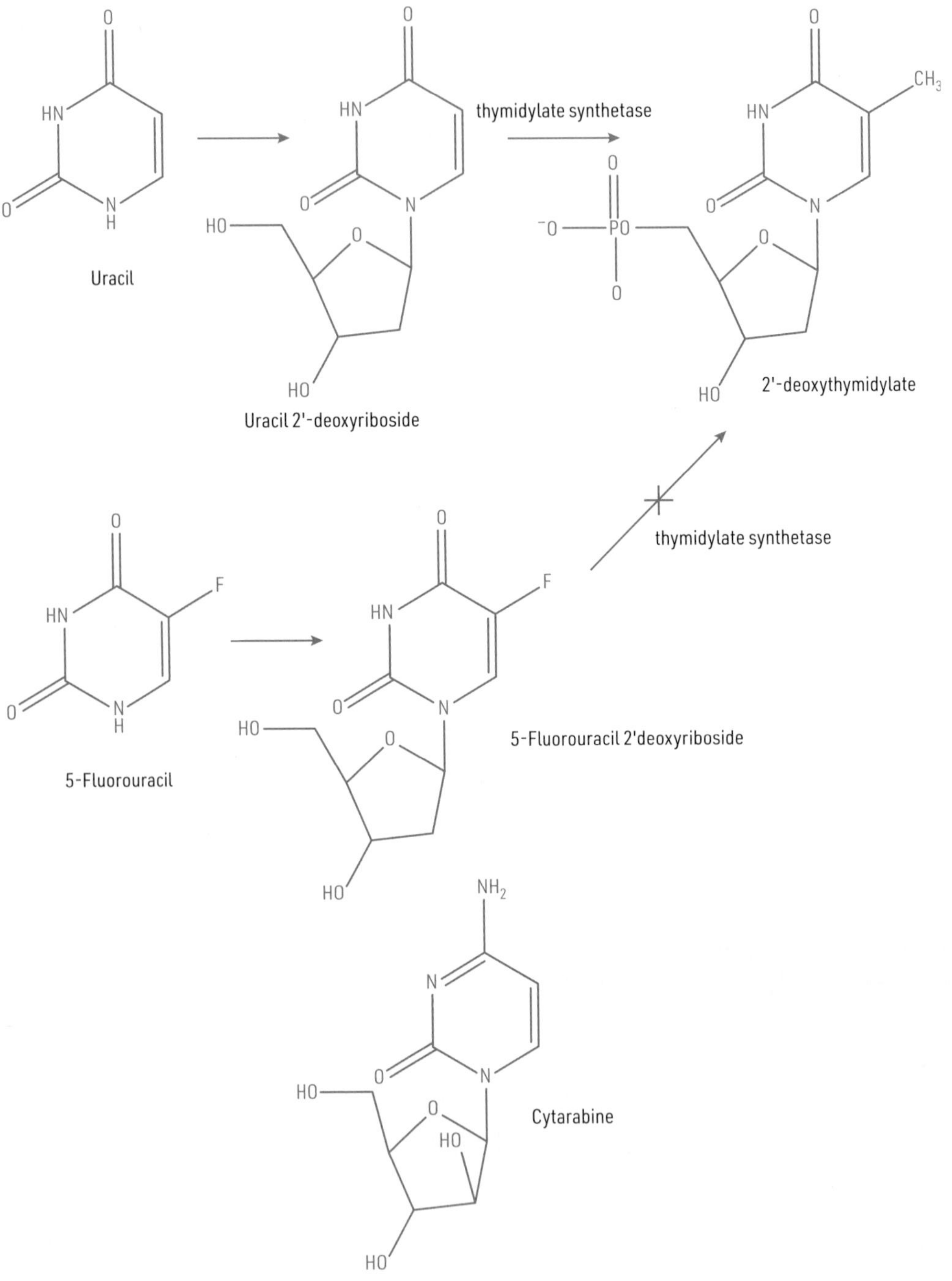

to the presence of the fluorine atom at position 5. This position is where subsequent methylation would take place, but the C-F bond is not susceptible to enzyme cleavage, preventing the formation of deoxy-thymidylate (see Figure 4.15).

Cytarabine is an analogue of the natural nucleoside 2'-deoxycytidine (see Box 4.4 The importance of small stereochemical differences). It undergoes the same phosphorylation reactions as 2'-deoxycytidine and can be incorporated, to some extent, into both DNA and RNA. Its main cytotoxic action, however, is the inhibition of DNA polymerase by the triphosphate. Serious toxic side effects are seen with both drugs, in particular **leukopenia** and gastrotoxicity.

BOX 4.4   THE IMPORTANCE OF SMALL STEREOCHEMICAL DIFFERENCES

We have already seen an example of the clinical effect of a change of stereochemistry at just one chiral centre in a molecule possessing several chiral centres (❯ **XR Box 4.2**). Cytosine arabinoside is another example. The 2'-hydroxy group of the sugar portion of the molecule is on the opposite side of the pentose ring in arabinose, compared to ribose.

There is a small group of drugs which act as enzyme inhibitors but not during the synthesis of DNA. Irinotecan, a drug derived from the natural product camptothecin, inhibits topoisomerase I which is in a group of enzymes responsible for the supercoiling, cleavage and re-joining of DNA during replication (❯ **XR Section 4.1.4**). However the clinical use of irinotecan (and related analogues) is limited by their toxicity and chemical instability. Drugs used as anti-cancer agents by acting against topoisomerase II include doxorubicin and mitoxantrone (❯ **XR Section 4.3.2**). Again the use of these drugs is limited by their cardiotoxicity. Also acting in a similar fashion but against bacterial DNA gyrase, rather than topoisomerases, are the fluoroquinolone antibacterial agents.

 The main pyrimidine antimetabolites are fluorouracil and cytarabine. Fluorouracil is converted into a false nucleotide which inhibits thymidylate synthetase. Cytarabine inhibits DNA polymerase.

4.3.2 Intercalators

Intercalators are planar molecules which interact with DNA molecules by insertion between the base pairs of the DNA double helix. This results in partial unwinding of the DNA helix thus inhibiting transcription. The mechanism of action is thought to be stabilization of the DNA-topoisomerase complex. In order to be able to insert themselves between the DNA bases, molecules need to possess a flat aromatic or **heteroaromatic** ring. Examples of such molecules with anti-cancer activity are doxorubicin and mitoxantrone (see Figure 4.16, both anthracycline derivatives.

 The most important anti-cancer drugs which act as intercalators are anthracycline derivatives. The planar nature of their structure allows them to insert themselves into the DNA double helix.

4.3.3 Alkylating agents

Alkylation can be defined as a nucleophilic substitution reaction. In the biological situation the nucleophile is a molecule such as a nucleic acid or protein, which displaces a leaving group from the alkylating agent. Most alkylating agents are bi-functional, i.e. have two alkylating groups. In this way they can form intra-strand cross-links within a DNA molecule or inter-strand cross-links between the two strands of the DNA double helix (see Box 4.5 The origins of alkylating agents in World War One). Because the N7 of guanine is highly nucleophilic this is the most likely target for alkylating agents, although N1 and N3 of

Figure 4.16 Examples of intercalators

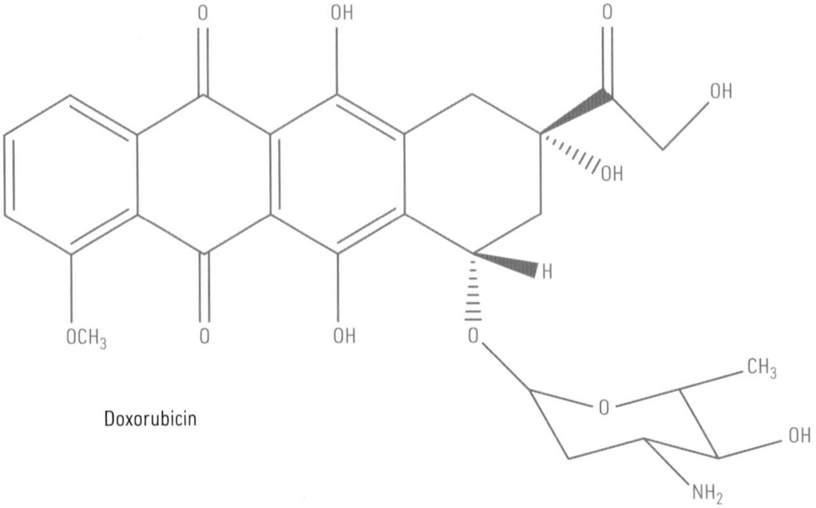

Doxorubicin

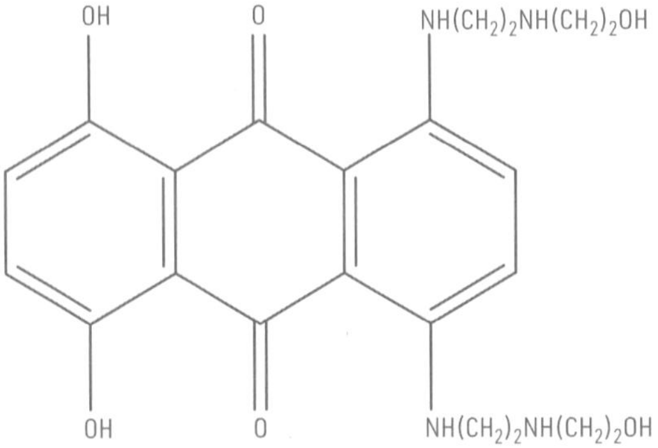

Mitoxantrone

adenine are also susceptible (see Figure 4.17). Many alkylating agents are used in cancer chemotherapy and the most common ones used clinically will now be considered.

| BOX 4.5 | THE ORIGINS OF ALKYLATING AGENTS IN WORLD WAR ONE |

Although the toxic effects of sulphur mustards were first observed in the nineteenth century, it was only during World War One that they were used militarily, as so-called 'mustard gas'. The pure form of mustard gas is the chemical bis(2-chloroethyl)sulphide. Observations on soldiers exposed to mustard gas showed significantly reduced white blood cell counts. This led to extensive research into related compounds, in particular nitrogen mustards. The first such drug to be used clinically was introduced in 1942. The term mustard arose from the smell of the gases used in World War One—their smell resembled that of mustard.

One of the problems with the initial nitrogen mustard (➤ XR Box 4.5) alkylating agents was their tendency to form **aziridinium** ions which are highly reactive and were responsible for many of the unwanted side effects. Chlorambucil (see Figure 4.18) was an attempt to reduce this possibility by the introduction of the electron-withdrawing aromatic ring. This meant that the molecule would only react with strong

Figure 4.17 Targets for alkylating agents

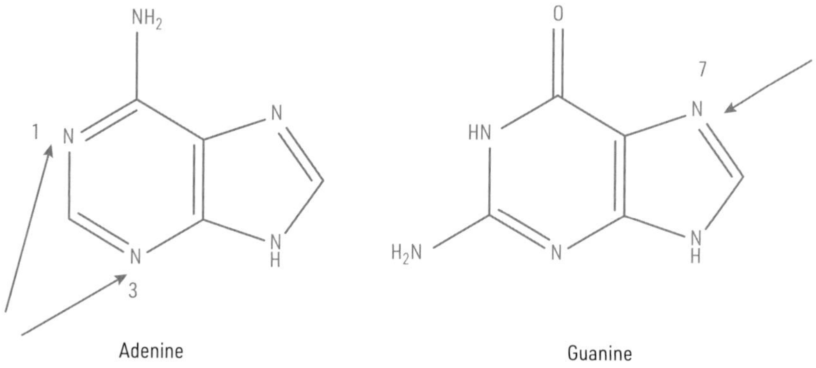

Adenine   Guanine

nucleophiles such as the N7 of guanine. The introduction of the aromatic ring also increases the stability of the nitrogen mustard and so chlorambucil can be taken orally.

The alkylating activity in busulfan results from the presence of the sulphonate esters, the leaving groups being mathylsulphonate (see Figure 4.18).

An alternative approach to reducing the general toxicity of alkylating agents led to the development of cyclophosphamide (see Figure 4.18). The observation that some tumours had high levels of **phosphoramidases** led to the development of cyclophosphamide as a prodrug (**❯ XR Section 12.6.4**) designed to be activated to an alkylating agent selectively in tumour cells. However the activation of the prodrug is by oxidation in the liver (see Figure 4.18).

A different type of alkylating agent is the nitrosoureas (see Figure 4.19 (a)). Again these are prodrugs (**❯ XR Section 12.6.4**) which give rise to the active alkylating agent by spontaneous degradation in aqueous solution under physiological conditions to produce a carbonium ion and an isocyanate, both of which can alkylate (see Figure 4.19 (a)). The drug temazolomide produces a methyldiazonium ion by reaction with water within the major groove of DNA (see Figure 4.19(b)).

Another prodrug (**❯ XR Section 12.6.4**) in this category is mitomycin (sometimes called mitomycin C) (see Figure 4.19(c)). In the body it is activated by reduction to a bi-functional alkylating agent which cross-links complementary DNA strands.

Cisplatin is an unusual alkylating agent in that it is a **square planar complex** containing platinum (see Figure 4.20 and Box 4.6 Geometrical isomerism). When it enters the cell the chloro groups are replaced by water molecules. The complex now possesses a positive charge, making the complex very reactive. This results in intra-strand cross-linking between N7 and O6 atoms of adjacent guanine residues. Related compounds such as carboplatin (see Figure 4.20) have been developed which have less general toxicity but are still **myelotoxic**.

BOX 4.6 **GEOMETRICAL ISOMERISM**

Geometrical isomerism occurs when atoms or groups of atoms are arranged asymmetrically across some element of rigidity, usually a double bond or a cyclic system. If similar atoms are on the same side, then this is the cis isomer; if the similar atoms are on opposite sides, this is the trans isomer (see Figure 4.21). This situation can also apply to organo-metallic complexes such as in cisplatin. In this complex the chlorine atoms are on the same side of the platinum atom, hence cisplatin. Transplatin does exist, but it is much less active. The cis arrangement of the chlorine atoms is the optimum one to allow cross-linking between DNA strands.

Figure 4.18 Examples of alkylating agents in clinical usage

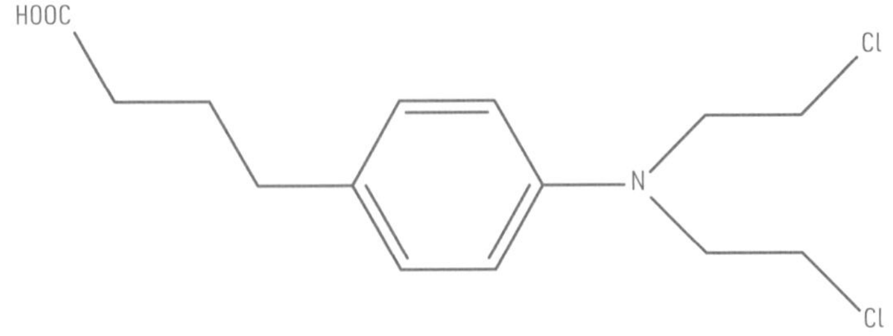

Chlorambucil

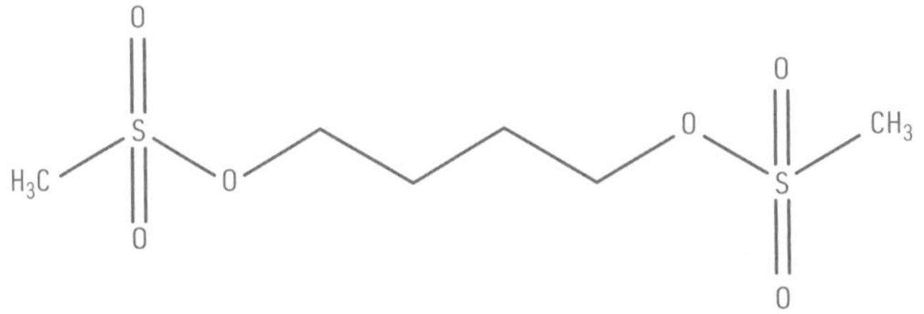

Busulfan

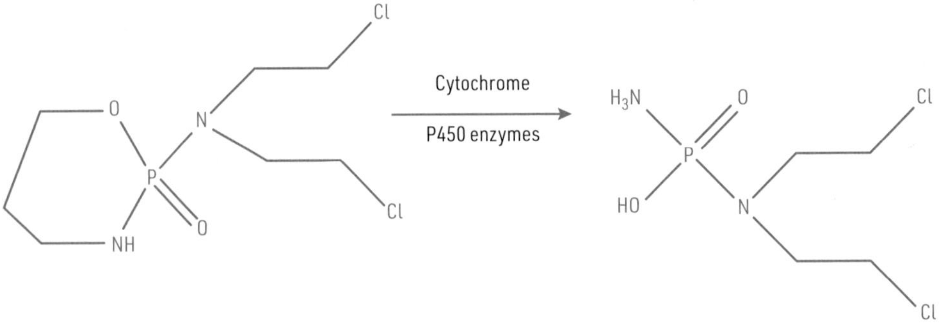

Cyclophosphamide - non-toxic

Cytochrome
P450 enzymes

Alkylating agent

Figure 4.19 (a) Nitrosoureas as prodrugs for alkylating agents

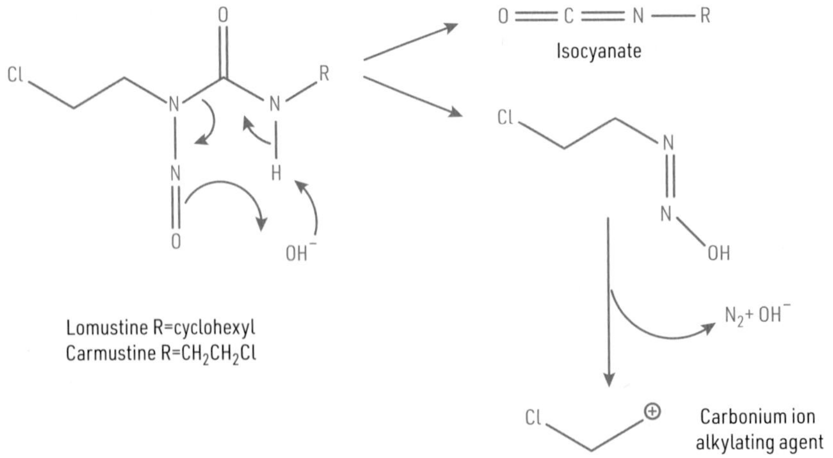

Isocyanate

Lomustine R=cyclohexyl
Carmustine R=CH₂CH₂Cl

N_2+ OH⁻

Carbonium ion
alkylating agent

Figure 4.19 (b) Temozolomide as a prodrug alkylating agent

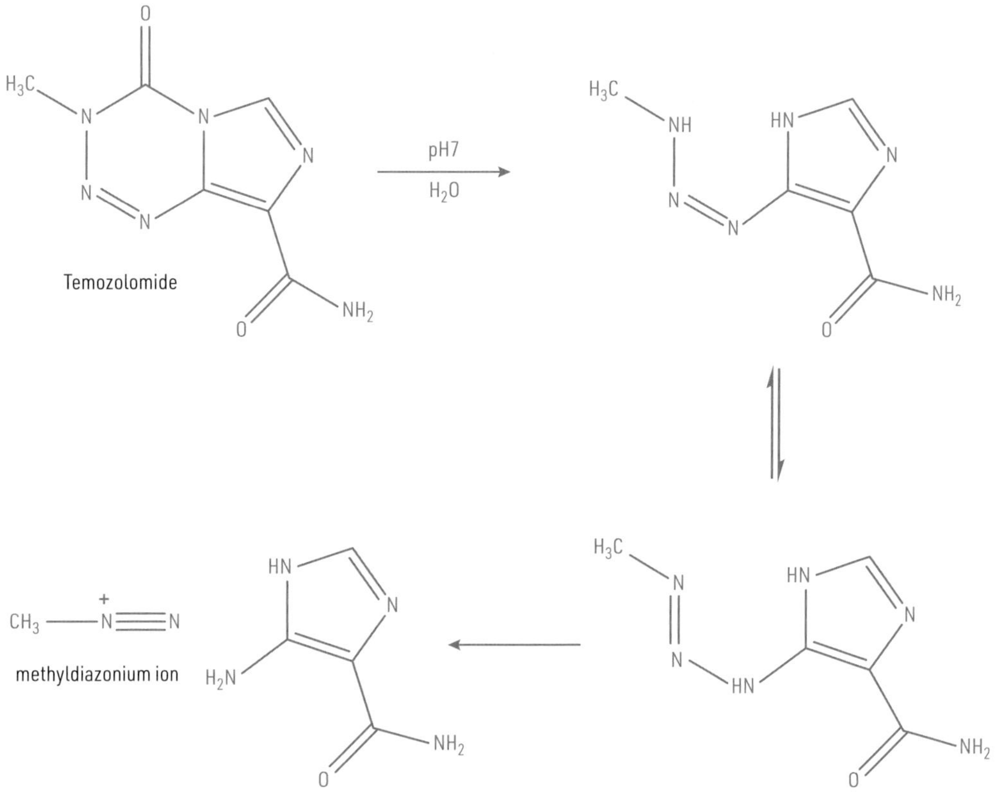

Temozolomide

$$\text{pH7} \quad H_2O$$

methyldiazonium ion

Figure 4.19 (c) Mitomycin C

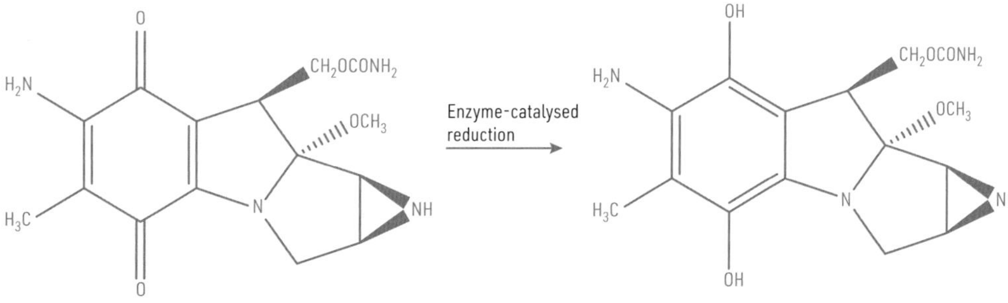

Enzyme-catalysed reduction

Mitomycin C

Because of the ability of these alkylating agents to react with any biological nucleophiles they do possess significant toxicity profiles. They are most toxic to rapidly proliferating cells and, therefore, will be active against rapidly growing tumours and are less effective against slow-growing tumours. As expected, they all cause bone marrow depression.

Alkylating agents form intra-strand or inter-strand cross-links within or between DNA strands. There are a wide variety of drug structures which are classed as alkylating agents, having different mechanisms for forming cross-links in DNA molecules.

Figure 4.20 Cisplatin and carboplatin

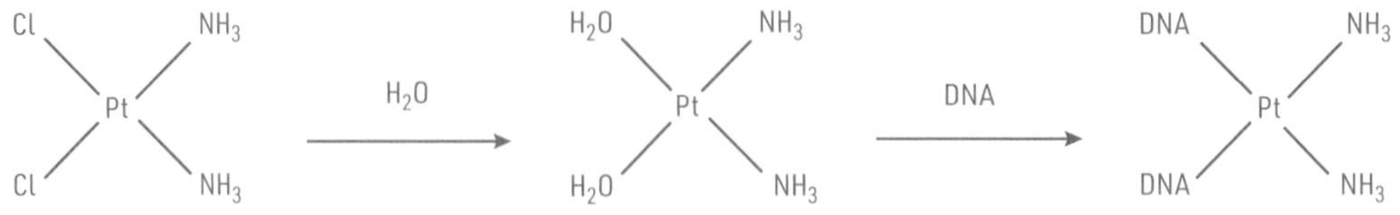

Cisplatin

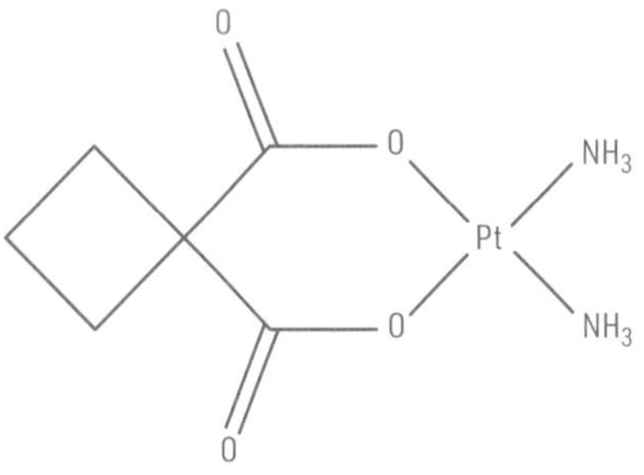

Carboplatin

Figure 4.21 Geometrical isomerism

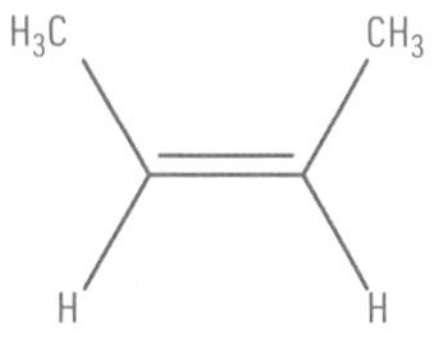

Cis isomer

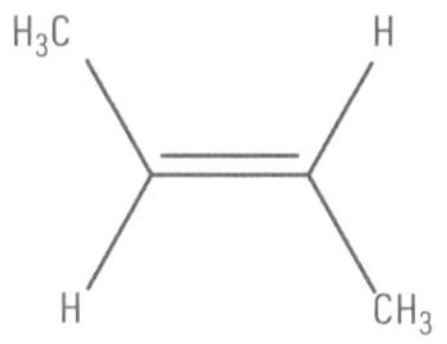

Trans isomer

4.3.4 Chain-cleaving agents

The final type of drug activity against nucleic acid molecules is that of chain cleavage, whereby the DNA molecules are broken into fragments. Currently the major drugs in this category are the bleomycins, which are actually a mixture of naturally occurring glycopeptides. They form complexes readily with metal ions. Within the cell bleomycin complexes with Fe(II) and molecular oxygen. This complex gives rise to free radicals such as hydroxyl radicals and superoxide. As these are generated within the DNA double helix, they cause cleavage of the phosphodiester bonds.

4.3.5 Drugs which target DNA repair mechanisms

DNA is under constant attack from endogenous and exogenous sources. Endogenous sources of damage include oxidation by reactive oxygen species, reactions such as hydrolysis and spontaneous mutations. Exogenous sources of damage can be ionizing radiation, UV light or exposure to chemicals such as are found in cigarette smoke. It has been estimated that cells experience as many as 10^5 DNA damage incidents per day.

Because this damage to DNA can alter transcription and replication, cells have evolved a number of repair processes known as the DNA damage response (DDR). DNA damage is recognized as a significant cause of cancer but has also been recognized as a useful target for cancer chemotherapy as well as radiotherapy. There are five major DNA repair pathways in human cells—base excision repair (BER), nucleoside excision repair (NER), mismatch repair (MMR), non-homologous end-joining (NHEJ), and homology-directed repair (HDR). An increased knowledge of these repair mechanisms presents future opportunities for cancer treatment.

While malfunction of the repair mechanisms can lead to tumour production, deliberate interference with the repair mechanisms presents a therapeutic opportunity. The most successful application to date is the use of poly-ADP ribose polymerase (PARP) inhibitors which act by suppressing the ability to repair single strand breaks (SSBs). Failure to repair single strand breaks leads to the formation of double strand breaks. If these breaks cannot be repaired, this leads to cell death. Because normal cells do not replicate as often as cancer cells this allows them to survive the PARP inhibition. The most successful drug of this class has been olaparib, which selectively targets cells that already have a reduced capacity to repair DNA strand breaks and has been used in treatment of types of breast cancer and ovarian cancer. Additionally, PARP inhibitors show increased anti-tumour activity when used in combination with other drugs which interfere with DNA repair mechanisms, such as cisplatin.

4.4 VIRUSES AS DRUG TARGETS

Viruses consist of nucleic acids (either DNA or RNA) encapsulated in a protein coat, although some have an additional lipoprotein envelope. Viruses have no metabolic processes of their own and, in order to replicate, have to enter a host cell and use the host cell's metabolic reactions. Viral replication requires viral nucleic acid synthesis and synthesis of viral proteins.

For DNA viruses, after entering the host cell, the viral DNA enters the host cell nucleus and is transcribed into mRNA by the host cell RNA polymerase. The mRNA is then translated into viral protein.

For RNA viruses, after entering the host cell, the viral RNA is translated into viral protein using the host cell ribosomes. For RNA retroviruses, after entering the host cell, enzyme systems known as reverse transcriptases, present in the virus, produce viral DNA from their RNA template. This viral DNA is incorporated into the host genome to produce a so-called 'provirus'. The provirus DNA is transcribed into new viral mRNA which is translated into viral proteins.

Because viruses utilize the metabolic processes of the host cell it is hard to find drugs that are virus-specific. However there are some virus-specific enzymes that can be used as targets for drug action. Most antiviral drugs, therefore, work by inhibiting viral nucleic acid synthesis or by inhibiting viral protein synthesis (see Table 4.1 and Figure 4.22).

 Viruses consist of either DNA or RNA encapsulated in a protein shell. Viruses enter a host cell and utilize the host cell's metabolic reactions to produce viral protein.

4.4.1 Viral nucleic acid synthesis as a drug target

All of the antiviral drugs active by inhibiting viral nucleic acid synthesis are required to be converted to a triphosphate by the host cell **kinases** before bringing about their action. Additionally, they are all analogues of purine or pyrimidine bases found in the nucleic acids. Aciclovir and ganciclovir are both guanosine analogues and vidarabine is an adenosine analogue. After conversion to the triphosphate they all inhibit DNA polymerase.

Table 4.1 Selected antiviral drugs and their mode of action

Drug	Mode of action
Aciclovir	Triphosphate inhibits DNA polymerase
Ganciclovir	Triphosphate inhibits DNA polymerase
Idoxuridine	Triphosphate inhibits DNA polymerase
Vidarabine	Triphosphate inhibits DNA polymerase and RNA reductase
Ribavirine	Triphosphate inhibits RNA polymerase
Zidovudine (AZT)	Triphosphate inhibits reverse transcriptase
Didanosine	Triphosphate inhibits reverse transcriptase

Aciclovir was the first effective antiviral agent to be introduced in the 1970s. It has low toxicity compared with vidarabine and ganciclovir which are exceedingly toxic. Ribavirin also is a guanosine analogue, but it inhibits viral RNA polymerase and is active against a wide range of both RNA and DNA viruses. Zidovudine (also known as AZT), a thymidine analogue, and didanosine, a purine nucleotide analogue, both inhibit viral reverse transcriptase and are incorporated into viral DNA causing chain termination. Idoxuridine is also a thymidine analogue. It appears to have a number of actions in inhibiting the replication of DNA viruses. It is, however, **mutagenic**, and is too toxic for systemic use and is only approved for topical use.

 Most antiviral drugs inhibit viral nucleic acid synthesis.

4.4.2 Viral protein synthesis as a drug target

The main drugs that act against viral protein synthesis are the interferons. These are a group of naturally occurring proteins produced by mammalian cells as part of the immunological response to viral (and non-viral) antigens. They are now produced by recombinant DNA technology (❯ **XR Chapter 11**). They work by inducing, in the host ribosomes, the production of enzymes which inhibit the translation of viral mRNA into viral protein. They are used mostly for treatment of hepatitis B and AIDS.

 Interferons are naturally occurring proteins which inhibit viral protein synthesis. They are now produced by recombinant DNA technology.

4.5 ANTISENSE DRUGS

An ongoing area of research into drugs that target nucleic acids is that of antisense **oligonucleotides**. These are synthetic nucleotides of short chain length (13–20 nucleotides) which bind to specific sections of mRNA by complementary base pair hydrogen bonding. This inhibits translation of the mRNA thus inhibiting synthesis of a specific protein which may be responsible for a particular disease state. Because of this specificity, antisense oligonucleotides have potential as anti-cancer and antiviral drugs and should exhibit fewer side effects than drugs in current usage.

Figure 4.22 Examples of antiviral drugs

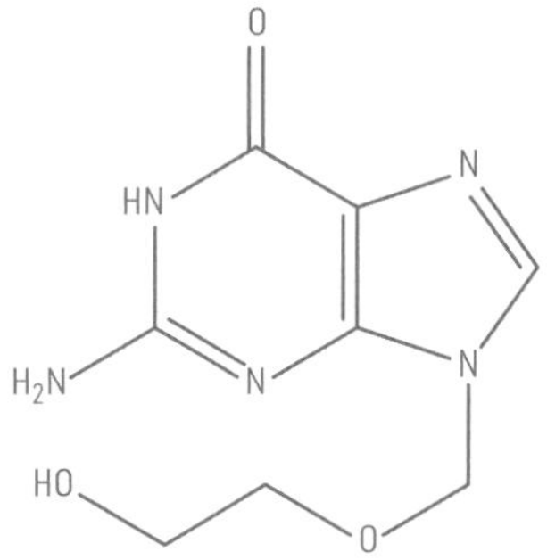

Aciclovir

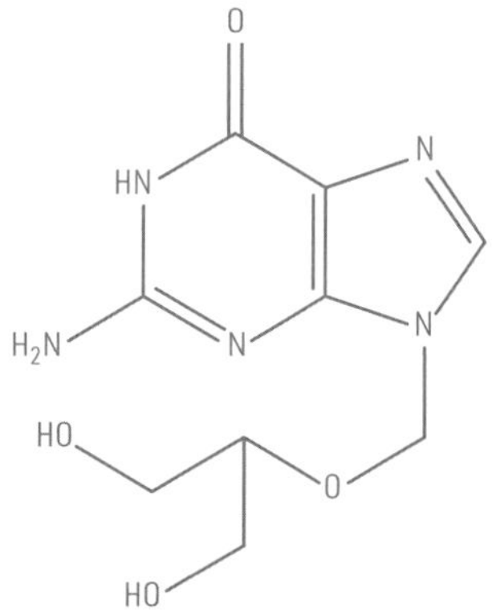

Ganciclovir

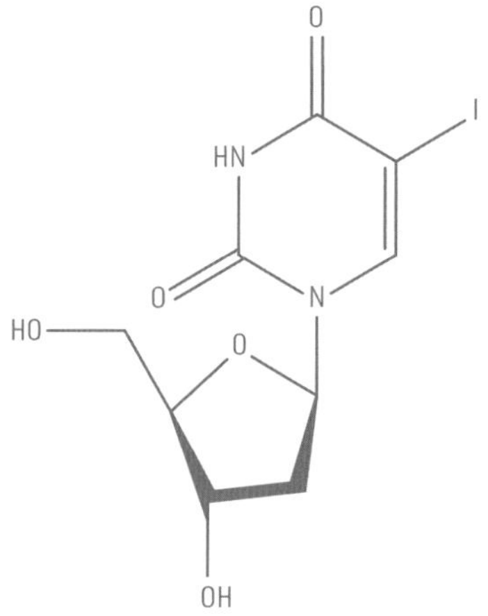

Idoxuridine

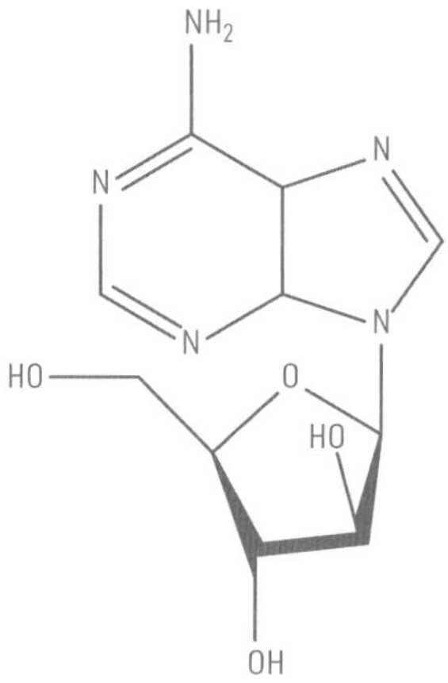

Vidarabine

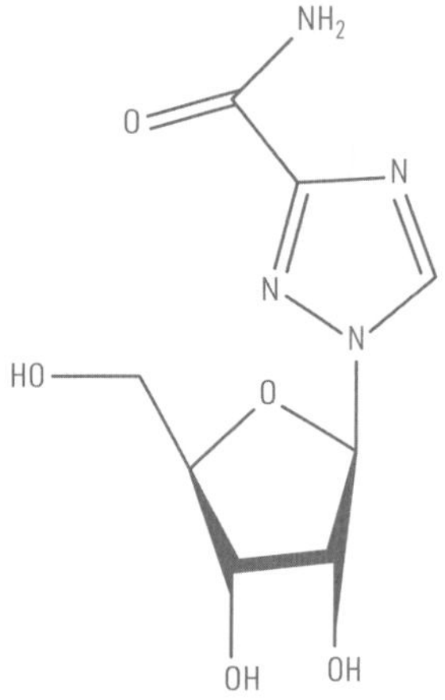

Ribavirin

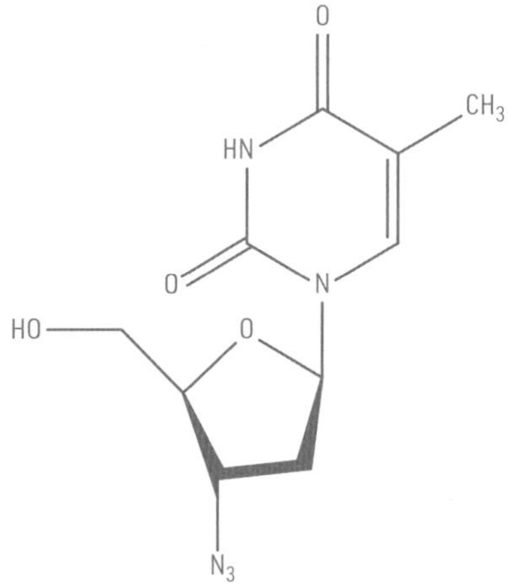

Zidovudine (AZT)

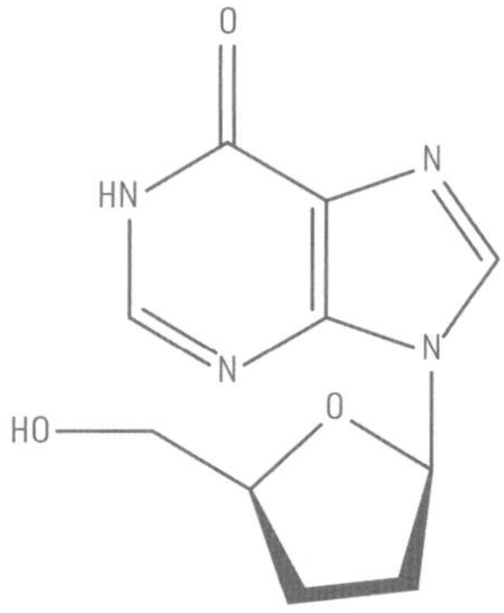

Didanosine

Figure 4.23 Phosphate to phosphothionate backbone modification

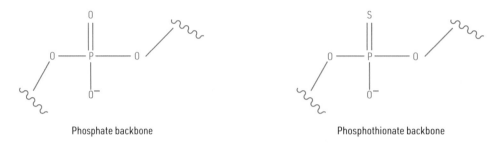

Phosphate backbone   Phosphothionate backbone

There are limitations to the use of antisense oligonucleotides themselves as drugs. They are relatively large molecules and so have poor uptake into cells. They are also susceptible to degradation by nucleases and so have short half-lives. Development is currently under way to modify the lead compounds to increase resistance to hydrolysis by modifying the backbone, by modifying the sugar residues, and by modifying the base. Modification of the backbone to increase stability towards nucleases has given rise to the phosphothionate oligonucleotides (see Figure 4.23). This resulted in the only antisense oligonucleotide to reach clinical usage, fomivirsen, used to treat retinal inflammation caused by cytomegalovirus infection in AIDS patients (but withdrawn due to a reduction in the number of patients requiring this treatment). Methods of improving cellular delivery have included liposome technology (➤ **XR Integration Box 11.4**) and the use of viruses to deliver oligonucleotides to cells (➤ **XR Chapter 11**).

 Antisense drug therapy uses oligonucleotides which are complementary to sections of mRNA. They bind to mRNA and prevent protein synthesis.

4.6 CHALLENGES OF USING NUCLEIC ACIDS AS DRUG TARGETS

The term chemotherapy includes drugs used to treat cancer and bacterial infections. While there is a problem with bacterial resistance to chemotherapy, cancer chemotherapy exhibits more fundamental difficulties with treatment. Often, cancer cells have their own unique characteristics and, as such, drugs active against one type of cancer are ineffective against other forms of cancer. There are other reasons why cancer chemotherapy is less successful than antibacterial chemotherapy. One reason for this is that human and bacterial cells are different. Bacterial cells have different cell walls and ribosomes compared to human cells. Because of these differences it is easier to target bacterial cells without significant toxic side effects. However there are little qualitative differences between normal and neoplastic human cells and thus anti-cancer drugs exhibit the significant toxic side effects previously referred to in this chapter.

Additionally, human immune defence systems recognize and kill bacterial cells, but cancer cells are not recognized as foreign cells and so immune systems have a much lesser role in destroying cancer cells. Having said this, much progress is being made in immunotherapy, particularly in the use of interferons, interleukins, monoclonal antibodies, and antisense oligonucleotides.

? Questions

1. Draw the structures showing how adenine and thymine and guanine and cytosine are hydrogen bonded to each other.

2. Briefly describe the roles of each of the principal types of RNA.

3. How does protein synthesis in prokaryotic cells differ from that in eukaryotic cells?

4. What are the differences between Gram-positive and Gram-negative bacteria?

5. Erythromycin is acid-labile. What is the nature of the reaction of erythromycin with acid?

6. Which groups are responsible for the polarity of the aminoglycosides?

7. Draw the structure of the chelate formed between tetracycline and calcium.

8. What are the structural features of chloramphenicol responsible for its antibacterial activity?

9. Proflavine is a topical antiseptic. What would you expect to be its mode of action?

10. Write the mechanism by which glutathione converts azathioprine to 6-mercaptopurine.

11. Why are antiviral drugs required to be converted to their triphosphate derivatives in order to be active?

12. Oligonucleotides are unsuitable as drugs because of their short half-lives. Why are their half-lives short?

↺ Chapter summary

- DNA carries the instructions for protein synthesis and RNA processes these instructions in order to make proteins. DNA is composed of two separate strands of nucleotides in the form of a double helix. RNA is composed of a single strand of nucleotides.

- The production of protein from the instructions contained in DNA involves transcription of the instructions from DNA to mRNA, followed by translation of this mRNA into a protein molecule. Additionally DNA is replicated when cells divide.

- The categories of drug which target one or more of these processes are antibacterial and anti-cancer agents.

- Bacterial protein synthesis is the target for a range of antibiotic drugs such as the macrolides, the aminoglycosides, the tetracyclines, and chloramphenicol.

- Anti-cancer drugs which target nucleic acid synthesis include antifolates and purine and pyrimidine antimetabolites.

- Anti-cancer drugs which target existing nucleic acid molecules are intercalators, alkylating agents, and chain-cleaving agents.

- Antiviral drugs which target viral nucleic acid synthesis are analogues of purine and pyrimidine bases and their nucleosides. They all require conversion to nucleotides to bring about their activity. They inhibit DNA polymerase, RNA polymerase, or reverse transcriptase.

- Interferons, which are naturally occurring immunological products, prevent viral protein synthesis by inhibiting translation of viral mRNA.

- Antisense oligonucleotides offer a new approach to designing drugs which target nucleic acids.

📖 Further reading

MacDougall, C. and Chambers, H.F. (2004) Macrolides and Ketides in *Goodmann and Gilman's The Pharmacological Basis of Therapeutics*, 12th edn. New York: McGraw Hill, pp. 1529–34.

An account of macrolide and ketide antibiotics.

Bhadra, P.K., Morris, and C.K., Barber, J. (2005) Design, synthesis and evaluation of stable and taste-free erythromycin prodrugs, *Journal of Medicinal Chemistry* 48: 3878–84.

An account of attempts to make erythromycin more pharmaceutically acceptable.

Mingeot-Leclercq, M.P., Glupczynski, Y., and Tulkens, P.M. (1999) Aminoglycosides: Activity and resistance, *Antimicrobial Agents and Chemotherapy* 43: 727–37.

A review of the antibacterial activity of and the development of resistance to aminoglycosides.

Chopra, I, Hawkey, P.M., and Hinton, M. (1992) Tetracyclines, molecular and clinical aspects, *Journal of Antimicrobial Chemotherapy* 29: 245–77.

A comprehensive review of many aspects of tetracyclines.

Opalinska, J.B. and Gewirtz, A.M. (2002) Nucleic acid therapeutics: Basic principles and recent applications, *Nature Reviews Drug Discovery* 1: 503–14.

A review of drugs acting upon nucleic acids.

De Clerq, E. (2004) Antiviral drugs in current clinical usage, *Journal of Clinical Virology* 30: 115–33.

A comprehensive review of antiviral drugs in clinical usage.

Other Drug Targets

The previous three chapters have concentrated on the role of proteins (as enzymes or receptors) and nucleic acids as targets for drug action. There are, however, other biomolecules which act as drug targets such as lipids, carbohydrates, and proteins other than those dealt with previously.

5.1 LIPIDS AS DRUG TARGETS

The majority of drugs which target lipids do so by interfering with the lipid structure of cell membranes, either human or bacterial. They do so in a variety of ways, although all disrupt the cell membrane in some respect.

5.1.1 General anaesthetics

There is still considerable debate about the mechanism by which general anaesthetics bring about their action. A number of theories have been proposed over the years, but they are all variations on a basic theme—that general anaesthetics cause reversible changes in nerve cell membranes. These theories concentrate on two components of cell membranes—lipids and proteins. Because of the structural diversity of molecules exhibiting general anaesthetic activity, it was suggested that this activity depends on physico-chemical properties, in particular lipid solubility. It was suggested that anaesthetic drugs dissolve in the lipid component of the cell membrane, thereby causing a volume increase or increasing membrane fluidity. This lipid theory of anaesthesia was derived originally from the hypothesis of Overton and Meyer published at the turn of the twentieth century. Their work on narcosis of tadpoles demonstrated an excellent correlation between the oil/water partition coefficients of a series of simple organic compounds and the concentration required to produce narcosis in the tadpoles. Almost 40 years later, Meyer proposed a theory that narcosis depends only on the molar concentration in the lipid components of the cell but is independent of the compound involved (see Figure 5.1(a)). Subsequently it has been confirmed that there is a relationship between anaesthetic potency and lipid solubility. However, it has also been observed that there is a point in a homologous series beyond which anaesthetic activity actually decreases although lipid solubility continues to increase. This, and other discrepancies, does cast doubt on the lipid theory of anaesthesia. For example the stereoisomers of an anaesthetic have different anaesthetic potencies, even though they have similar lipid solubilities. Additionally, some drugs that are highly soluble in lipids exert only one component of anaesthesia (amnesia). Membrane fluidity is affected by an increase in temperature but does not cause anaesthesia. A more recent version of the lipid hypothesis is that general anaesthetics change the lateral pressure within the lipid bilayer of the nerve membrane, and this affects the conformation of certain membrane proteins, such as ion channels (see Figure 5.1(b)).

In an extension to this theory, it was demonstrated in the 1980s that general anaesthetics may interact with hydrophobic sites of certain membrane proteins. To date, no one theory of anaesthesia has proved entirely satisfactory. It seems that the mechanism of anaesthesia, far from being explained by the simple hypothesis proposed by Meyer and Overton, is actually much more complex and still requires much more research.

Inhalational (gaseous) anaesthetics are used to maintain anaesthesia and should be highly volatile, lipid soluble, chemically stable, and non-toxic. Diethyl ether fulfils most of these criteria but is dangerous because of its flammability. Nitrous oxide and chloroform have also been used but all have been super-seded by the halogenated anaesthetics such as halothane and enflurane (see Figure 5.2(a)). Intravenous anaesthetics are used mainly to induce anaesthesia and act much more rapidly than gaseous anaesthetics, producing unconsciousness in a matter of seconds after administration. Thiopentone is most commonly used (see Figure 5.2(b) and Integration Box 5.1 Ketamine).

Figure 5.1 (a) Meyer–Overton correlation

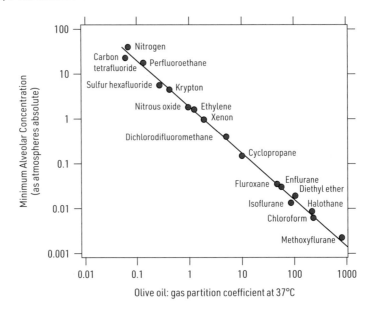

Figure 5.1 (b) Lipid bilayer expansion hypothesis

Lipid bilayer expansion hypothesis of anaesthetic effect

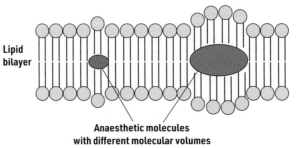

Figure 5.2 (a) Examples of gaseous anaesthetics

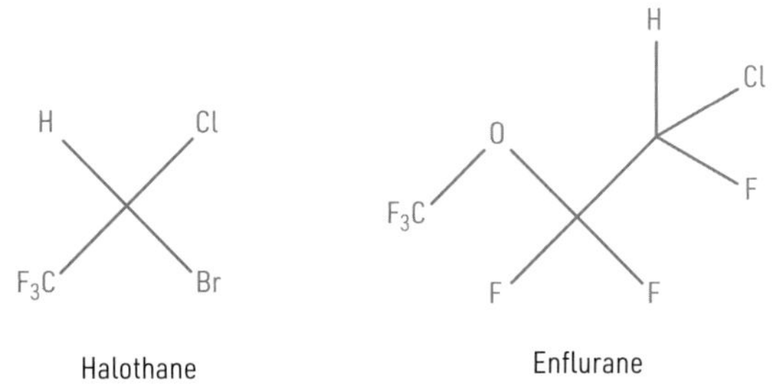

Halothane

Enflurane

Figure 5.2 (b) Examples of intravenous anaesthetics

Thiopental

Ketamine

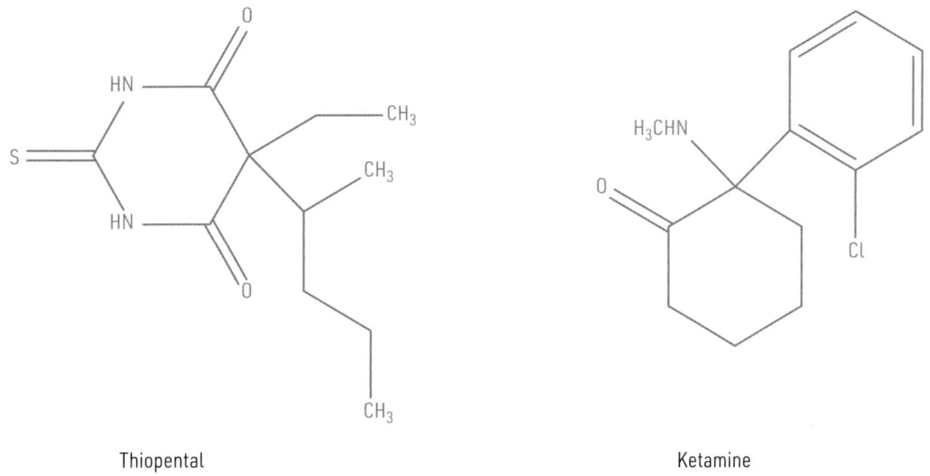

Anaesthetics cause changes in nerve cell membranes. There is still a debate as to the mechanism by which they do this—by dissolving in the lipid compartment or by binding to the protein component.

INTEGRATION BOX 5.1   KETAMINE

Another intravenous anaesthetic is ketamine, but this drug has a different mode of action to other intravenous anaesthetics. It acts by blocking N-methyl-D-aspartate (NMDA) receptors. This is a sub-type of excitatory amino acid receptor in the CNS. It is coupled to an ion channel and ketamine blocks this channel. It produces a type of anaesthesia known as dissociative anaesthesia where the patient can remain conscious although insensitive to pain and often amnesic. Ketamine was synthesized as a replacement for phencyclidine which has similar pharmacological properties but produces serious hallucinations and disorientation on recovery of consciousness. Phencyclidine found more use as a drug of abuse and as a possible model for schizophrenia than as an anaesthetic drug. Ketamine has also found its way into the drug abuse culture where it is known as 'special K'. Interestingly, ketamine is a chiral molecule, but the two enantiomers have different activity profiles. The S-isomer is an anaesthetic, but the R-isomer has poor anaesthetic activity but has psychotic activity. However, the commercially available drug (Ketalar) is a racemic mixture.

5.1.2 Tunnelling molecules

Tunnelling molecules are molecules which can insert themselves into the cell membrane of fungi and bacteria. Because of their structure, which renders them part hydrophilic and part hydrophobic, they can act as false membrane components, binding avidly to ergosterol, causing membrane disruption and loss of cellular components, particularly potassium ions.

Amphotericin B and nystatin can insert themselves into the cell membrane of fungi (see Figure 5.3 (a)) and gramicidin and polymyxin B into the cell membrane of bacteria (see Figure 5.3 (b)), making them leaky and allowing the contents of the cell to drain away thus causing cell death.

Amphotericin B and nystatin are both polyene macrolide antifungal drugs. They bind avidly to fungal cell membranes hence their use as antifungal agents. However, they can also bind to mammalian cell membranes (although less avidly) and hence are quite toxic. Their activity is thought to be due to their binding to ergosterol in the fungal cell membrane (the equivalent of cholesterol in mammalian cell membranes), thus forming an ion pore. Because of their toxicity and poor oral bioavailability, their use is mainly limited to topical usage. Amphotericin B and nystatin are both used against skin infections caused by *Candida*, such as thrush and athlete's foot. Amphotericin B, however, can be used systemically to treat severe life-threatening fungal infections such as cryptococcal meningitis.

Gramicidin, a polypeptide antibiotic, acts in a similar way on bacterial cell membranes. It is effective primarily against Gram-positive bacteria because it is a neutral molecule and cannot penetrate the outer envelope of Gram-negative bacteria. Polymixin B also acts on the bacterial cell membrane. Unlike gramicidin, however, it can penetrate the outer envelope of Gram-negative bacteria and act on the inner cell membrane, thus causing leakage of small molecules. It is seriously neurotoxic as it shows only slight selective toxicity for bacterial cells over mammalian cells. As such it is largely limited to topical use.

Although, strictly speaking, not tunnelling molecules, the azole antifungal agents (see Figure 5.3 (c)) do cause a change in fluidity of fungal cell membranes. Azole antifungal agents have a mechanism of action which confers selectivity for the infecting fungus over the human host. They do so by blocking the synthesis of ergosterol which is a vital component of fungal cell membranes but not mammalian cell membranes. Unlike amphotericin, nystatin, gramicidin, and polymixin B which are obtained from bacteria, the azoles are purely synthetic drugs and available in a wide range of structures. Because of this variety of structures, the azoles can be used, depending on the drug chosen, for treatment of simple topical fungal infections (clotrimazole), or against life-threatening systemic fungal infections (ketoconazole).

 Tunnelling molecules insert themselves into the cell membranes of fungi and bacteria. By doing so, they cause leakage of the cell contents leading to cell death.

5.1.3 Ion carriers

Ion carriers, also known as ionophores, are molecules that can increase the permeability of cell membranes to ions. They are molecules which transport ions from one side of the cell membrane to the other side. They are specific for individual ions.

Valinomycin, for example, is a specific carrier of potassium ions. Valinomycin is obtained from *Streptomyces* species and has a cyclic structure, consisting of three molecules of L-valine, three molecules of D-valine, three molecules of lactic acid, and three molecules of D-hydroxyisovalerate (see Figure 5.4). These constituent molecules are arranged such that the polar carbonyl groups point inwards

Figure 5.3 (a) Examples of antifungal tunnelling molecules

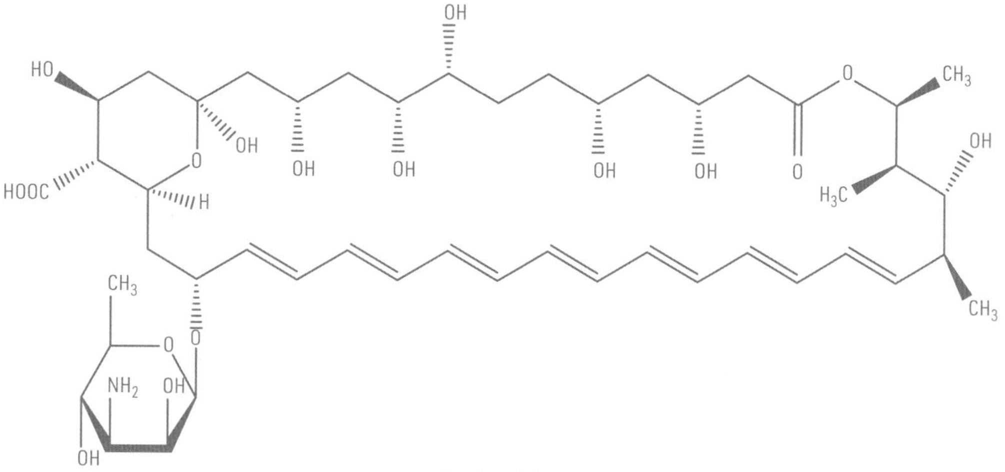

Amphotericin

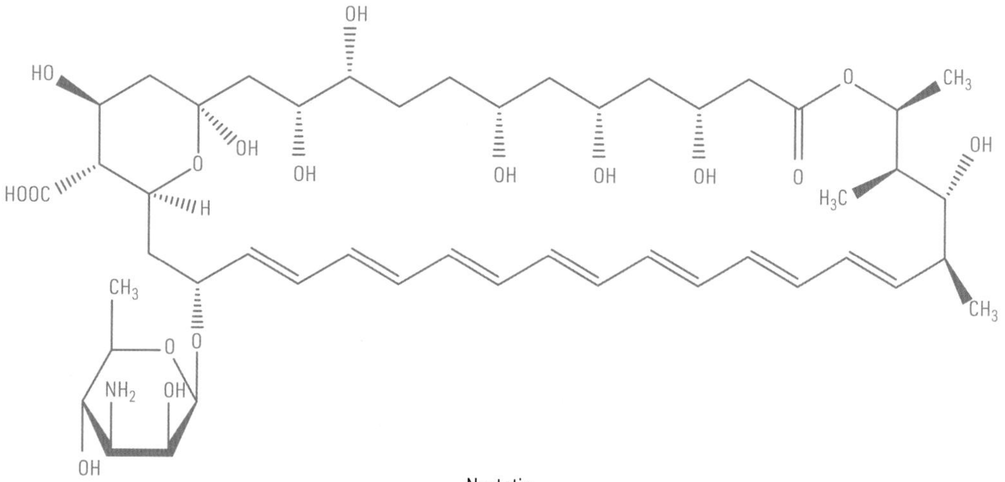

Nystatin

Figure 5.3 (b) Examples of antibacterial tunnelling molecules

Val-Gly-Ala-Leu-Ala-Val-Val-Val-Trp-Leu-Trp-Leu-Trp-Leu-Trp-NH-CH₂-CH₂-OH

Gramicidin

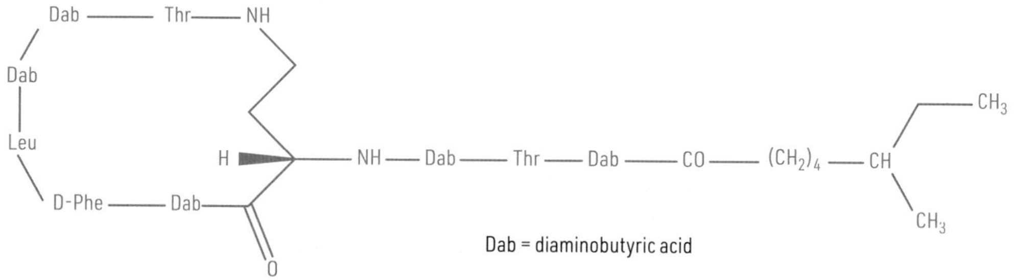

Dab = diaminobutyric acid

Polymixin B

Figure 5.3 (c) Examples of azole antifungal drugs

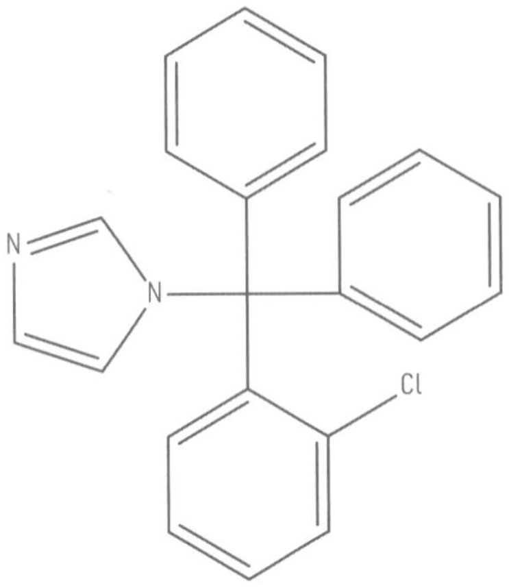

Clotrimazole

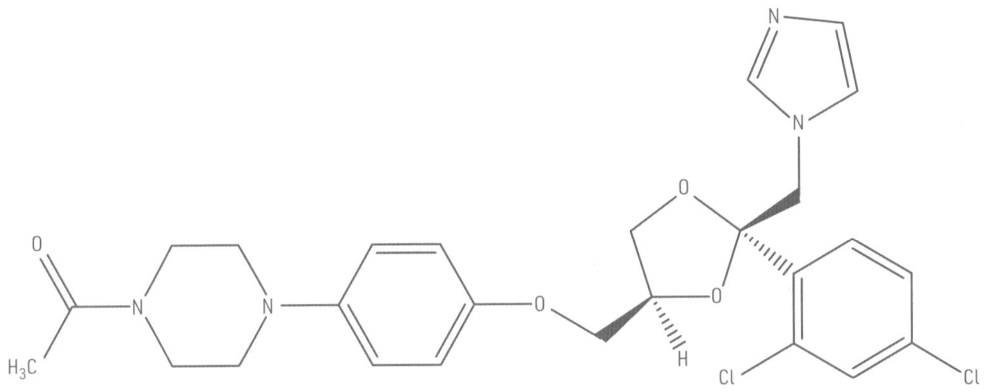

Ketoconazole

and the hydrocarbon chains point outwards. This hydrophobic exterior allows the complex to inter-act with the lipid membrane, whilst the hydrophilic interior can accommodate a potassium ion. Valinomycin, therefore, can pick up a potassium ion from the inner side of the cell membrane, carry it across the membrane and release it outside the cell, thus disrupting the ionic equilibrium of the cell. The cavity within the valinomycin molecule fits only the non-hydrated potassium ion and not the more readily hydrated sodium ion.

Because ion carriers like valinomycin do not distinguish between mammalian and bacterial cell membranes to any significant extent, they have not been of much clinical value. Valinomycin, however, has recently been shown to be highly active against cells infected with the SARS virus.

 Ion carriers transport ions, typically potassium ions, across the cell membrane, disrupting the ionic equilibrium of the cell.

Figure 5.4 Valinomycin

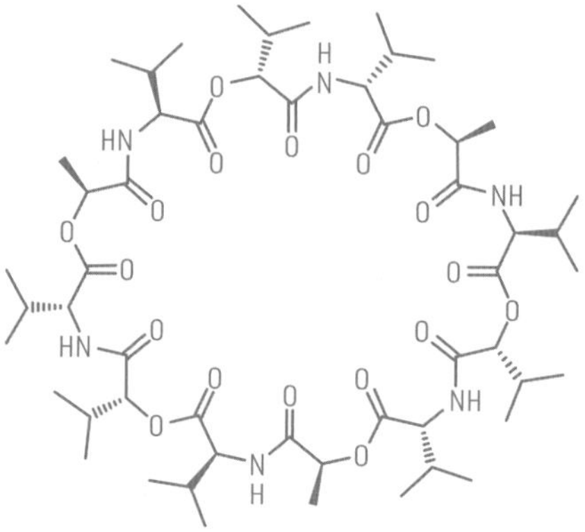

5.2 CARBOHYDRATES AS DRUG TARGETS

For many years, the role of carbohydrates was regarded as structural (cellulose) or energy storage (glycogen, starch). As such carbohydrates were not regarded as suitable drug targets. More recently, however, it has become apparent that carbohydrates have roles in cell recognition. Bacteria and viruses need to recognize host cells before they can invade them. These recognition processes, and the carbohydrate molecules involved in them, have become a focus for drug research. In addition to antibacterial and antiviral activity, drugs which target these carbohydrate molecules may also be of use in cancer and autoimmune diseases which often show changes in cell surface recognition carbohydrates.

The carbohydrates involved in cell recognition are not simple carbohydrates but are more complex **glycoproteins** and **glycolipids**. The protein or lipid parts of the molecules are embedded in the cell membrane, with the carbohydrate part projecting from the cell surface, thus enabling the recognition role. Drug research in this area is still at an early stage as attempts are made to fully understand the role of carbohydrates in these processes. One particular area of progress has been in the treatment of the influenza virus which contains the glycoprotein neuraminidase. Neuraminidase assists with penetration of the virus through mucus and the release of the virus from infected cells. Neuraminidase has been used as an antigen to allow the production of flu viral inhibitors (zanamivir, oseltamivir). However, because of the ease with which the flu virus can mutate, new vaccines are required each year.

Carbohydrates have only recently become regarded as potential drug targets. The role of carbohydrates in cell recognition is now regarded as important in the design of new drugs with potential activities against bacteria, viruses, cancer, and autoimmune diseases.

5.3 NON-ENZYMATIC PROTEINS AS DRUG TARGETS

Enzymes, which are protein in nature, as drug targets have already been dealt with (❯ XR Chapter 3) but there are other types of protein which can act as drug targets, namely structural proteins, transport proteins, cell membrane protein building blocks, ion channel proteins, cell signalling proteins, and viral proteins.

5.3.1 Structural proteins

Microtubules are involved in cell division and in the maintenance of cell structure. They are formed by polymerization of a structural protein tubulin. In the preparation for cell division, the microtubules depolymerize and then re-polymerize to produce a spindle which forms the frame on which the chromosomes can be transferred to the daughter cells. Drugs which target tubulin act by binding to it, inhibiting the polymerization into microtubules thus preventing **mitosis**.

The drugs which act in this way have largely been developed from natural sources. The first drug to be discovered in this category was colchicine (see Figure 5.5 (a)), isolated from the autumn crocus plant. It has been long known as an anti-tumour agent but has serious side effects and has been largely replaced (see Integration Box 5.2 Colchicine and gout).

INTEGRATION BOX 5.2   **COLCHICINE AND GOUT**

Colchicine is a natural product derived from the autumn crocus (*Colchicum autumnale*). Its mode of action is by binding to tubulins preventing their polymerization. Colchicine does possess anti-tumour activity, but its primary use is as a treatment for **gout**, where it prevents the migration of neutrophils into the joints. Colchicine has numerous side effects and is now used only to relieve acute attacks of gouty arthritis.

Another class of natural products which prevent tubulin polymerization are the Vinca alkaloids (see Figure 5.5 (b)), isolated from the Madagascar periwinkle (*Vinca rosea*). Three closely related compounds have anti-tumour activity—vincristine, vinblastine, and vindesine. Of these, vincristine and vinblastine are used clinically. Another plant product that targets tubulin is taxol (see Figure 5.5 (c)), isolated from the bark of Pacific yew trees. Unlike the Vinca alkaloids, the taxol derivatives inhibit depolymerization of microtubules, but the pharmacological effect is the same—halting cell division (see Box 5.1 Semisynthetic replacement for taxol—saving the yew trees).

Figure 5.5 (a) Colchicine

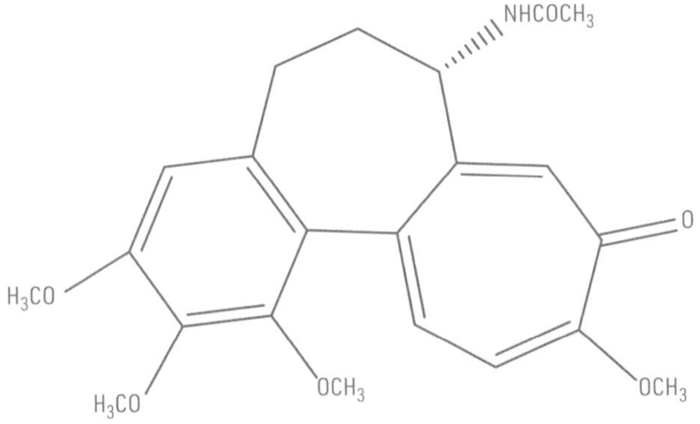

Colchicine

Figure 5.5 (b) Vinca alkaloids

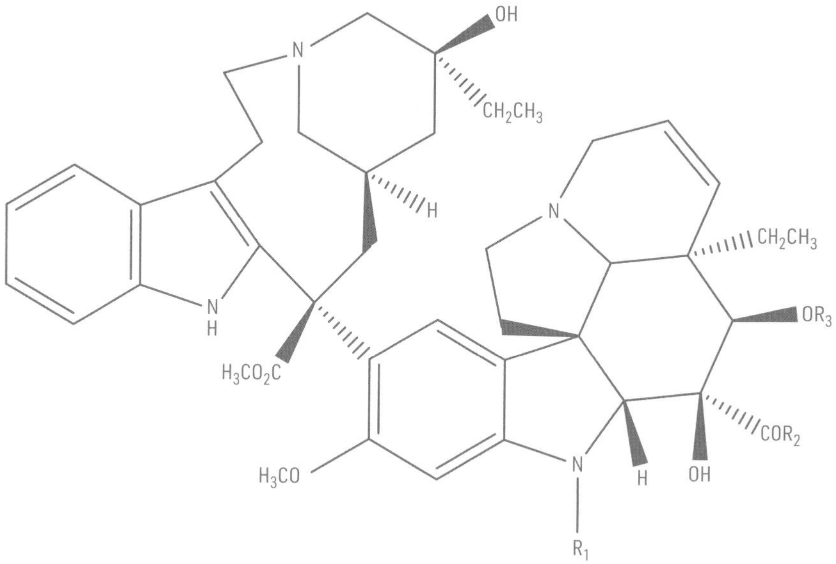

Vincristine R_1 = CHO, R_2 =OCH$_3$, R_3 = COCH$_3$
Vinblastine R_1 = CH$_3$, R_2 =OCH$_3$, R_3 = COCH$_3$
Vindesine R_1 = CH$_3$, R_2 = NH$_2$, R_3 = H

Figure 5.5 (c) Paclitaxel and docetaxel

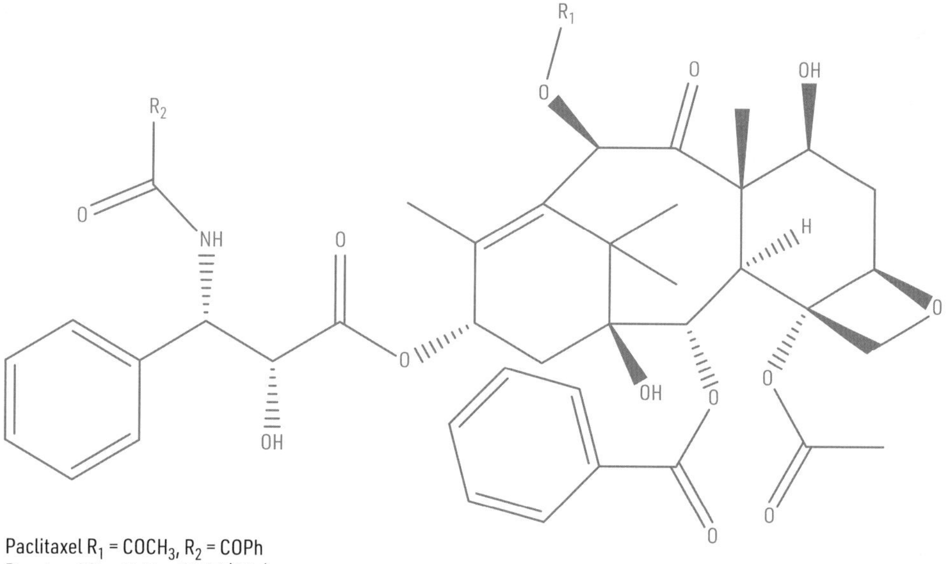

Paclitaxel R_1 = COCH$_3$, R_2 = COPh
Docetaxel R_1 = H, R_2 = COOC(CH$_3$)$_3$

Drugs which target the structural protein tubulin prevent its polymerization to microtubules, thus preventing cell division. Most of the drugs which act in this way, at present, are natural products or semi-synthetic derivatives of natural products.

5.3.2 Transport proteins

Transport proteins are cell membrane proteins whose role is to transport endogenous molecules across the cell membrane. Generally, they facilitate the uptake of endogenous molecules from outside the cell, resulting in their reduced contact and interaction with the relevant receptors on the target cell. Therefore, drug molecules that bind to transport proteins and inhibit this process can have a therapeutic effect as they prolong the presence of the endogenous molecules within the vicinity of the receptor. Such drug molecules are referred to as re-uptake inhibitors.

Examples of such drugs are the tricyclic antidepressants (see Figure 5.6 (a)) which block the re-uptake of endogenous amines such as noradrenaline and 5-hydroxytryptamine (serotonin). Selective serotonin re-uptake inhibitors (SSRIs) (see Figure 5.6 (b)), which exhibit selective serotonin re-uptake inhibition relative to noradrenaline, have a similar clinical profile but with reduced toxicity, particularly with respect to anticholinergic and cardiovascular effects.

Levodopa (see Figure 5.6 (c)), a drug used in the treatment of Parkinsonism, is targeted towards the transport protein normally used by phenylalanine. Levodopa is, in fact, a prodrug (❯ XR Section 12.6.4) for dopamine, a molecule which is too polar to be transported across the blood-brain barrier. Once in the brain levodopa is converted to dopamine by dopa decarboxylase. In this way, the deficiency of dopamine, which is the primary cause of Parkinsonism, is addressed.

Many drugs which target transport proteins bring about their activity by binding to the transport protein and prevent the binding of the endogenous substrates normally transported. They are referred to as re-uptake inhibitors.

5.3.3 Protein building blocks

The glycopeptide antibiotic, vancomycin (see Figure 5.7), targets the mucopeptide building blocks of the bacterial cell wall, preventing cell wall synthesis. Vancomycin caps the building block preventing its incorporation into the bacterial cell wall (see Box 5.2 Chiral centres—nature vs chemists).

Vancomycin prevents bacterial cell wall synthesis by capping the developing mucopeptide building blocks.

Figure 5.6 (a) Examples of tricyclic antidepressants

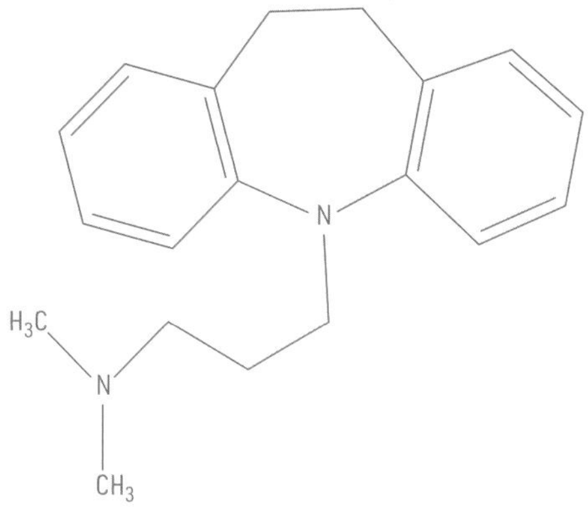

Imipramine

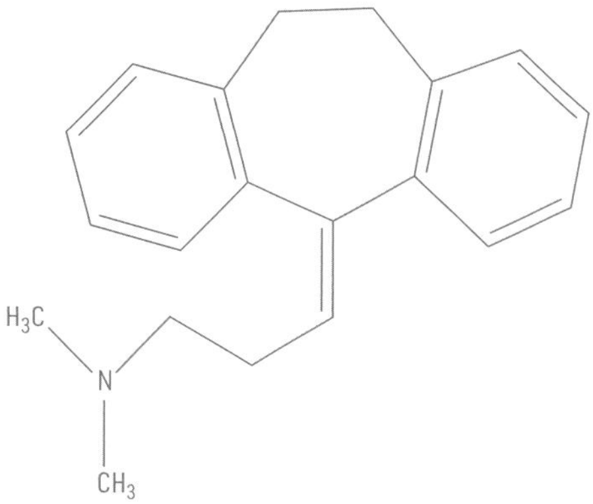

Amitriptyline

Figure 5.6 (b) Examples of selective serotonin reuptake inhibitors (SSRIs)

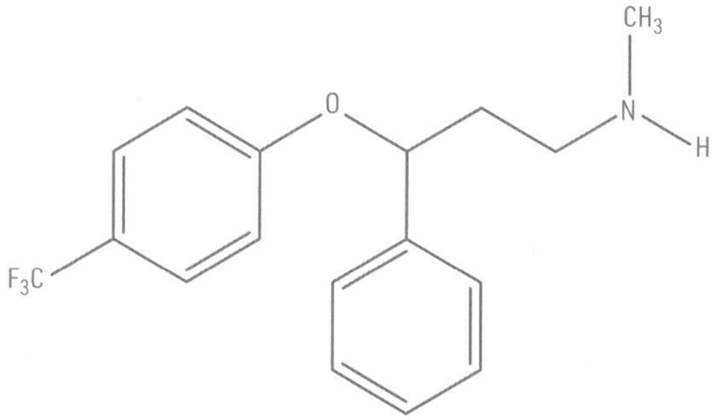

Fluoxetine

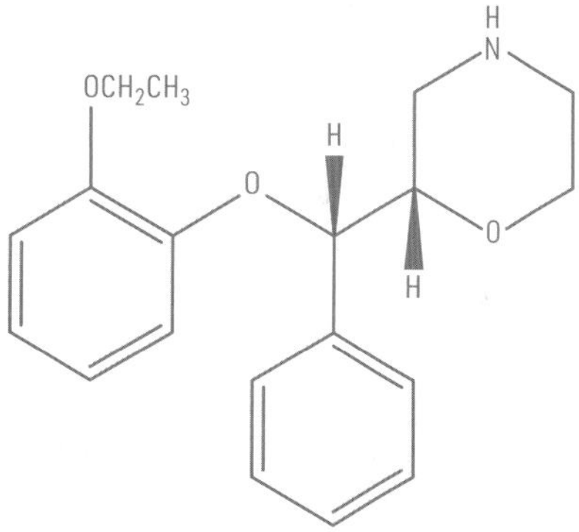

Reboxetine

Figure 5.6 (c) Levodopa

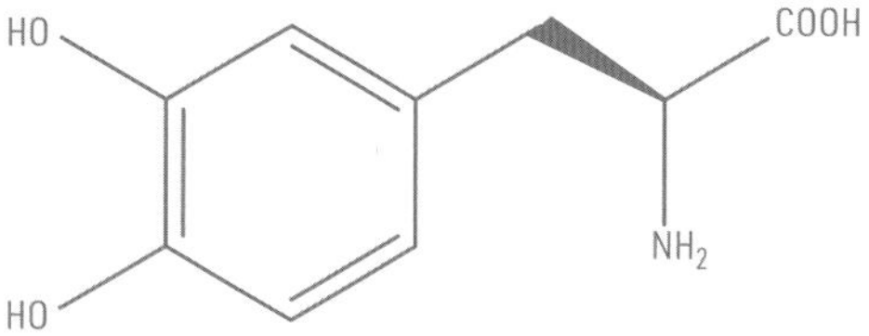

Levodopa (L-DOPA)

Figure 5.7 Vancomycin

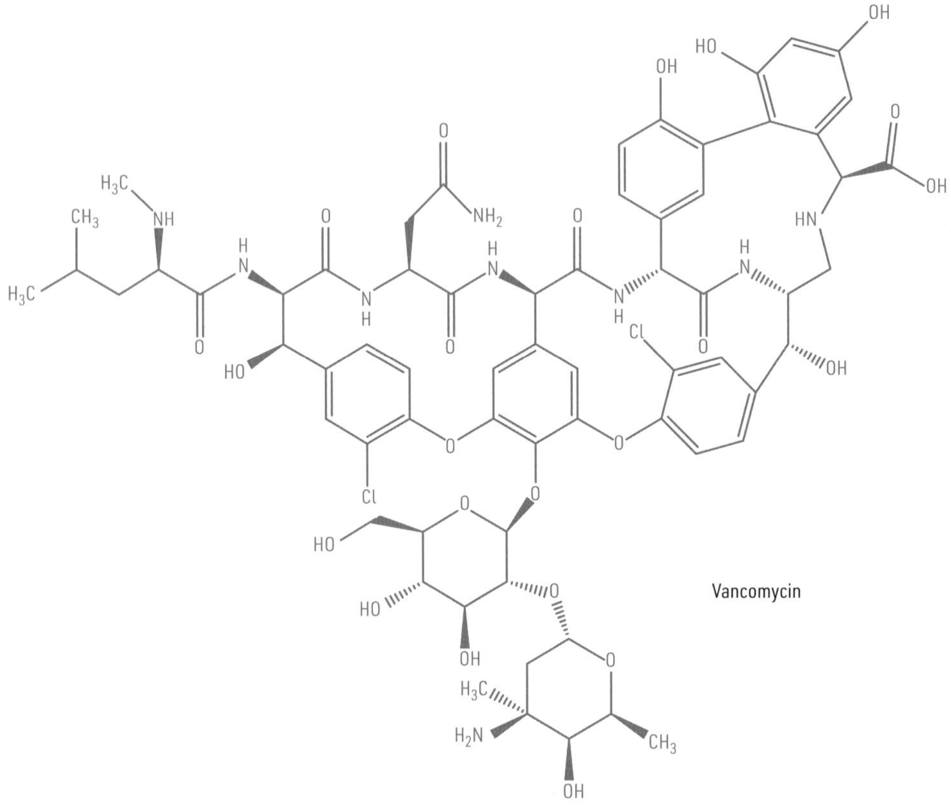

Vancomycin

BOX 5.2   CHIRAL CENTRES—NATURE vs CHEMISTS

If you examine the structure of vancomycin (see Figure 5.7), you will find that it possesses 18 chiral centres. This means there are potentially 2^{18}, that is 262164, possible isomers. But the natural source of vancomycin, a soil bacterium *Streptomyces orientalis*, produces only one isomer—remarkable! Although first isolated in the 1950s, it took chemists until 1998 to produce a synthetic version of vancomycin. However, the synthesis is not economic, and vancomycin continues to be isolated from the natural source.

Puromycin is another antibiotic and one which terminates the growth of protein chains during translation (▶ **XR Section 4.1.3**). Structurally it resembles the terminus of an aminoacyl tRNA molecule (see Figure 5.8), the molecule which transports an amino acid to a ribosome for addition to the growing peptide chain. Puromycin enters the ribosome and prevents the aminoacyl tRNA molecule from binding. Puromycin binds to the growing peptide chain, causing chain termination and premature release of the incomplete protein.

 Puromycin interferes with bacterial protein synthesis.

Figure 5.8 Puromycin and aminoacyl-tRNA

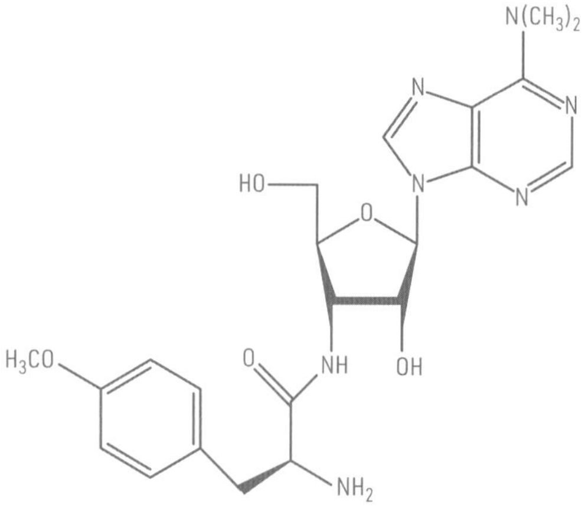

Puromycin

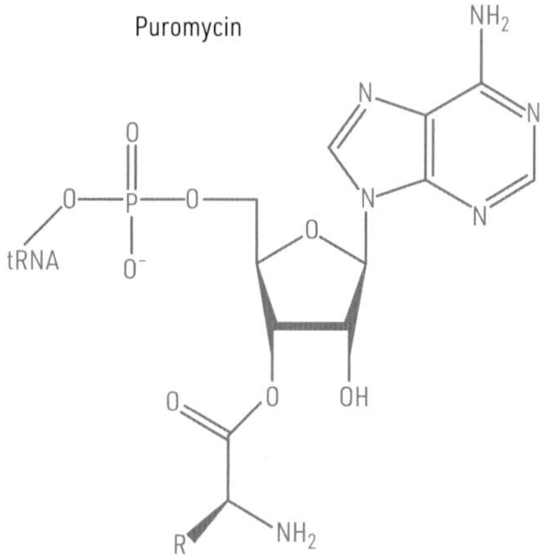

Aminoacyl-tRNA

5.3.4 Ion channel proteins

Ion channel receptors (❯ **XR Section 2.2.3**) are pore-forming proteins that allow the passage of ions across cell membranes. These receptors are responsive to either ligands (ligand-gated) or changes in voltage (voltage-gated). Ligand-gated ion channels are operated by the binding of a specific ligand and include the nicotinic acetylcholine (nAch), $5HT_3$ and glutamate receptors which are excitatory receptors. $GABA_A$ and glycine ion channels are inhibitory receptors. Drugs which act blocking agents at these receptors include tubocurarine (nAch), ondansetron ($5HT_3$), and ketamine (glutamate). Gabapentin, a drug used to treat **neuropathic pain**, inhibits the $GABA_A$ ion channel.

Voltage-gated ion channels are classified according to the ions which they allow across the membrane—Ca^{2+}, Na^+, K^+ and Cl^-. Calcium channel blockers act at the L-type calcium channels, are used to treat hypertension, and include such drugs as amlodipine, felodipine and verapamil. Sodium channel blockers include class I antiarrythmic drugs such procainamide and local anaesthetics like lidocaine. Also used as antiarrhymic agents are potassium channel blockers such as sotolol, known as class III antiarrhymics. There are currently no drugs used to block chloride channels.

Different ion channel blockers act on either ligand-gated or voltage-gated ion channels, preventing the passage of specific ions across cell membranes.

5.3.5 Cell signalling proteins

Cytokines are cell signalling peptides (**⏵ XR Section 2.2.5**). They are generally small proteins (usually ~ 20 kD) and are a vital part of the immune system. They are released by certain cells of the immune system and interact with cell surface receptors to alter cell function and are often referred to as immunomodulators. Normally they circulate in very low concentrations (10^{-12}M), but significantly increase in concentration, by up to 1000X, when the immune cells are stimulated. Cytokines include interferons, interleukins, lymphokines and tumour necrosis factor (TNF). Cytokines are different from hormones which are secreted by specialized glands whereas cytokines are produced by single cells, especially those of the immune system. Cytokines are used to treat cancer (interleukin 2), multiple sclerosis (interferons alpha and beta), and as adjuvants to cancer treatment to prevent neutropenia (various cytokines).

Growth factors are also cell signalling molecules and are often classified as cytokines. However, while growth factors always have a positive effect on cell division and growth, responses to cytokines can be positive or negative on cell proliferation. Growth factors may be protein in nature (e.g. colony stimulating factors, erythropoietin) and also include some hormones (e.g. insulin). Growth factors have found a variety of medical uses, such as wound healing and treatment of blood disorders (**neutropenia**, leukaemias, aplastic anaemia).

 Cytokines are small peptides released by cells of the immune system and may have a positive or negative effect on cell proliferation. Growth factors always stimulate cell proliferation.

5.3.6 Viral membrane fusion proteins

Although viruses are composed largely of nucleic acids (**⏵ XR Section 4.4**), these nucleic acids are encapsulated in a protein coat called a capsid. When a virus enters a host cell, the protein coat has to fuse with the host cell proteins present in the host cell membrane. This fusion triggers a sequence of events which allow the virus to enter the host cell. Enfuvirtide is an example of the class of drugs, known as fusion inhibitors, which can prevent this fusion.

Enfuvirtide is a peptide containing thirty-six amino acids and is very complicated to synthesize, requiring over a hundred synthetic steps. Not surprisingly, therefore, research is focused on the development of simpler molecules which can act as fusion inhibitors. Because of the expense of production, enfuvirtide use is restricted to the treatment of HIV patients who have failed to respond to other drug treatments.

 Fusion inhibitors prevent the entry of viruses into a host cell by preventing the fusion of the viral protein coat with the host cell proteins.

？ Questions

1. Do local anaesthetics work in the same way as general anaesthetics?
2. The structure of amphotericin (see Figure 5.2 (a)) has a lipophilic portion and a hydrophilic portion. How do these two parts of the molecule contribute to its antifungal activity?
3. Why are the flu vaccines only active against viral cells and not active against human or bacterial cells?
4. What are the clinical indications for the Vinca alkaloids?
5. Cocaine is a re-uptake inhibitor—for which endogenous substances?

⟳ Chapter summary

- The mechanism by which anaesthetics bring about their pharmacological activity is still a matter of debate.
- The lipid theory suggests that they disrupt the nerve cell membrane by dissolving in the lipid component of the membrane.
- The protein theory suggests that they interact with the hydrophobic parts of membrane proteins.
- Tunnelling molecules insert themselves into the cell membrane of fungi and bacteria. This causes the membrane to become leaky and cell contents are lost.
- Ion carriers can transport specific ions across the cell membrane disrupting the ionic equilibrium of the cell.
- Carbohydrates are becoming the focus for much drug research, only recently being regarded as drug targets. Complex carbohydrates, such as glycolipids and glycoproteins, are important molecules in cell recognition processes.
- A variety of natural products have been found to target the protein tubulin, preventing its conversion into microtubules, thus preventing cell division. These compounds, and their derivatives, are active against a variety of cancers.
- Drugs which resemble the endogenous substrates of transport proteins can bind to the protein and prevent binding of the endogenous substrate. Such drugs have proved particularly useful in preventing the re-uptake of neurotransmitters such as noradrenaline and serotonin.
- Valinomycin and puromycin are antibiotics which terminate the construction of the bacterial cell wall and bacterial protein synthesis respectively.
- Ion channel proteins may be ligand-gated or voltage-gated and allow the passage of certain ions across the cell membrane. Ion channel blockers prevent the passage of these ions.
- Cytokines and growth factors are cell signalling peptides, which have effects on the growth and proliferation of cells.
- Fusion inhibitors prevent the entry of viruses into a host cell by preventing the fusion of the viral protein coat with the host cell proteins.

📖 Further reading

Mechanism of action of inhaled anaesthetic agents (2005) *Anaesthesia UK*, https://www.frca.co.uk/article.

A very good concise review.

Jordan, M.A. (2002) Mechanism of action of antitumour drugs that interact with microtubules and tubulin, *Current Medicinal Chemistry–Anticancer Agents* 2: 1–17.

A comprehensive account of the mechanism of action of the various natural products that interact with these structural proteins.

Fu, Y., Li, S., Zu, Y., Yang, G., Yang, Z., Jiang, S., Wink, M., and Efferth, T. (2009) Medicinal chemistry of paclitaxel and its analogues, *Current Medicinal Chemistry* 16: 3966–85.

An in-depth account of the medicinal chemistry of paclitaxel and its analogues.

Anderson, I.M. (2000) Selective serotonin re-uptake inhibitors vs tricyclic antidepressants: a meta-analysis of efficacy and tolerability, *Journal of Affective Disorders* 58: 19–36.

A comparison of the clinical usefulness of these two groups of re-uptake inhibitor drugs.

Lee, S. and Margolin, K. (2011) Cytokines in cancer immunotherapy, *Cancers* 3: 3856–93.

Comprehensive review of the role of cytokines in cancer treatment.

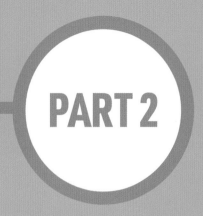

PART 2

Origins of Drug Molecules

Part 1 of this book introduced the types of targets at which potential drug molecules are aimed. Part 2 will deal with the origins of potential drug molecules, so-called lead compounds (▶ XR Chapters 6 and 7), the ways in which the biological activity of these lead compounds can be improved (▶ XR Chapters 8 and 9), the means by which large numbers of potentially biologically active molecules can be synthesized and tested (▶ XR Chapter 10), and the role of biotechnology in drug design and drug development (▶ XR Chapter 11).

6

Sources of Lead Compounds

A lead compound is one that exhibits a desired pharmacological property which can then be developed further to optimize its biological activity. It provides a starting point for further structural modifications in order to achieve greater potency, greater selectivity, and more appropriate pharmacokinetic parameters. Identification of a lead compound is an important feature of the drug design process. But from where do we obtain these lead compounds? This chapter will identify the many and varied sources of lead compounds that have been exploited and those that continue to be used by academic researchers and the pharmaceutical industry.

6.1 NATURAL SOURCES

For thousands of years man has used materials from the natural world to treat various illnesses and conditions. The first written records of medicines used by man, called herbals or pharmacopoeias, were composed entirely of materials from nature. It is only to be expected, therefore, that the natural world has proved to be a rich source of lead compounds. Of 1,073 new drugs discovered between 1981 and 2010, 6 per cent are natural products, 28 per cent are modified natural products, and 30 per cent mimic natural products.

6.1.1 Plant sources

The plant kingdom has been the source of a wide variety of the drugs that are in use today, for example morphine from the opium poppy, quinine from Cinchona bark, paclitaxel from the Pacific yew tree (❯ XR Section 5.3.1 and Box 5.1), vincristine from the Madagascar periwinkle (❯ XR see Section 5.3.1), digoxin from the foxglove (*Digitalis purpurea*) (see Figure 6.1). Having said that, how does one identify the active component in the plant and hence a lead compound? Ancient civilizations have used a comprehensive 'trial and error' system of investigations and this has led, in some cases, to the establishment of very detailed written records (Box 6.1).

BOX 6.1   DOCUMENTATION OF NATURALLY-SOURCED MEDICINES

Some communities have been producing documentation relating to the use of natural (in particular plant) sources as medicines for thousands of years. The oldest written records belong to the Ayurvedic medicine system which dates back to around 2500 BC. This system has been used by the Persians, Moghuls, and Indians, where it continues to be used to the present day. However there is a certain amount of controversy associated with these medicines which often include toxic metal ions. The ancient Egyptian civilization was recording the use of plant materials as medicines as early as 1700 BC. Amongst the plants documented were garlic (for many uses), ganja (for eye problems), and poppies (as a sedative, particularly for children!). Probably the most extensive use of natural sources as medicines is in traditional Chinese medicine (TCM) which first produced written records in the first century AD and continues to this day. In India the Unani Canon of Medicine was written in the eleventh century AD and has considerable similarities to Ayurvedic medicine, often utilizing similar natural products as therapy. The number of plants recorded for use in these documents is very large, Chinese *materia medica* consisting of around 5800 plants and India's *materia medica* around 2,500 plants. In Africa and South America written records are not available to the same extent as in the Middle East and Asia, there being a greater reliance on the oral tradition of tribal healers.

One of the first moves away from 'trial and error' methodology to a more scientific basis was an investigation by William Withering in 1785. It was his work on treatment of dropsy (congestive heart failure) with extract of digitalis that heralded the modern era of the use of plants as a source of lead compounds. Even today, however, the potential for plants to provide lead compounds has barely begun to be exploited. It is estimated that we have only been able to fully explore 0.5 per cent of the higher plants on Earth for their chemical composition and their pharmaceutical potential. Despite this it is estimated that about 25–30 per cent of the drugs currently available are derived from plants.

Bioprospecting is a recently introduced term used to describe the centuries-old process of collecting and screening plant (and other biological) material for commercial purposes. In addition to collecting plant samples, indigenous knowledge is utilized to assist in discovery and exploitation of plant resources. Researchers could, theoretically, take thousands of plant samples and subject them to biological screening—a process which would be time-consuming and economically inefficient. Useful discoveries could be accelerated by collecting and using local knowledge regarding plant species and their indigenous usage. Random screening of samples has an estimated success rate of producing a lead compound of about one in 10,000 which could be converted to a much-improved hit rate of about one in 5,000 by use of traditional knowledge.

6.1.2 Marine sources

In contrast to the extensive historical usage of plant sources, marine sources have only recently begun to be investigated as a source of lead compounds. Despite having given rise to large numbers of biologically active compounds, few have resulted in the development of clinically useful drugs. The only real success to date is the introduction of eribulin for the treatment of metastatic breast cancer. This was derived from halichondrin B isolated from a marine sponge. Of more significance has been the isolation of some of the most toxic compounds known to man, for example tetrodotoxin isolated from the puffer fish (Figure 6.2). This molecule has found use in neurochemical research into the molecular basis of the action of sodium channels.

Figure 6.1 Examples of drugs from plant sources

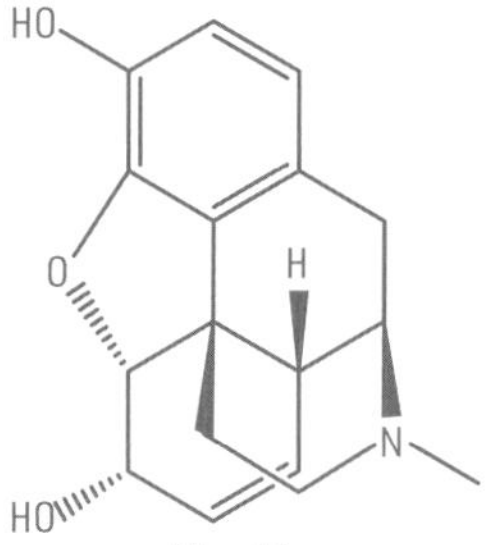

Morphine

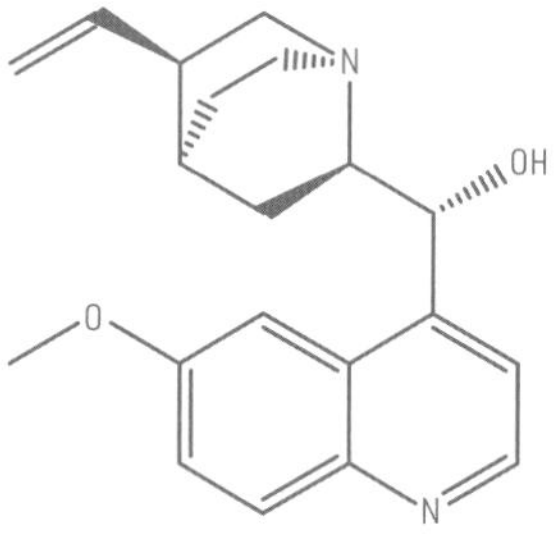

Quinine

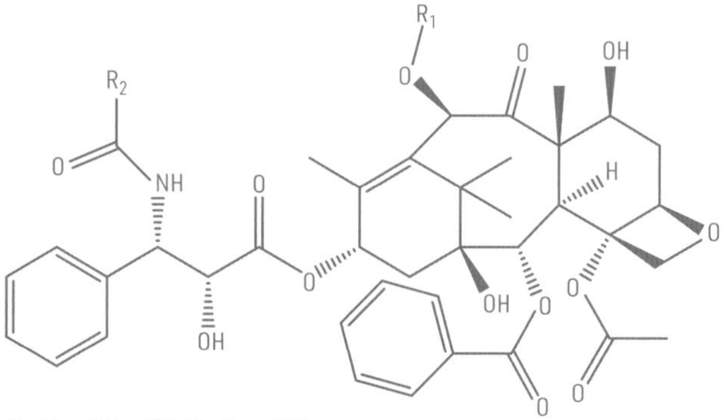

Paclitaxel R$_1$ = COCH$_3$, R$_2$ = COPh
Docetaxel R$_1$ = H, R$_2$ = COOC(CH$_3$)$_3$

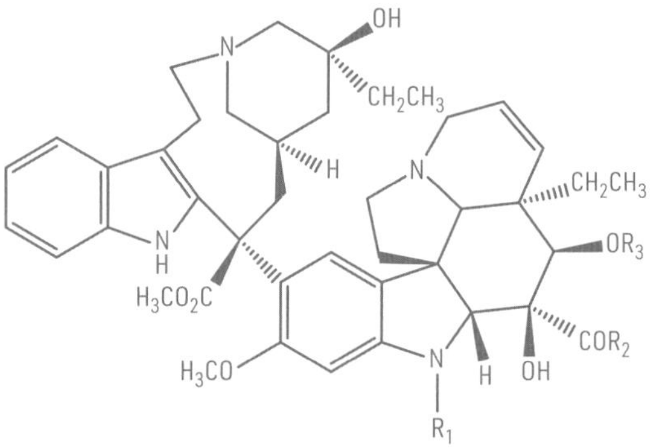

Vincristine R$_1$=CHO, R$_2$=OCH$_3$, R$_3$=COCH$_3$
Vinblastine R$_1$=CH$_3$, R$_2$=OCH$_3$, R$_3$=COCH$_3$
Vindesine R$_1$=CH$_3$, R$_2$= NH$_2$, R$_3$= H

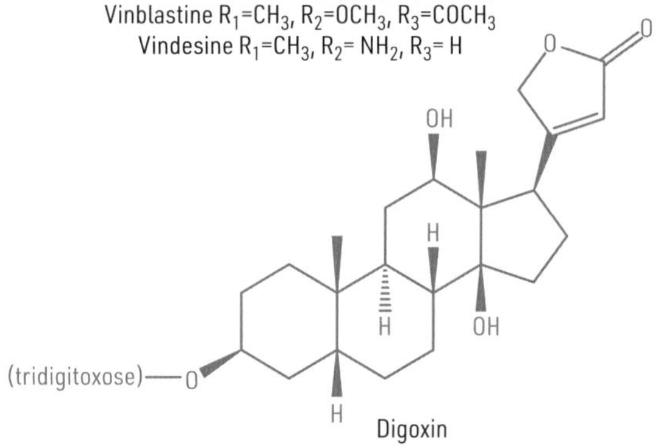

(tridigitoxose)—O

Digoxin

Figure 6.2 Tetrodotoxin

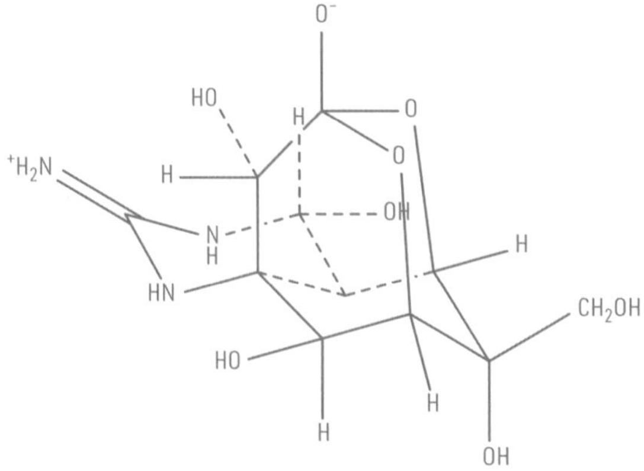

Tetrodotoxin

6.1.3 **Microorganisms**

Microorganisms have proved to be an excellent source, not only of lead compounds, but also of clinically used drug molecules. After the isolation of penicillin in 1940, samples of bacteria and fungi were collected worldwide and biologically tested providing, largely, molecules with antibiotic activity. These include, in addition to penicillins (➤ **XR Section 3.2.2**), cephalosporins (➤ **XR Section 3.2.2**), chloramphenicol (➤ **XR Section 4.2.4**), tetracyclines (➤ **XR Section 4.2.3**), aminoglycosides (➤ **XR Section 4.2.2**) and vancomycin (➤ **XR see Section 3.2.2**). The lead compound for the **statin** group of drugs, lovastatin, was isolated from a fungus (➤ **XR see Box 3.1** and Case Study 6.1), as was the **immunosuppressant** ciclosporin (Figure 6.3) (Integration Box 6.1).

Figure 6.3 Ciclosporin

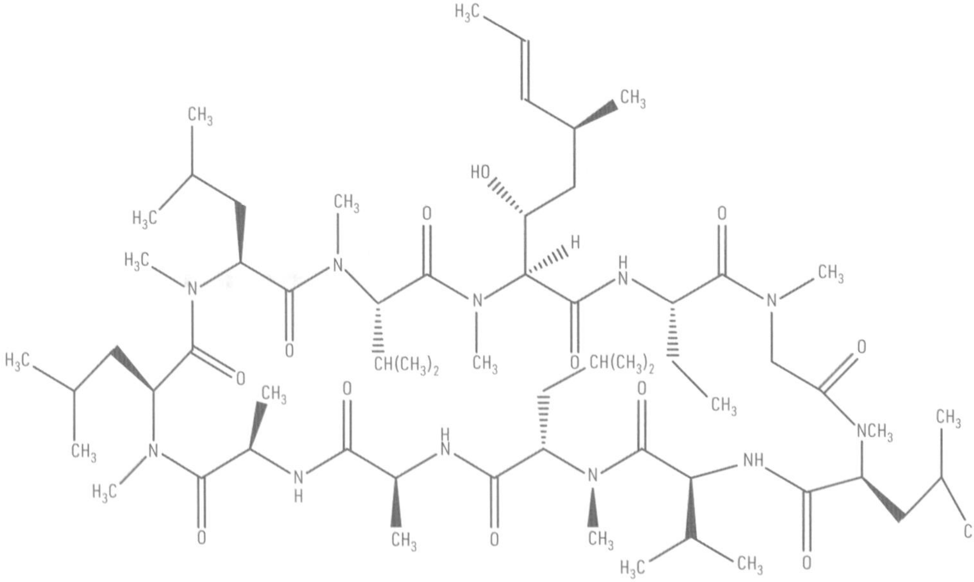

Ciclosporin

CICLOSPORIN AS AN IMMUNOSUPPRESSANT

Ciclosporin, also known as ciclosporin A, is used to suppress the immune response after organ transplant in order to prevent rejection of the transplanted organ. Ciclosporin was first isolated from the fungus *Tolypocladium inflatum* found in a soil sample in Norway in 1969. Originally tested for antibiotic activity, the immunosuppressant activity was discovered in 1972 as a result of general *in vitro* biological screening. In humans, ciclosporin is extensively metabolized, however the metabolism is much reduced for a short period following consumption of grapefruit juice (❯ **XR see Section 12.5.4**).

6.1.4 Venoms and toxins

Venoms and toxins have been evolved by species for protection from predators. As such, they are expected to be highly toxic and, therefore, not particularly useful as lead compounds. However a significant number of venoms and toxins have proved extremely useful tools for pharmacological research (❯ **XR Section 6.1.2**) (Integration Box 6.2 α-Bungarotoxin). An example, however, where a venom has provided a lead compound is in the development of a particular class of antihypertensive drugs. The venom from the Brazilian pit viper provided a peptide which led to the development of the ACE inhibitors such as captopril, enalopril, and related compounds (❯ **XR Case Study 3.1**).

α-BUNGAROTOXIN

α-Bungarotoxin, isolated from the venom of the many-banded krait *Bungarus multicinctus* (a snake found in Asia) (see Figure 6.2.1), is a polypeptide containing seventy amino acids. It irreversibly blocks the nicotinic cholinergic receptor by binding to both the α and β subunits of the receptor. This irreversible binding has assisted in the investigation of the structure of the nicotinic cholinergic receptor and its mode of action.

Figure 1 Many-banded krait

(Credit: Fearingpredators/Wikimedia Commons (CC BY-SA 3.0)).

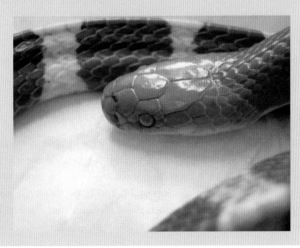

6.1.5 Animal sources

Animals have been used as sources of medicines for thousands of years but have provided relatively little in the way of lead compounds for development of new drugs. Because animals have, generally speaking, body chemistry broadly similar to humans it is unlikely that they will provide new compounds for investigation as drug substances. From time to time new natural ligands for drug targets have been discovered but these discoveries have not provided, until recently, any significant examples of new drug developments (Integration Box 6.3 Enkephalins and endorphins). Although there are many traditional medicines based on animal tissues this does raise ethical and ecological issues. The demand for certain animal body parts for use in traditional medicine has led to the near extinction of some species and this is not acceptable, particularly in view of the unproven efficacy of many such medicines.

INTEGRATION BOX 6.3   **ENKEPHALINS AND ENDORPHINS**

Although morphine has been known for its powerful analgesic activity since the nineteenth century, it was over a hundred years before it was elucidated how it brought about this activity. Morphine is now known to bind to opioid receptors in the central nervous system. There are three main types of opioid receptor, μ, κ, and δ, and they are inhibitory G-protein coupled receptors. Morphine is an **agonist** at all these receptors. Knowing the existence of these opioid receptors raises the question—what is the **endogenous** ligand at these receptors? In 1975 two pentapeptides were isolated which exhibited opiate-like activity. They were named enkephalins—methionine-enkephalin and leucine-enkephalin (see Figure 6.3.1). Subsequently, larger peptides, termed endorphins, were also isolated and these also exhibited opiate-like activity. The duration of action (of the order of a few minutes) of these natural ligands is much shorter than morphine, as might be expected with endogenous ligands. Additionally, like morphine, they can induce tolerance and dependence and, to date, have not led to the introduction of any drug derived from them.

Figure 2 Enkephalins

Tyr ——— Gly ——— Gly ——— Phe ——— Met   Met-enkephalin

Tyr ——— Gly ——— Gly ——— Phe ——— Leu   Leu-enkephalin

 The natural world has proved to be a valuable source of lead compounds and drugs derived from them.

6.2 SYNTHETIC SOURCES

In the early days of drug research, most lead compounds were derived from natural sources. However, with the rapid development of synthetic organic chemistry in the early twentieth century, the emphasis shifted from lead compounds obtained from natural sources to lead compounds generated in the laboratory. Although, initially, there was an element of 'hit and hope' about the early attempts to produce synthetic lead compounds, the synthetic products rapidly became more rationally based in a number of ways (❯ **XR Chapter 7**).

6.2.1 Semi-synthesis

Semi-synthesis is the chemical manipulation of the structure of a (usually complex) natural product in the laboratory. As these natural products were produced by plants and microorganisms to give them some kind of evolutionary advantage, it is unlikely that they will be an ideal drug candidate in terms of their human pharmacological activity, selectivity, toxicity and availability. It makes sense, therefore, to manipulate their structures to try and improve their suitability for human usage. This process can sometimes lead to molecules which can be converted to the original natural product more efficiently thus not having to rely on the natural source (❯ **XR see Box 5.1**) or the production of analogues which have potential for improved biological activity (Integration Box 6.4 Semi-synthetic penicillins).

INTEGRATION BOX 6.4   **SEMI-SYNTHETIC PENICILLINS**

Although the introduction of penicillins in the 1940s was correctly regarded as an enormous medical breakthrough, the original penicillins were by no means ideal. Benzylpenicillin (Penicillin G) is orally inactive because it is degraded by gastric acid and so had to be injected. It also had a narrow spectrum of antibacterial activity and was inactive against a wide range of bacteria. The development of more effective analogues was, therefore, of great importance. This proved difficult, however, as penicillin G was only available from fermentation and a synthetic method of production had not yet been achieved. The synthesis of penicillin was eventually achieved in 1957 and, shortly afterwards, a biosynthetic intermediate of penicillin was isolated–6-aminopenicillanic acid (6-APA). This intermediate could now be used as the starting material for an enormous range of penicillin analogues–the semi-synthetic penicillins. 6-APA produced by fermentation, when reacted with a range of acyl chlorides, yielded the large number of penicillin analogues available today, such as ampicillin, amoxicillin and flucloxacillin (see Figure 6.4.1).

Figure 3 Formation of semi-synthetic penicillins from 6-APA

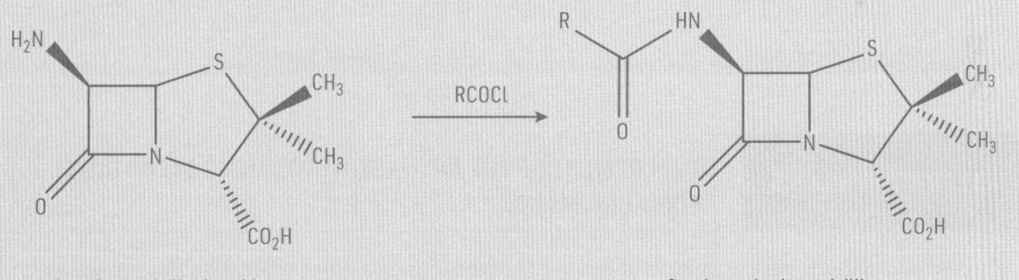

6-aminopenicillanic acid   Semi-synthetic penicillin

6.2.2 Synthesis based on the natural ligand

As biochemical and pharmacological investigations became more sophisticated, many of the natural ligands for drug targets were discovered and isolated. These endogenous molecules thus became the starting point for synthesis of new lead compounds. For example the anti-asthmatic drug salbutamol was developed using the endogenous ligand adrenaline as a lead compound (Integration Box 6.5). Histamine, an endogenous agonist, was used as the lead compound for the development of ranitidine which is a histamine H_2 antagonist (❯ **XR Case Study 8.1**). The anti-migraine sumatriptan was synthesized using the endogenous compound 5-HT as the lead compound (Figure 6.4).

Figure 6.4 Examples of drugs developed from endogenous ligands

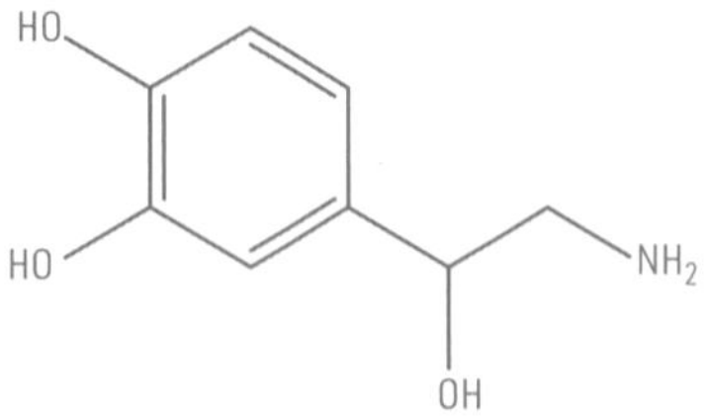

Noradrenaline

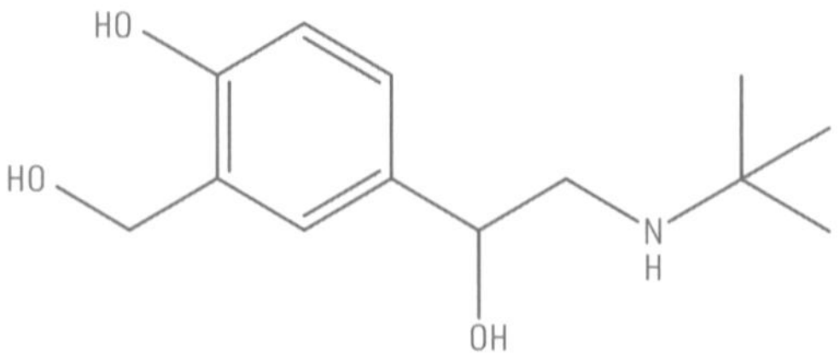

Salbutamol

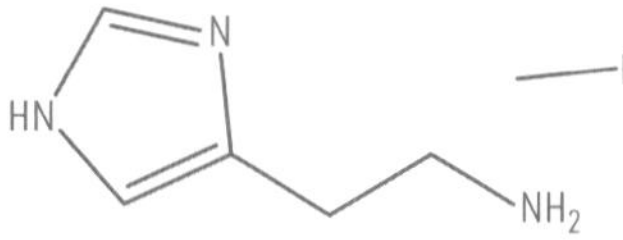

Histamine

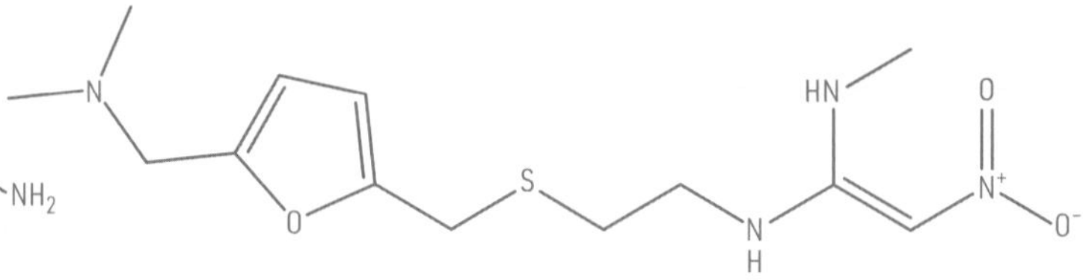

Ranitidine

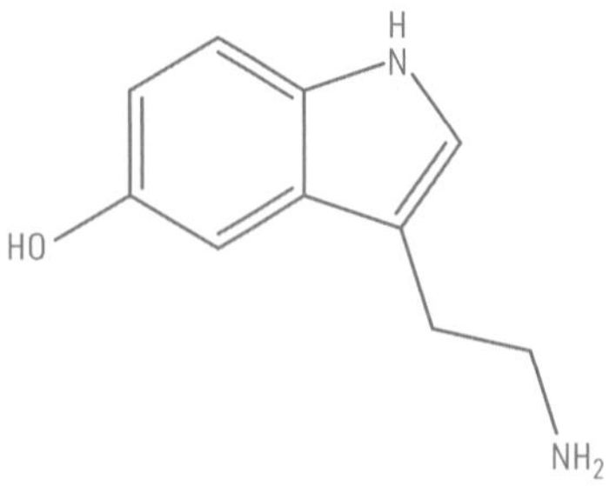

5-hydroxytryptamine

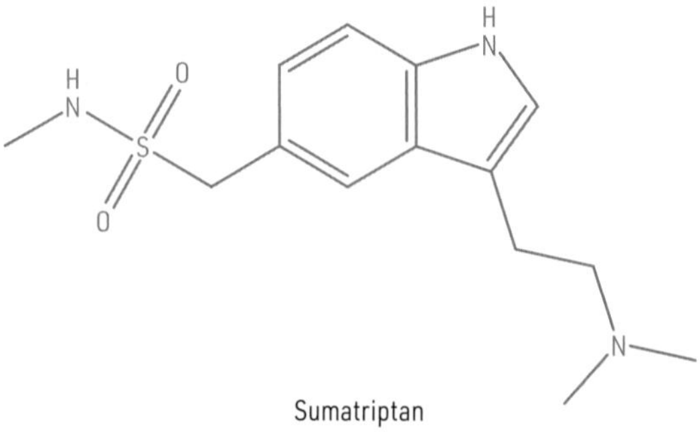

Sumatriptan

| INTEGRATION BOX 6.5 | **DEVELOPMENT OF THE ANTI-ASTHMATIC DRUG SALBUTAMOL FROM ADRENALINE** |

The main clinical use for adrenergic agonists is in the treatment of asthma. Adrenaline can be used to dilate airways in an emergency situation but is unsuitable for long-term use because it is rapidly metabolized and interacts with all types of adrenergic receptors causing significant unwanted side effects. Ideally, therefore, a molecule with a longer duration of action and which is selective for β_2-adrenergic receptors (present in the lungs) is required for use in the treatment of asthma. It was found that bulky N-substituents increased the selectivity for β-adrenergic receptors over α-adrenergic receptors. This led to the synthesis of isoprenaline. Unfortunately isoprenaline stimulated not only β_2-receptors but also β_1-receptors (found in the heart), producing unwanted cardiovascular effects. The real advance came as a result of trying to increase the duration of action by making a molecule more resistant to metabolism. The metabolism of adrenaline (and isoprenaline) takes place via action of the enzyme catechol-O-methyltransferase (COMT). Both adrenaline and isoprenaline are catecholamines, i.e. they both possess the 1,2-benzenediol (catechol) ring system. COMT acts by methylating the meta phenolic hydroxyl group to produce an inactive ether. Replacing this phenolic group proved difficult because it is necessary for adrenergic activity, in particular β-adrenergic activity. What was required was a substituent that could still interact by hydrogen bonding with the

→

Figure 4 Adrenaline, isoprenaline, and salbutamol

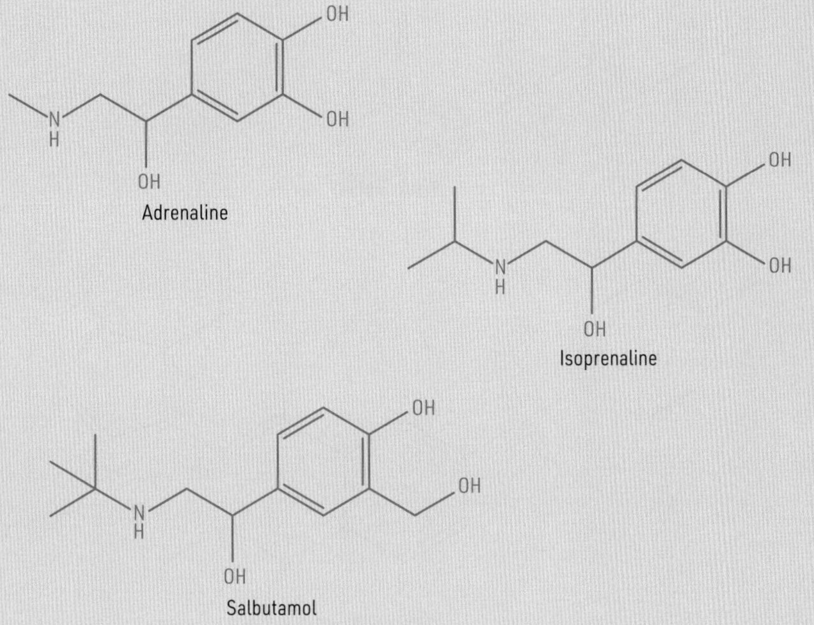

Adrenaline

Isoprenaline

Salbutamol

β_2-receptor, but which was not rapidly metabolized. Several substituents were tried but the most successful was replacement of the meta phenolic hydroxyl group by hydroxymethylene, producing salbutamol. Salbutamol has equal activity to isoprenaline at the β_2-receptor but is 2,000 times less active at β_1-receptors in the heart. In addition, it is not metabolized by COMT and has a longer duration of action (a half-life of around 4 hours).

6.2.3 Modification of existing drugs

Drugs that are already in clinical usage are often used as lead compounds for the development of new drugs. Because a drug is in clinical usage, a great deal of biological testing data, clinical trials data, and regulatory data is already available. This makes it relatively easy to modify the existing drug molecule to produce another drug molecule with, hopefully, improved properties compared to the original drug molecule. Such molecules are often referred to as 'me-too' drugs and may be produced by the same manufacturer as the original drug molecule in an attempt to extend the patent life of the existing drug. Alternatively, an existing drug may be used by a different pharmaceutical company to produce a new drug with similar and, hopefully, improved properties (so-called 'me-better' drugs).

A different approach to modify an existing drug is to concentrate on the side effects, which may have some benefit in a different therapeutic area. The aim would be to modify the existing drug to increase the side effect activity and to reduce the original clinically useful activity. A good example of this approach is the development of the anti-diabetic drug tolbutamide derived from the observed hypoglycaemic activity of some sulfonamides (Figure 6.5). An often-quoted example of this approach is the development of sildenafil (Viagra®) which is marketed as a treatment for male impotence. It was developed as a result of observations during investigations into its use as a vasodilator used to treat hypertension (Figure 6.5).

Figure 6.5 Examples of drugs developed by exploitation of side effects

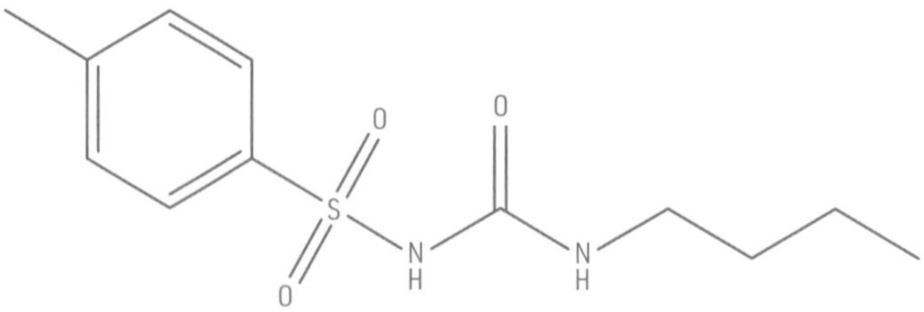

Tolbutamide

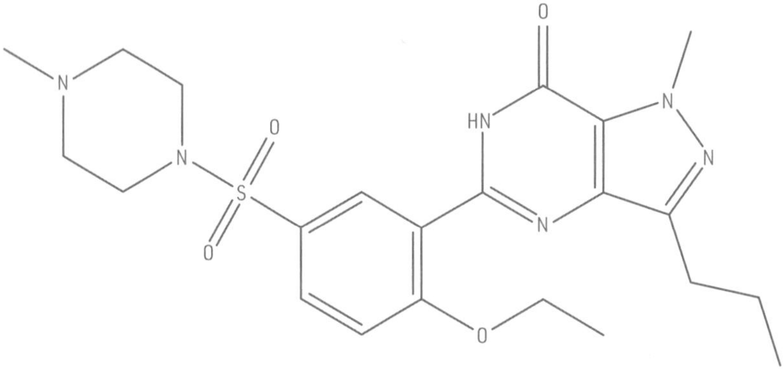

Sildenafil

6.2.4 Rational drug design

Many lead compounds are now produced as a result of research on disease states. An assessment is made of the biochemistry of the medical condition or invading microorganism, leading to decisions about where an intervention is likely to be most successful, i.e. the drug target. Based on this information medicinal chemists will decide on the most suitable structure for a lead compound which is then synthesized together with structurally related analogues.

A more recent approach that has resulted from high throughput screening (❯ XR Section 10.10) is the development of large libraries of compounds (known as combinatorial libraries (❯ XR Section 10.9), where minute quantities of many structurally-related compounds are synthesized and tested for biological activity with the aim of identifying a lead compound.

 Synthetic organic chemistry has been a vital tool in the production of lead compounds and the development of drugs from these lead compounds.

6.3 SERENDIPITY

In terms of drug discovery, serendipity is regarded as the occurrence of a chance discovery together with the necessary understanding to take advantage of that chance discovery. We have already seen an example of this with the development of sildenafil (❯ XR Section 6.2.3).

Probably the most famous example of serendipity is the discovery of the antibacterial activity of a *Penicillium* fungus by Alexander Fleming in 1928, which eventually led to the development of the penicillin antibiotics.

The anti-cancer activity of the Vinca alkaloids (❯ **XR Section 5.3.1**) was discovered during a search for anti-diabetic lead compounds in *Vinca rosea*. The original rationale for the search was based on the (erroneous) use of an extract of *Vinca rosea* by Madagascan natives as a treatment for diabetes.

The pharmacological activity of two important classes of antidepressants was also discovered by chance. Patients suffering from tuberculosis, when treated with isoniazid, showed an improved mood which eventually led to the introduction of iproniazid, the first monoamine oxidase inhibitor used to treat depression (Figure 6.6). Imipramine, the first tricyclic antidepressant to be used, was originally synthesized as an anti-psychotic because of its resemblance to chlorpromazine—which itself was originally synthesized as an antihistamine (Figure 6.6).

All the previous examples of serendipity arose from a chance discovery of biological activity. The introduction of propranolol, the original β-blocker, arose because of a lack of availability of a starting material. The programme to develop a β-blocker began with the endogenous ligand noradrenaline (Figure 6.7). This first developed the drug pronethalol which was then modified to produce propranolol. Note the position of the sidechain in pronethalol. The sidechain in propranolol is attached at a different position. This situation arose because, in synthesizing the original target structure, 2-naphthol was not available in the chemical stores so 1-naphthol was used instead.

 Chance observations and the realization of their significance have given rise to the introduction of a significant number of lead compounds and drugs derived from them.

Figure 6.6 Examples of antidepressant drugs discovered as a result of serendipity

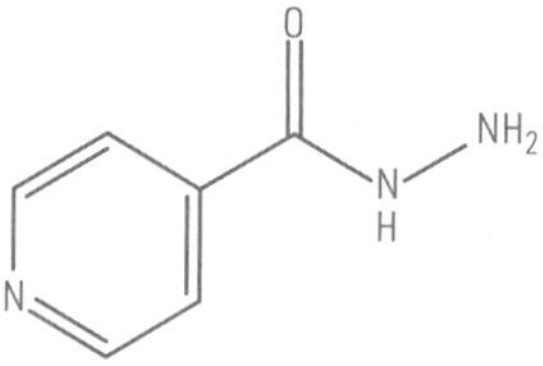

Isoniazid

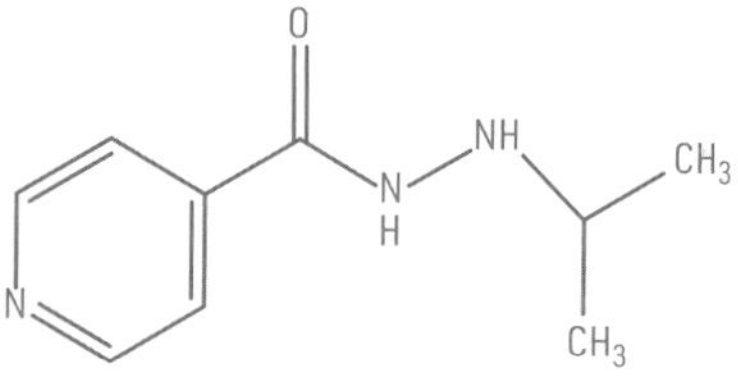

Iproniazid

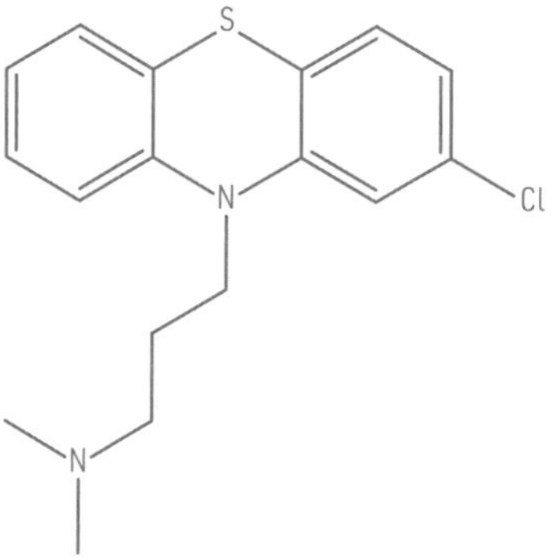

Chlorpromazine

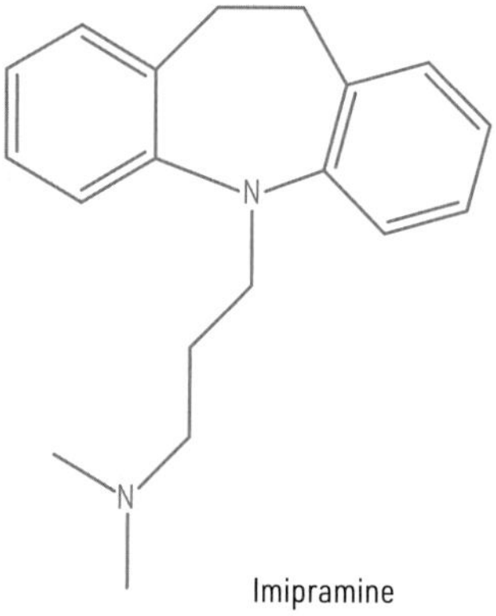

Imipramine

Figure 6.7 Serendipitous development of propranolol from noradrenaline via pronethalol

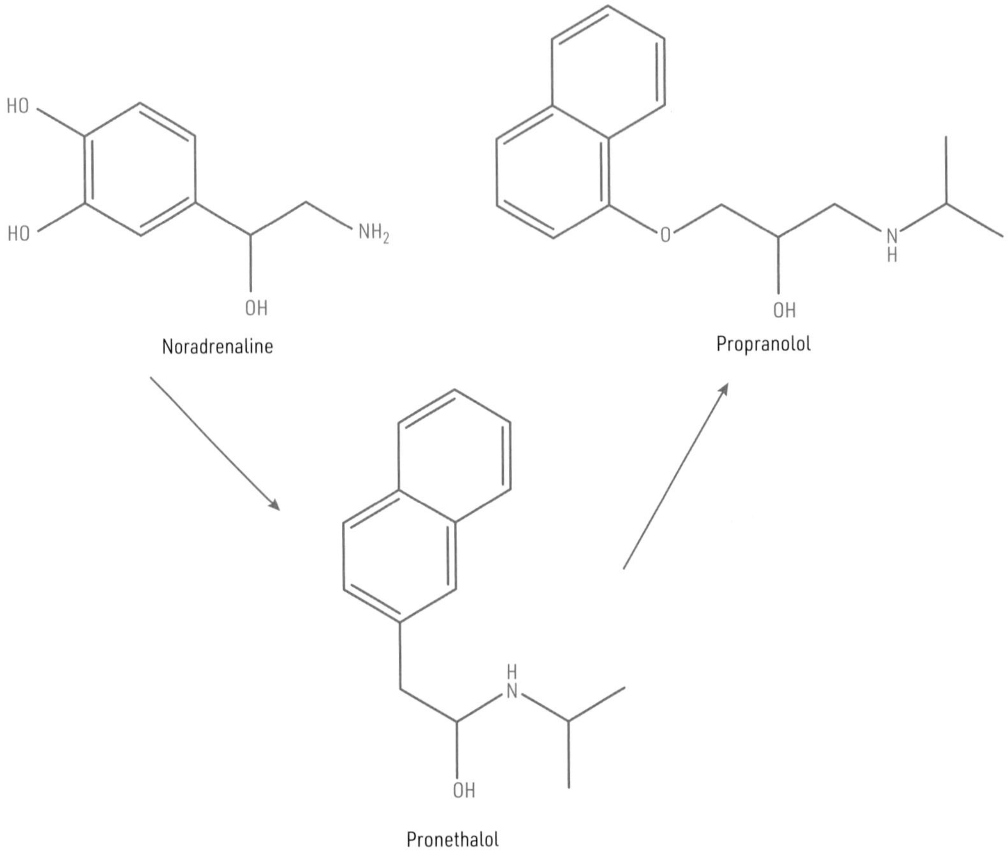

Noradrenaline

Propranolol

Pronethalol

6.4 SCREENING PROCEDURES

In order to identify lead compounds it is necessary to be able to screen new compounds (from whatever source) for appropriate biological activity. These screening programmes can be designed to identify several types of pharmacological activity or to identify activity against a specific target. An appropriate screening programme is vital in the search for a new or more effective drug. Rarely will a screening programme involve a single test. Usually the screening programme will involve a variety of *in vitro* tests and *in vivo* tests in order to determine as much information about the biological activity of the lead compounds. Not only is it necessary to identify activity at a desired target but also activity at any other targets which may give rise to undesirable side effects (see however ❯ XR Section 6.3).

6.4.1 *In vitro* tests

In vitro tests utilize isolated receptors, enzymes, cells, or tissues but do not use live animals. In the past these test materials had to be obtained from animals but advances in genetic engineering (❯ XR Chapter 11) mean that the difficulties of isolation and purification of such materials can be avoided. Enzymes can now be produced by **cloning** the gene for a particular enzyme into a yeast or bacterium, allowing the determination of inhibitory activity both qualitatively and quantitatively in terms of IC_{50}

values. Receptors can also be cloned into rapidly dividing cells, allowing the affinity of new ligands for these receptors to be measured often using radiolabelled molecules. Isolated cells and tissues can be utilized to identify higher level physiological effects such as muscle contraction or relaxation.

In more recent years *in vitro* tests have been computerized and miniaturized to allow vast numbers of compounds to be tested on a number of systems simultaneously. This is known as high throughput screening (HTS) and will be dealt with in Chapter 10 (**>> XR Section 10.10**).

6.4.2 *In vivo* tests

Although *in vitro* tests have the advantages of being more rapid, cheaper and easier to carry out, *in vivo* tests are also necessary. Demonstrated biological activity in an *in vitro* test is no guarantee of *in vivo* activity. Because *in vivo* tests are usually more expensive and more controversial, they are usually only carried out if the *in vitro* results indicate a positive response. Often *in vivo* tests use **transgenic** animals in which the animals have been genetically allowed to be susceptible to a particular disease or condition. *In vivo* testing is also utilized to identify pharmacokinetic properties such as absorption, distribution, metabolism and excretion (see, however, Integration Box 6.6).

INTEGRATION BOX 6.6 | **BIOLOGICAL TESTING AND THALIDOMIDE**

Thalidomide was licensed as a sedative in 1957, and was released as an 'over the counter' medicine in 1960 as a treatment for morning sickness in pregnancy. Subsequently, in the early 1960s, thalidomide was shown to be responsible for the formation of malformed foetuses, i.e. it had teratogenic activity. This property had not been identified during initial biological testing. The *in vivo* testing had only utilized mice and thalidomide does not exhibit teratogenicity in mice, but only in rabbits and humans. However, if rabbits had been used for the *in vivo* testing, the teratogenicity may still not have been apparent as thalidomide, which has a chiral centre, was only tested as the racemate—there was no requirement to test individual isomers at this time. The S-isomer of thalidomide, which has sedative activity, is also teratogenic whereas the R-isomer, also a sedative, has no teratogenic activity. The teratogenicity of the S-isomer may have been masked by the presence of the R-isomer. Incidentally, the non-teratogenic R-isomer is racemized *in vivo*, leading to the production of some of the teratogenic S-isomer. The positive outcome from this tragedy has been the development of the stricter regulations relating to the efficacy and safety of drugs currently in operation.

 In vitro and *in vivo* biological testing is utilized to determine as much information as possible about the biological activity of lead compounds and their analogues.

? Questions

1. What do you think are the advantages and disadvantages of using compounds from natural sources as lead compounds?

2. Divers and snorkellers must avoid fire coral which can cause painful stings. Try and discover the mechanism of this toxic effect.

3. How would you synthesize the following semi-synthetic penicillins from 6-APA: meticillin, ampicillin, flucloxacillin, amoxicillin?

4. Why do you think that fungi have been such a valuable source of antibiotic lead compounds?

Chapter summary

- Plant sources have been, and continue to be, a valuable source of lead compounds, with an estimated 25–30 per cent of drugs currently available derived from plants.

- Marine sources have only recently begun to be examined as a source of lead compounds.

- Many of the antibiotics currently available have been derived from lead compounds isolated from microorganisms.

- Venoms and toxins, from a variety of natural sources, have provided useful molecules for pharmacological research.

- As animals have, generally speaking, the same body chemistry as humans it is not surprising that they have not been very productive source of new lead compounds.

- Synthetic organic chemistry has been utilized in producing lead compounds by chemical manipulation of natural products, endogenous ligands, and existing drugs.

- Serendipity has had a significant role in the generation of lead compounds.

- Lead compounds are screened for biological activity, both desirable and undesirable, utilizing both *in vitro* and *in vivo* tests.

Further reading

Newman, D.J. (2008) Natural products as leads to potential drugs: An old process or the new hope for drug discovery? *Journal of Medicinal Chemistry* 51, 2589–99.

    A concise review of the influence of natural products on drug discovery.

Houlton, S. (2014) Chemistry in bloom, *Chemistry World* October 11: 46–9.

    An account of the role of botanical gardens in drug discovery.

Mann, J. (2000) *Murder, Magic and Medicine.* 2nd edn, Oxford: Oxford University Press.

    A very readable book outlining the evolution of modern drugs from their origins in nature and their use as poisons and medicines.

Megget, K. (2011) Of mice and men, *Chemistry World* April 8: 42–5.

    A discussion about the use of transgenic animals in drug research.

(T) CASE STUDY 6.1   **DRUGS INSPIRED BY NATURE–DEVELOPMENT OF STATINS**

Arteriosclerosis has been known about since the nineteenth century, but it was not until 1910 that the involvement of cholesterol in arteriosclerosis was recognized. Even then, it wasn't until the 1950s that high blood levels of cholesterol could be correlated with heart attacks. This discovery led to a significant effort to determine the pathway by which cholesterol is synthesized in the body. In 1960, it was confirmed that the synthesis takes place in four stages. The third reaction stage is the first rate-limiting step and this is the major regulatory point in the cholesterol biosynthetic pathway. This step is the reduction of hydroxymethylglutarate-Coenzyme A (HMG-CoA) to mevalonate, controlled by the enzyme HMG-CoA reductase (Figure CS6.1). What are the other three stages of cholesterol biosynthesis? As more evidence began to accumulate linking cholesterol levels to heart disease, the search for drugs which would lower blood cholesterol levels intensified.

The first class of drugs to be successful in this regard were the fibrates, which came into use in the 1960s (Figure CS6.2). The fibrates were thought to reduce cholesterol levels in a number of ways. They inhibit cholesterol synthesis by

→

Figure CS6.1 HMG-CoA reductase reaction

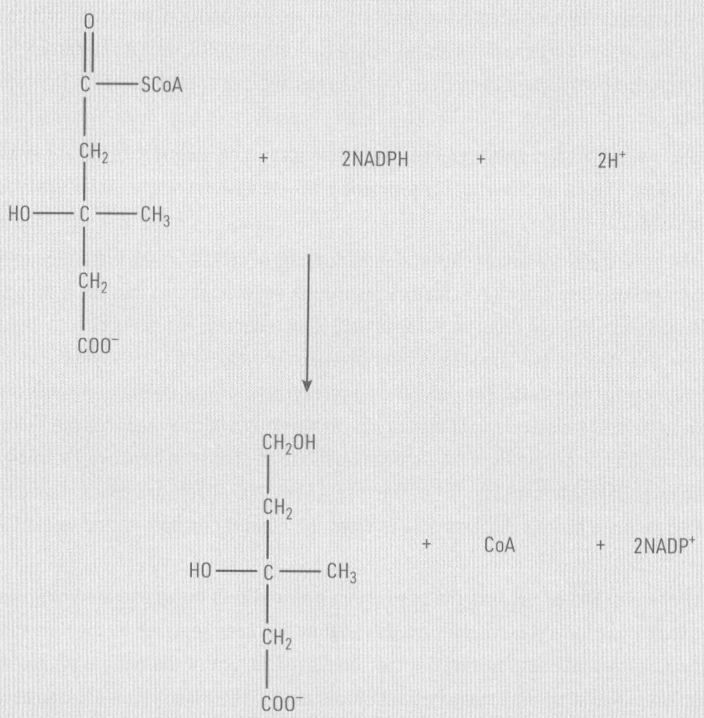

Figure CS6.2 Examples of fibrate drugs

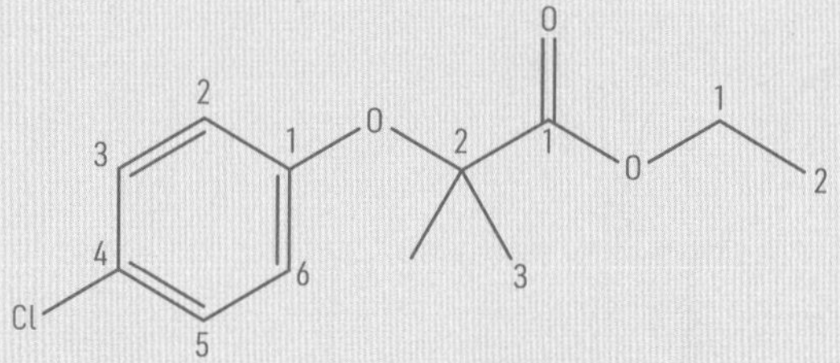

Clofibrate

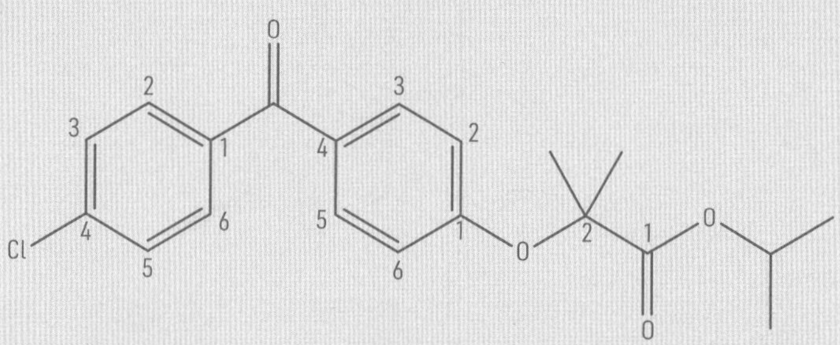

Fenofibrate

→

→

inhibiting incorporation of acetate, by increasing secretion of bile acids and, most significantly, by inhibiting HMG-CoA reductase. In the 1970s, Japanese workers isolated natural products which were more powerful inhibitors of HMG-CoA reductase and the first product, compactin (mevastatin), was isolated from a fermentation broth of *Penicillium citinium*. However, it was too toxic in animal studies to be used clinically. In 1978, workers at Merck Research Laboratories isolated a novel product from *Aspergillus terreus* which was named lovastatin (Figure CS6.3), which finally gained FDA approval in 1987.

Since lovastatin was isolated, six more statins have been introduced—two semi-synthetic ones (simvastatin and pravastatin) (Figure CS6.4), and four totally synthetic ones (fluvastatin, atorvastatin, rosuvastatin, and pitavastatin), (Figure CS6.5).

Simvastatin and pravastatin are simply chemical modifications of lovastatin and are structurally similar. They are known as type 1 statins. Simvastatin is actually a prodrug as the lactone ring must be hydrolysed to the hydroxyl acid to be inhibitory to HMG-CoA reductase. These HMG-CoA reductase inhibitors directly block the active site of the enzyme which is the rate-limiting step in the conversion of HMG-CoA to mevalonic acid which is part of the biosynthetic pathway of cholesterol. The open-chain hydroxyl acid form of the statins mimics the normal substrate of the enzyme and blocks the active site of the enzyme. Pravastatin, which already has the hydroxyl acid sidechain, was developed for this reason. Firstly, if the lactone ring has to be opened to be active, then why not give the open-chain form anyway? Secondly, simvastatin has significant CNS side-effects and it was argued that the open-chain molecule would be more hydrophilic, less able to cross the blood-brain barrier, and would have less CNS side-effects.

The totally synthetic stains all possess the open-chain hydroxyl acid group and are known as type 2 statins. In all these molecules, the butyryl group of the type 1 statins has been replaced by the fluorophenyl group. These synthetic structures are attempts to simplify the complex structure of the natural product lovastatin (do you consider them simplified structures compared with lovastatin?). The essential differences between them are the

Figure CS6.3 Structure of lovastatin

Lovastatin

Figure CS6.4 Simvastatin and pravastatin

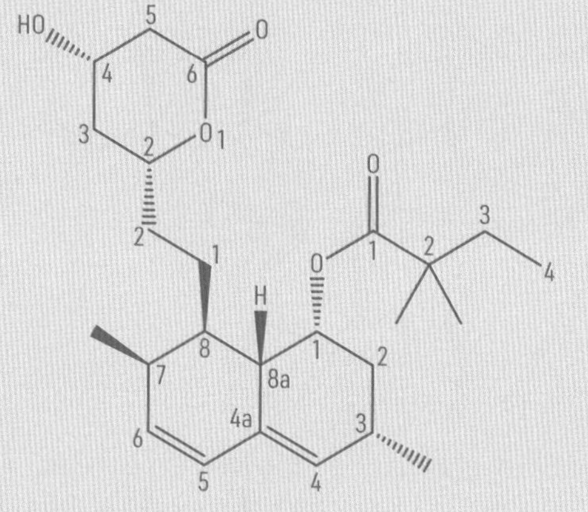

Simvastatin

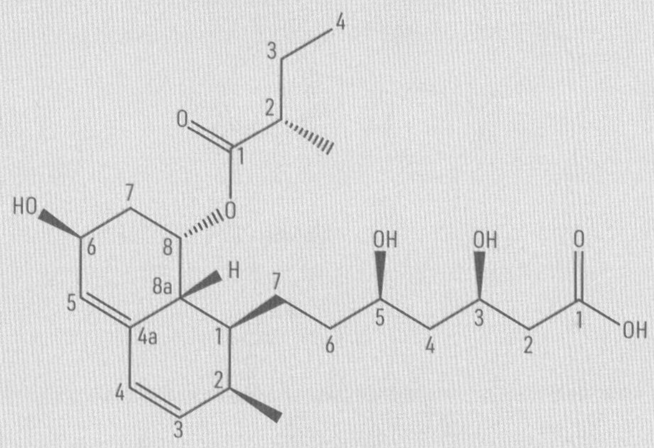

Pravastatin

Figure CS6.5 Type 2 statins

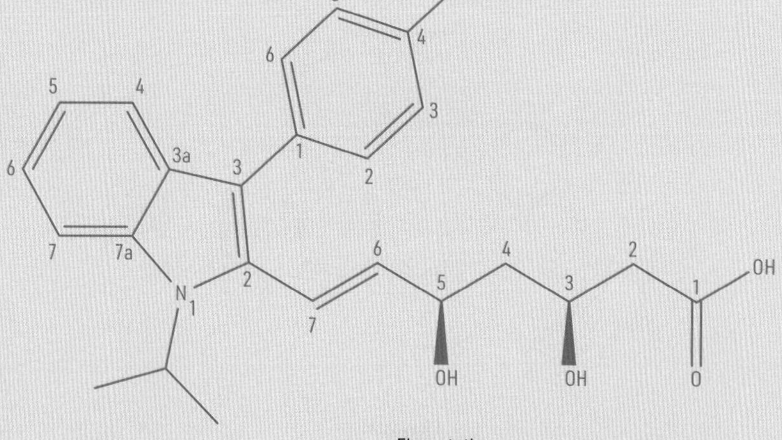

Fluvastatin

→

Figure CS6.5 (*Cont.*)

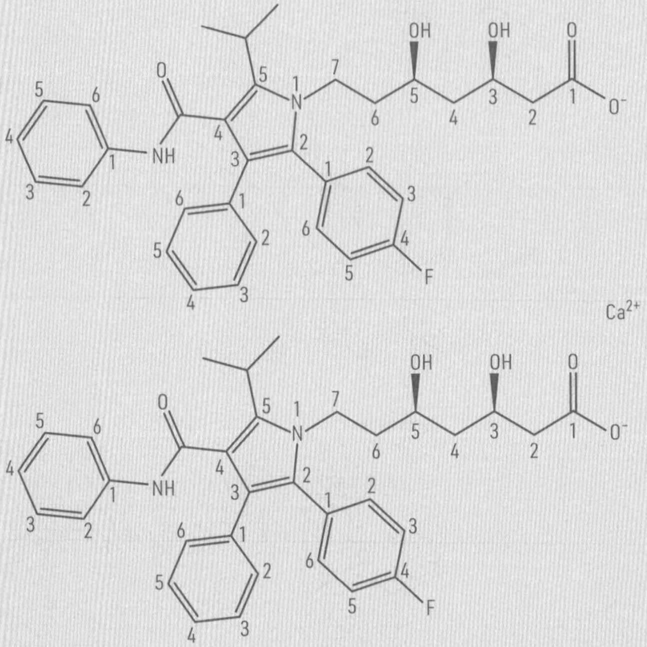

Ca²⁺

Atorvastatin

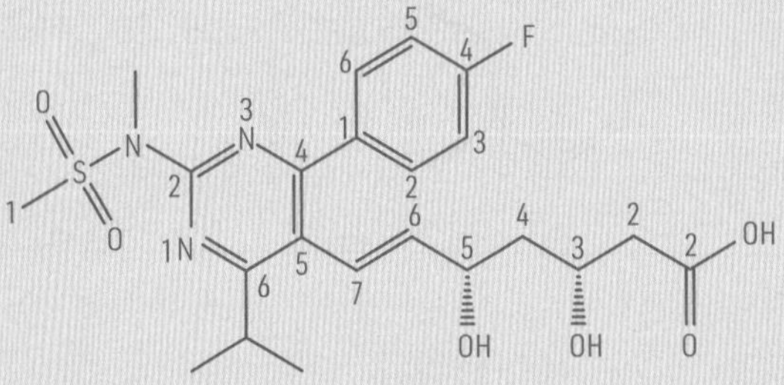

Rosuvastatin

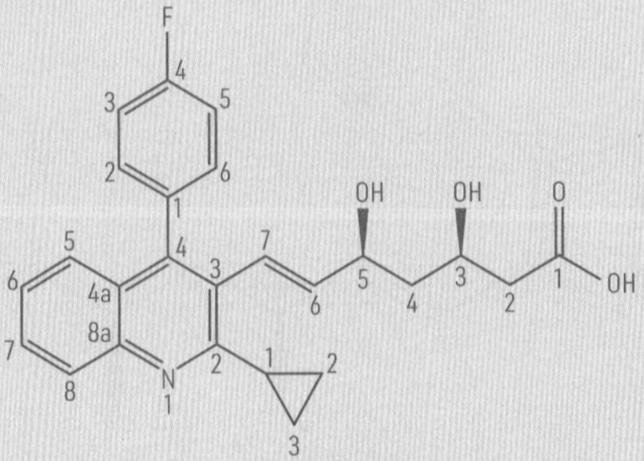

Pitavastatin

nature of the central ring system, being indole in fluvastatin, pyrrole in atorvastatin, pyrimidine in rosuvastatin, and quinolone in pitavastatin. Can you identify all the functionalities?

Today an estimated 30 million patients worldwide take statins and worldwide sales are estimated at 19 billion dollars—an eminently successful drug development.

Suggested reading

K.J. Lyons, and M. Harbinson (2009) Statins: In the beginning, *Journal of the Royal College of Physicians Edinburgh*. 39: 362–64.

    A detailed account of the development of statins.

T.P. Stossel (2008) The discovery of statins, *Cell* 134: 903–05.

    An account which concentrates on the scientists involved in the development of statins.

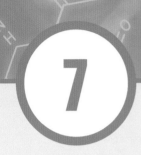

Drug Synthesis

In the infancy of drug development all the drugs utilized were of natural origin. The biological effects of these natural products often had been known for some considerable time, in some cases for thousands of years. As the science of medicinal chemistry began to develop it was recognized that semi-synthetic or totally synthetic molecules could potentially provide improved therapeutic outcomes—increased potency and/or reduced toxicity. Thus the use of organic synthesis in drug development began largely by the production of analogues of existing natural products, in order to improve their therapeutic effect (⯈ **XR Section 6.2**). However, because of the structural complexity of many natural products and their semi-synthetic analogues, medicinal chemists soon began to produce completely synthetic analogues which generally possessed simple structural characteristics. The identification of drug targets (⯈ **XR Part 1**) also promoted the synthesis of organic molecules specifically designed to interact with these targets.

Drug synthesis, therefore, has become an integral component, not only of drug development, but also of drug design. Numerous approaches to drug synthesis are used by the pharmaceutical industry. Organic synthesis can be used to produce a range of structurally diverse molecules in the search for new lead compounds (⯈ **XR Section 6.2**) or for the optimization of an existing lead compound (⯈ **XR Section 6.2**). There are a number of synthetic strategies which can be used such as **retrosynthesis** (⯈ **XR Section 7.2.1**), combinatorial synthesis (⯈ **XR Chapter 10**), partial synthesis (⯈ **XR Section 7.6**) and, more recently, the use of biotechnology for drug production, particularly of proteins (⯈ **XR Section 7.7**). In many cases, drugs are required to possess chiral centres in order to be therapeutically active and so the processes of chiral synthesis are important (⯈ **XR Section 7.5**).

7.1 GENERAL CONSIDERATIONS FOR DRUG SYNTHESIS

Key to any synthetic method is the nature of the starting materials. Wherever possible, a balance must be achieved between the availability and cost of starting materials and the relative probability of them giving rise to the required final product. In addition to the starting materials, the nature of the chemical reactions involved in the synthetic pathway need to be taken into consideration. The reaction yield, at each stage in the pathway, should be as high as possible, particularly if the pathway has numerous steps. As many potential drug molecules are required to be **chiral**, it is important that, wherever possible, reactions which yield a stereospecific product are utilized and chiral synthesis is often a vital component of drug synthesis (❯ **XR Section 7.5**).

From a production point of view, the intermediates and the final product need to be easy to isolate and purify. It is also important, in the initial research synthesis that, wherever possible, reactions and reagents are utilized which are compatible with the large-scale manufacturing process which may be required for a successful drug candidate.

 There are numerous factors which need to be considered in the design of the synthesis of a new drug: availability and cost of starting materials, reaction yield at each step in the synthesis, chirality of products, isolation and purification of intermediates, and ease of scale-up for manufacturing.

7.2 DESIGN OF DRUG SYNTHETIC PATHWAYS

The synthesis of potential drug molecules, like any organic synthesis, can be a linear synthesis (Figure 7.1) or a convergent synthesis (Figure 7.2). A linear synthesis is one in which the product of each reaction in the pathway is used in the subsequent step. A convergent synthesis involves the formation of individual sections of the target molecule being produced separately and then combined to yield the final product. Because each potential drug molecule will have a different structure, there needs to be a process to devise a synthetic route appropriate to that structure. The design process that is most commonly used in synthetic design is retrosynthetic analysis, also known as the disconnection method.

 Drug synthesis may be a linear or a convergent process.

Figure 7.1 Linear synthesis

$$A \longrightarrow B \longrightarrow C \longrightarrow D \longrightarrow E \longrightarrow F \longrightarrow G \longrightarrow \text{Target}$$

Figure 7.2 Convergent synthesis

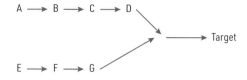

7.2.1 Retrosynthetic analysis

In order to ensure that the best synthetic route to a target molecule is chosen from the enormous number of potential synthetic routes, the process of retrosynthesis is used. This involves working backwards (on paper) from the target molecule until cheap, commercially available starting materials are reached.

Table 7.1 Examples of synthons

Type of synthon	Examples
C_2 unit	Ethyne
C_2O unit	Ethylene oxide
Carbocation	Alkyl halide, alcohols, amides
Carbanion	Grignard reagent, enolate

The process involves starting with the structure of the target molecule and theoretically breaking the structure into smaller sections which are called **synthons** (Table 7.1). Each of these synthons can be theoretically related to a real molecule known as a reagent, having a structural similarity to the synthon. As a number of potential disconnection steps may be possible, the ones which are ultimately chosen are the ones which provide the most likely possibility for a reconnection reaction. This retrosynthetic process is continued until cheap available starting materials are reached.

Disconnection can be achieved by disconnecting functional groups or carbon-carbon bonds. It is usually more appropriate to disconnect functional groups because the reaction to reconnect functional groups is usually easier than to reform a carbon skeleton. Examples of disconnections along with their reagents and reconnection reactions are shown in Figure 7.3.

The retrosynthetic or disconnection approach to the synthesis of target molecules requires a great deal of careful planning. When deciding on a suitable disconnection approach it is important to consider the order of the disconnection processes as each disconnection will influence subsequent disconnections. It may also be necessary to take into account the stereochemistry of reconnection reactions to ensure the required chiral centre(s) in the target molecule. It may also be necessary to include a protecting group (**> XR Section 7.4**) to ensure the reaction of one particular functional group in the presence of, potentially, several reactive centres. While the use of retrosynthesis will, of necessity, be different for each target molecule, some guidelines have been developed to assist in the process.

 Retrosynthesis involves theoretically disconnecting the molecular structure of the target molecule into smaller sections known as synthons, which eventually can be related to real molecules, which can act as reagents for the synthesis.

7.2.2 Convergent synthesis

The retrosynthetic approach to drug target synthesis can lead to a suggested linear pathway or a convergent pathway. One potential difficulty with a linear synthesis may arise if this produces a multi-step process. Even if the yield of product at each individual stage is good, the overall yield of the final product is likely to be much reduced. For example a 10 step linear synthesis with 90 per cent yield at each step produces a final product yield of only about 33 per cent (and a 90 per cent yield is unlikely at all stages). In order to reduce the number of steps in a synthetic process, convergent synthesis can be used. The more convergent pathways that are used the higher the overall product yield will be, compared to a linear synthesis (Figure 7.4).

 The use of convergent synthesis, as opposed to linear synthesis, can often improve the overall yield of the final product.

Figure 7.3 Examples of disconnections, reagents, and reconnection reactions

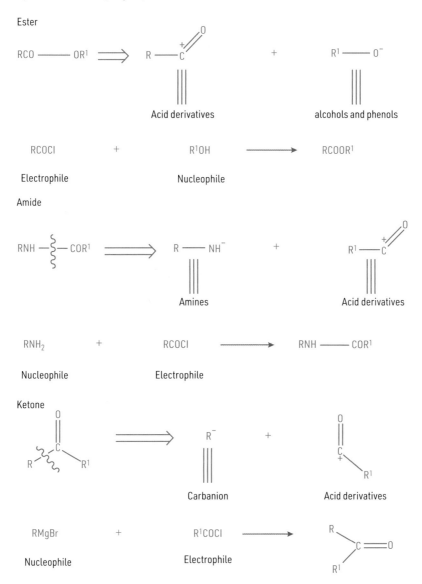

Ester
RCO — OR1
R — C
O
R1 — O−
Acid derivatives
alcohols and phenols
RCOCl
R1OH
RCOOR1
Electrophile
Nucleophile
Amide
RNH — COR1
R — NH−
R1 — C
O
Amines
Acid derivatives
RNH2
RCOCl
RNH — COR1
Nucleophile
Electrophile
Ketone
O
C
R
R1
R−
Carbanion
Acid derivatives
RMgBr
R1COCl
C = O
Nucleophile
Electrophile

Figure 7.4 Percentage yield of convergent vs linear synthesis

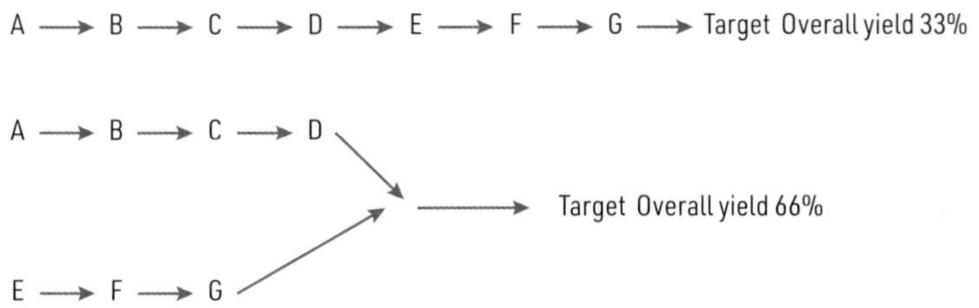

A → B → C → D → E → F → G → Target Overall yield 33%
A → B → C → D
E → F → G
Target Overall yield 66%

7.3 DIVERSITY-ORIENTED SYNTHESIS

A vital part of drug design is the optimization of the structure of a lead compound and this process involves the production of as wide a range of analogues as possible. It makes sense, therefore, to design a synthetic process that allows the production of such a range of analogues. This is diversity-oriented synthesis. Strategies that can be employed are modification of functional groups and/or side chains or the introduction of new substituents (Figure 7.5). The design of the synthetic process should, if possible, allow for such structural changes without any significant changes to the overall synthetic process.

Figure 7.5 Examples of diversity-oriented synthesis

6-aminopenicillanic acid

Amoxicillin

6-aminopenicillanic acid

Meticillin

6-aminopenicillanic acid

Oxacillin

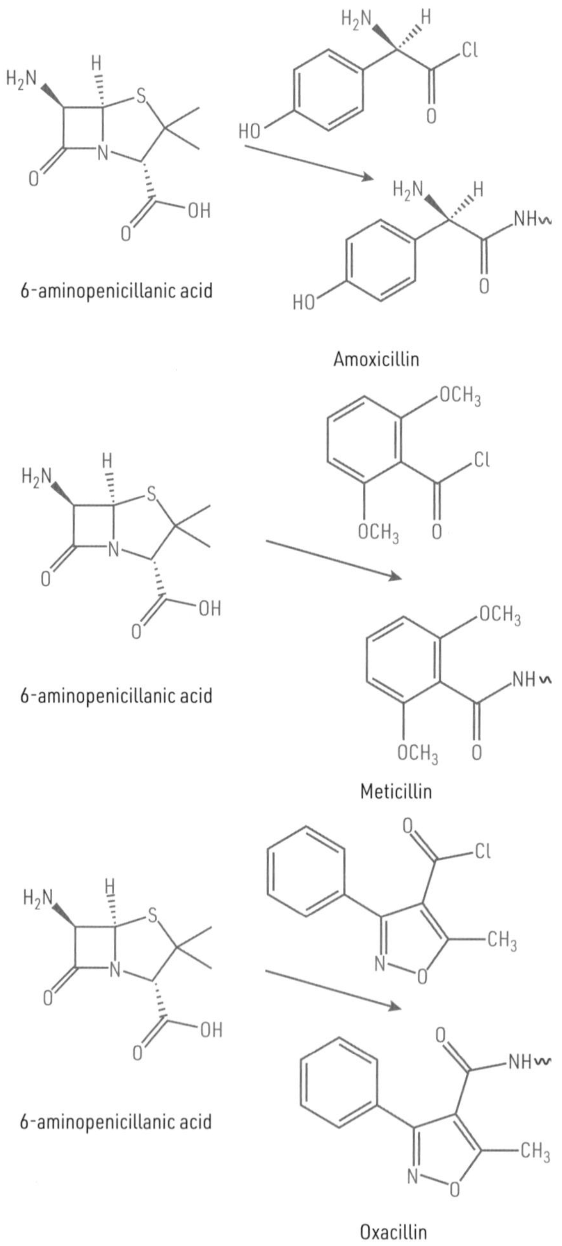

The ability to produce a wide range of structural analogues by variation of the lead compound is a common desirable feature of drug synthesis.

7.4 PROTECTING GROUPS

Most synthetic pathways require, at some stage, the reaction of one particular point of a molecule (usually a functional group), whilst avoiding reaction at another point in the molecule. Usually this will involve the use of a protecting group. A protecting group is attached to the molecule where reaction is undesirable, preventing reaction when the primary reaction site is acted upon. The nature of a protecting group should be such that reaction at the relevant point of the structure is easy, produces a stable structure that does not react under the primary reaction conditions and can be easily removed after the primary reaction is complete. Examples of protecting groups can be seen in Table 7.3.

 The use of protecting groups is often utilized within drug synthesis to ensure that reaction takes place only where it is required.

Table 7.2 Examples of protecting groups

Functional group to be protected	Protecting group	Method of removal
Alcohol	Trityl (triphenylmethyl) ether	Acid treatment
	Trifluoroacetate	Aqueous base treatment
Amine	Ethanamide	Hydrolysis
	Benzylchloromethanoate	Hydrogenolysis
Carboxylic acid	t-Butyl ester	Acid hydrolysis
	Trichloroethyl ester	Zn elimination
Phenol	Benzyl ether	Catalytic hydrogenation

Table 7.3 Examples of differences in activity between enantiomers

Enantiomeric drug	Enantiomer	Pharmacological activity
Promethazine	S	Antihistamine
	R	Antihistamine
Verapamil	S	Potent Ca channel blocker
	R	Weak Ca channel blocker
Propranolol	S	β-blocker
	R	Inactive
Oxazepam	S	Anxiolytic
	R	Inactive
Ketamine	S	Hypnotic/analgesic
	R	Psychotic

7.5 CHIRAL SYNTHESIS

Possession of the correct three-dimensional shape of a drug molecule is now universally recognized as vital for interaction at a target receptor. The chirality of a potential drug molecule must, therefore, be carefully controlled during the synthetic process. Often synthetic pathways will lead to the production of **stereoisomers**, only one of which possesses the appropriate therapeutic activity (see Table 7.3). In instances where the target molecule possesses one or more chiral centre(s), obtaining a single isomer entails the use of a non-stereospecific reaction followed by resolution (separation) of the isomer, or the use of a stereospecific reaction which produces (mainly) only one isomer.

 It is often important to ensure the correct chirality of the final product of a drug synthesis.

If a reaction produces a mixture of **diastereoisomers**, which have different physical properties, the individual isomers can be separated by methods such as chromatography or **fractional crystallization**. If a reaction produces a **racemic mixture**, where the isomers have identical physical properties, more complex methods have to be employed to separate the individual isomers (resolution). This usually involves the reaction of the racemic mixture with a **resolving agent** (an enantiomerically pure compound) to form diastereoisomers which can then be separated. The individual isomers are then regenerated (see Figure 7.6). Of course, such processes essentially reduce the yield of this particular synthetic

Figure 7.6 Resolution of enantiomers via formation of diastereoisomers

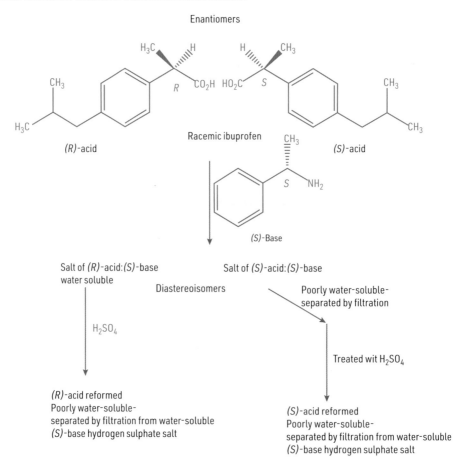

step to 50 per cent at best and, usually, significantly less than this value. It makes sense, therefore, to utilize, if possible, a stereospecific reaction which gives rise, mainly, to the single desired isomer (see Figure 7.7). There are a number of strategies by which stereospecific reactions can be achieved: use of enzymes as catalysts, use of non-enzyme catalysts, use of chiral starting materials, and use of **chiral auxilliaries** (Figure 7.8).

 The correct chirality of the final product of drug synthesis may be achieved by the use of separation techniques or the use of stereospecific reactions.

Figure 7.7 Example of use of stereospecific reactions to produce a single isomer

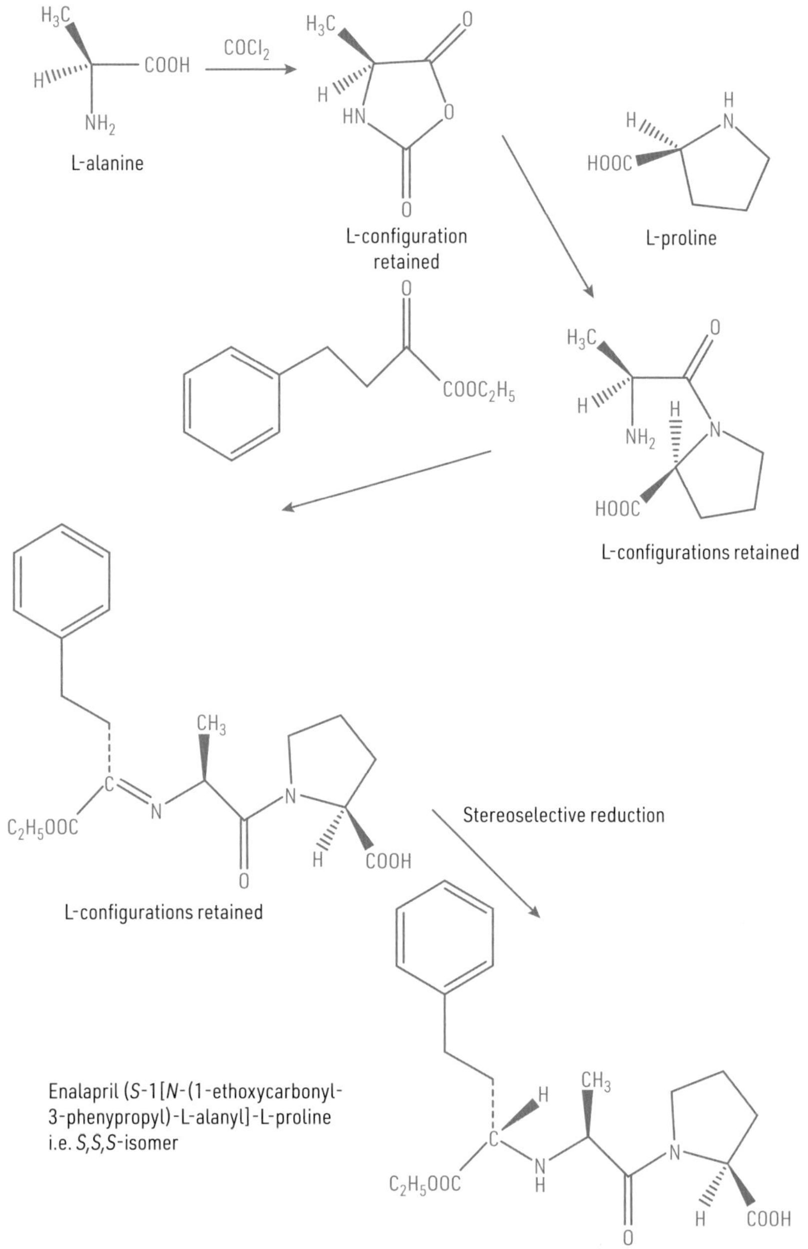

L-alanine

L-configuration retained

L-proline

L-configurations retained

L-configurations retained

Stereoselective reduction

Enalapril (S-1[N-(1-ethoxycarbonyl-3-phenypropyl)-L-alanyl]-L-proline i.e. S,S,S-isomer

Figure 7.8 Example of use of chiral auxiliary

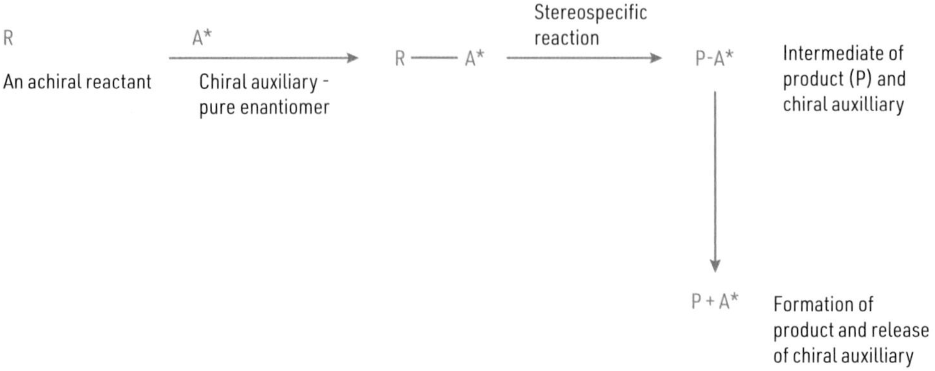

| R | A* | Stereospecific reaction | | |
| An achiral reactant | Chiral auxiliary – pure enantiomer | R — A* → P-A* | | Intermediate of product (P) and chiral auxilliary |

P + A*   Formation of product and release of chiral auxilliary

7.6 PARTIAL SYNTHESIS OF XENOBIOTICS (SEMI-SYNTHETIC DRUGS)

Many drugs and potential drugs have been isolated from natural sources. Such compounds, however, are present in relatively small quantities which do not make their extraction a viable economic process (see Box 5.1). Additionally, natural products are often limited by their toxicity. Consequently, organic synthesis is used to produce reasonable quantities of the drug or, more commonly, to chemically alter the structure of the natural product to produce analogues with improved therapeutic activity and/or re- duced toxicity. This process is known as semi-synthesis. Often, the total synthesis of a natural product is not feasible, the structure being too complex or containing too many chiral centres (Figure 7.9). In these instances, biochemical methods are used to produce molecules possessing the required basic molecular structure, which can then be converted into the target molecule and appropriate analogues (Figure 7.5 and Box 7.1 Semi-synthetic penicillins for example).

 Organic synthesis is often used to produce analogues of natural products in attempts to improve the therapeutic activity or reduce the toxicity of the original natural material.

Figure 7.9 Example of complex structure where total synthesis is not feasible

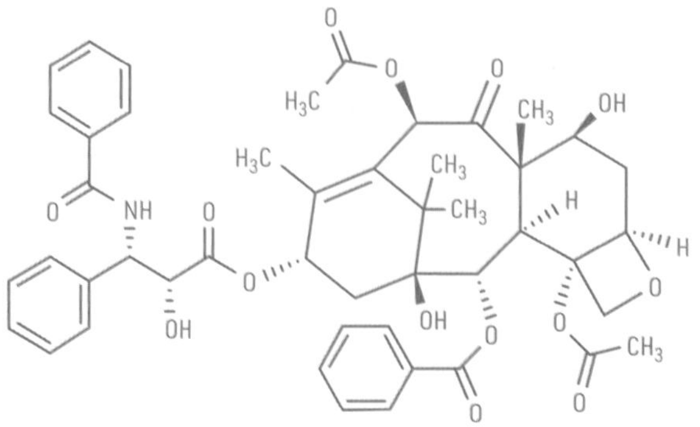

SEMI-SYNTHETIC PENICILLINS

The presence of the four-membered ring and the numerous chiral centres in the structure of the penicillin antibiotics makes their laboratory synthesis extremely difficult. Although benzylpenicillin (penicillin G) (see Figure 7.10) was isolated from natural sources in 1940, it was not until 1957 that a laboratory synthesis of a penicillin derivative (phenoxymethylpenicillin (penicillin V)—see Figure 7.5) was achieved by an American chemist, John Sheehan. Unfortunately, this brilliant organic synthetic method is not an economical way of producing penicillin derivatives. When the isolation of 6-aminopenicillanic acid (6-APA) from *Penicillium* fungi was reported this allowed the semi-synthesis of a large number of penicillin derivatives (see Figure 7.5). The free amine function of 6-APA is a good nucleophile, and can be used to prepare a wide range of the necessary amide derivatives, leading to the large number and variety of semi-synthetic penicillins currently on the market.

Figure 7.10 Benzylpenicillin (penicillin G)

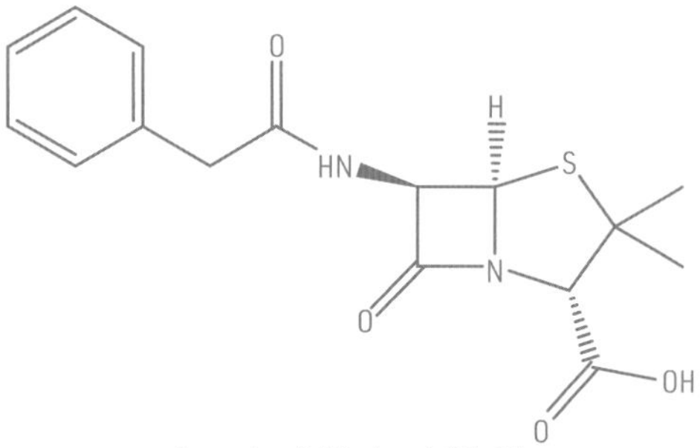

benzylpenicillin (penicillin G)

7.7 GENETICALLY ENGINEERED SYNTHESIS

Advances in molecular biology (**> XR Chapter 11**) have led to the use of genetically modified organisms for the production of, in particular, protein drugs. Genetic engineering allows the cloning of specific genes and the incorporation of these genes into the DNA of rapidly-growing organisms such as bacteria and yeasts. Such genetic engineering can lead to the synthesis of relatively large quantities of proteins and other potential drugs. Such processes are already used for the production of biopharmaceuticals such as insulin (Box 7.2 Genetically engineered insulin), human growth hormones and **monoclonal antibodies**.

GENETICALLY-ENGINEERED INSULIN

Insulin is a protein that most humans and other mammals produce successfully in the pancreas. Individuals with type 1 diabetes cannot synthesize sufficient insulin and are required to take replacement therapy. For many years, patients were treated with pig insulin, which differs from human insulin by only one amino acid (in fifty-one amino acids). Some people can develop an allergic reaction to pig insulin because it is not identical to human insulin and is recognized as foreign by the immune system. Insulin is now produced by inserting the human gene for insulin into bacterial cells using genetic engineering. The bacteria are then able to produce human insulin cheaply, and in a state that can be more easily purified than insulin from mammalian sources. This reduces the risk of contamination by viruses and other, disease-causing, proteins. The introduction of genetically-engineered insulin has allowed the manipulation of the human gene to produce insulin analogues such as insulin lispro (a fast-acting insulin) and insulin glargin (a long-acting insulin).

Advances in genetic engineering have allowed the more efficient production of so-called biopharmaceuticals.

? Questions

1. Devise a feasible retrosynthetic route, using readily available starting materials, for the local anaesthetic benzocaine.

2. Atorvastatin can be synthesized by either a linear synthesis or a convergent synthesis. Investigate and compare the relative yields of each type of synthesis.

3. What are considered to be the requirements for a good protecting group?

4. Represent, diagrammatically, the resolution of a pair of acidic enantiomers using the resolving agent phenylethylamine.

5. Identify a drug in common usage which has been produced by structural modification of the following natural products: morphine, cocaine, lovastatin, adrenaline, histamine.

↺ Chapter summary

- Availability and cost of starting materials, reaction yield, isolation, and purity of intermediates are all factors to be considered when devising a synthetic route to a drug candidate.

- The chirality of products and the ease of scale-up of reactions also need to be taken into consideration.

- Linear synthesis involves the product of each reaction being used in the subsequent reaction.

- Convergent synthesis involves the construction of separate sections of the target molecule which are joined together to form the final product.

- The overall reaction yield is usually better for a convergent synthesis than a linear synthesis.

- Retrosynthesis is the theoretical process of constructing a molecular structure from smaller sections known as synthons.

- Synthons are ultimately related to readily available reagents.

- Retrosynthesis is also known as the disconnection approach to synthetic design.

- A synthetic approach that allows the production of a wide range of structural analogues is a desirable feature for drug design.

- The use of protecting groups ensures that reactions take place at only the required point within the molecule.

- It is important, within drug synthesis, to ensure the appropriate chirality of the final product.

- Achieving the correct chirality of the final product can utilize a variety of techniques such as resolution of enantiomers or the use of stereospecific reactions.

- Synthetic methods are often used to improve the availability, the therapeutic activity and the toxicity profile of a molecule isolated from natural sources.

- Biotechnological methods are increasingly being used to produce new drug substances, particularly biopharmaceuticals.

Further reading

Patrick, G.L. (2015) *An Introduction to Drug Synthesis*. Oxford: Oxford University Press ISBN 9780198708438.

An extremely comprehensive treatment of the role of organic synthesis in drug design and development.

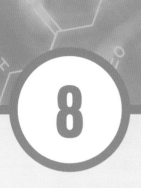

8

Optimization of Lead Compounds

Once a lead compound has been identified, from whatever source, the next step in the drug design and development process is the optimization of this lead compound. There are two main aspects to this optimization process, improvement in the interaction of the molecule with the appropriate drug target (pharmacodynamics) (▶ **XR Section 8.1**) and improvement in the ability of the molecule to be available to that target (pharmacokinetics) (▶ **XR Section 8.2**). These two processes are carried out simultaneously because it would be pointless identifying a molecule that is highly active at the target only to find that it cannot be absorbed or is very rapidly metabolized. It should also be mentioned that during this improvement process *in vitro* (and possibly *in vivo*) testing will continue on any molecules so produced in order to further inform the optimization process. Once this optimization process has given rise to a molecule which shows particular promise in pharmacological tests it will be necessary to investigate the conversion of the putative drug into a medicine suitable for administration to patients. This is known as formulation science and is dealt with in Part 4 of this volume.

8.1 OPTIMIZATION OF INTERACTION WITH THE DRUG TARGET

The purpose of this optimization is to try and ensure the most effective interaction of the potential drug molecule with the appropriate drug target. Hopefully achieving this will improve the pharmacological activity of the lead compound by improving the binding efficiency of the lead compound, by improving the selectivity for a particular target, and reducing the unwanted side effects. This process usually involves the development of structure-activity relationships which are designed to identify those parts of the structure of the lead compound that are important for its biological activity. This is known as the identification of the **pharmacophore** for that particular drug target.

Optimization of the lead compound is carried out to try and improve binding efficiency and selectivity at the desired receptor.

There are a number of strategies which can be used in the development of structure-activity relationships (SARs) and one or more of these may be used in the design of a new drug. Construction of a traditional structure-activity relationship involves the synthesis of a number of structural analogues of the lead compound in order to see what effect these structural variations have upon the biological activity. The choice of which analogues to synthesize is not random but is based upon a set of established criteria. These criteria have been developed over the years by observation of the general biological effects resulting from certain structural changes. These criteria are often referred to as rules but are, in fact, only guidelines (see Table 8.1).

The starting point for any SAR development is the identification, in the lead compound, of those functionalities which could be involved in interaction with the target receptor. The various types of drug-receptor interactions were detailed in Chapter 2 (**> XR Table 2.1** and **Figure 2.2**). Identification of the various groups present in the lead compound can be categorized in respect of the type of potential interaction with the target receptor.

Ionic bonds are likely to be formed if, at physiological pH, the lead compound possesses any charged atoms or groups. Quaternary ammonium salts are positively charged and could form ionic bonds with a receptor. Amines, including heterocyclic amines, are very likely to be protonated at physiological pH and, as such, could form ionic bonds with an anionic site of the receptor. Carboxylic acids, on the other hand, may form carboxylate anions at physiological pH and thus could form ionic bonds with a cationic site at the receptor.

Whereas the number of functionalities able to form ionic bonds are relatively few (although extremely important), there are significantly more that can interact the target receptor by hydrogen bonding. Alcohols, phenols, amines, amides, carboxylic acids, thiols, and some heterocyclic ring systems can potentially act as both hydrogen bond donors and acceptors. Carbonyl groups (such as ketones), esters and ethers are only able to act as hydrogen bond acceptors.

Interaction by hydrophobic bonding, including Van de Waals forces, can occur with aromatic rings, alkenes, alkyl groups and heterocyclic rings. Dipole-dipole interaction tends to occur mainly with carbonyl groups. Covalent bond formation tends to occur only with reactive alkyl halides. Because covalent bond formation between the ligand and the receptor causes permanent attachment, such groups are usually only present in alkylating agents, used mainly in cancer chemotherapy (**> XR see Section 4.3.3**).

Table 8.1 SAR guidelines

Structural variation	Anticipated outcome
Identification of pharmacophore	Identification of drug-receptor interactions
Isosteric replacement	Possible change in selectivity/toxicity/metabolism
Change size/shape of lead compound	Produce more rigid/flexible analogues
Introduction of alkyl substituents	Improve lipophilicity/selectivity/change metabolism
Introduction of halogen substituents	Increase lipophilicity
Introduction of hydroxyl groups	Increase hydrogen bonding capacity/hydrophilicity
Introduction of acidic or basic group	Improve subsequent formulation
Simplification of structure	Increase ease of synthesis
Rigidification of structure	Increase in affinity/selectivity
Investigation of stereochemistry	Provide information about chiral environment of receptor

It is important in lead optimization to identify the nature of the interactions at the receptor.

An important method used to determine the nature and importance of functional groups in the lead compound is the use of **isosterism**. This involves the introduction of substituents or groups which have similar physical and chemical properties and, therefore, would be expected to produce broadly similar biological effects. A significant change in potency is unlikely but there may be a significant change in selectivity, toxicity or metabolism. Classical isosteres have approximately the same size, shape and **electronic configuration** and are *like for like* replacements in terms of the number of atoms, valency, aromaticity or degree of unsaturation (Figure 8.1). Non-classical isosteres retain properties such as pKa and **electrostatic potential** (Figure 8.1). The term **bioisosteres** is used to include both classical and non-classical isosteres. It is important to remember that almost always more than one property will be affected by isosteric replacement. For example, the change from CH_2 to O to S affects size, shape, electronic distribution, water/lipid solubility, pKa, hydrogen bonding, and metabolism.

The nature of hydrogen bonding between lead compound and receptor can often be clarified by isosteric replacement. If a lead compound contains a secondary amide (CONH) group where the primary interaction is as a hydrogen bond acceptor, replacement by ester, ketone or a tertiary amide will retain potency. If the primary interaction is as a hydrogen bond donor, the same changes are likely to lead to reduced potency (Integration Box 8.1). It is also important to remember that a successful bioisosteric replacement is specific to a particular type of ligand-target interaction and is not guaranteed to have the same effect in a different type of ligand-target interaction (guidelines NOT rules!).

 The use of isosteric replacement is widely used in optimization of lead compounds.

Figure 8.1 Classical and non-classical isosteres

Classical isosteres - approximately the same size, shape and electronic configuration

Like for like replacement in terms of number of atoms, valency, aromaticity, degree of unsaturation

Non-classical isosteres - retain properties such as pKa, electrostatic potential

CONH COO COCH$_2$

CO SO

COOH SO$_2$NH

Cl CF$_3$

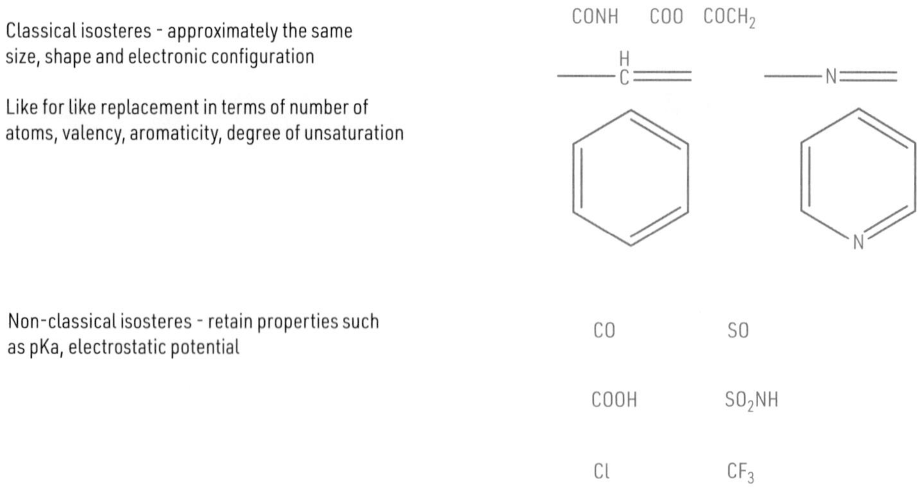

INTEGRATION BOX 8.1 **ISOSTERIC REPLACEMENT AS A SOURCE OF NEW DRUGS**

Hypoxanthine is a naturally occurring purine derivative sometimes found as a constituent of nucleic acids and exists in a tautomeric equilibrium with 6-hydroxypurine. Isosteric replacement of the 6-hydroxy group with a thiol group yields 6-mercaptopurine which is an immunosuppressant used mainly to treat acute leukaemia and Crohn's disease. It has a very short duration of action and so a prodrug, azathioprine, is used instead (❯ XR Integration Box 4.6).

Uracil is one of the pyrimidine nucleosides found in RNA. Replacement of the hydrogen in the 5 position by fluorine produced 5-fluorouracil (5-FU) which is active against several solid tumours. 5-FU inhibits thymidylate synthase and its co-factor N^5, N^{10}-methylenetetrahydrofolate. A key step in thymidine biosynthesis is the loss of the proton at position 5 of uracil. The 5-fluoro group of 5-FU cannot, however, be lost as it would require the formation of a positively charged fluorine ion and this cannot happen because fluorine is too electronegative. Consequently, 5-FU remains covalently attached to the enzyme active site, blocking the synthesis of thymidine and the synthesis of DNA (❯ XR Figure 4.15).

8.1.1 Changing the size and shape of the lead compound

This is a process in drug design which doesn't necessarily alter the functional groups of the lead compound but leads to a change in the overall size and/or shape of the lead compound. One method of changing the size and shape of a molecule is the introduction or removal of a ring system. In particular, the introduction of an aromatic ring system increases the size of the molecule in addition to increasing its rigidity. The π-system of an aromatic ring may increase the binding to the target site by increased hydrophobic interactions. Often this change will convert an agonist to an antagonist (Integration Box 8.2).

A change that is used less frequently is the introduction of a double bond. The effect of this change is more difficult to predict. It introduces an extra element of rigidity into the lead compound (❯ **XR Section 8.1.4**) and this may cause a change in potency and/or type of activity. Such a change can also cause potential problems. The introduction of a double bond can lead to the formation of Z and E (i.e. geometrical) isomers which often vary significantly in biological activity. Additionally, a carbon-carbon double bond is more susceptible to metabolism by oxidation (❯ **XR Section 12.4.1**)—this may or may not be desirable.

Introduction of additional methylene groups into a chain or ring increases the size of the lead compound and also increases its flexibility. This change will also increase the lipid solubility, which will allow a wider distribution across lipid membranes. However, addition of extra methylene units beyond a certain number will result in reduced distribution because of decreased water solubility.

 The size and shape of a lead compound can be changed in order to make the structure more rigid or more flexible depending on the groups added.

8.1.2 Substituent variation

It is an unfortunate fact that rarely does a lead compound possess ideal drug characteristics. The drug design process is usually concerned with production of analogues in order to change the potency, the duration of action, the metabolic profile and reduce toxic side effects. In each individual case the particular desired property will drive the choice of substituent variation. The variations will be chosen based upon guidelines established from previous usage, but there will inevitably be outcomes which do not fit the established patterns.

INTEGRATION BOX 8.2   **CONVERSION OF AN AGONIST TO AN ANTAGONIST**

In the search for drugs with β-blocking activity, i.e. antagonists at β-adrenergic receptors in the heart, isoprenaline was chosen as the lead compound. Although isoprenaline was an agonist rather than an antagonist, it was selective for β-adrenergic rather than α-adrenergic receptors. The next step in the drug design process was to replace one of the groups known to be necessary for agonist activity at adrenergic receptors. Replacement of the phenolic groups by chloro substituents produced dichloroisoprenaline. This molecule blocked the β-receptors, but still had some agonist activity, i.e. it was a partial agonist. A common structural change that converts agonists to antagonists is the addition of an aromatic ring. This provides an additional hydrophobic interaction at the receptor, which is not involved in agonist action. The first molecule of this nature to be produced was pronetholol, which was a much better antagonist but was still a partial agonist. This molecule did reach clinical trials but was subsequently withdrawn due to toxicity issues. Further molecular modification led to the production of propranolol, the first successful β-blocker to be introduced (➤ XR see Section 6.3). James Black was awarded the Nobel Prize for medicine in 1988 for this and his work on the H_2-antagonist cimetidine.

Figure 1 Isoprenaline was chosen as the lead compound

Isoprenaline

Dichloroisoprenaline

Pronethalol

Propranolol

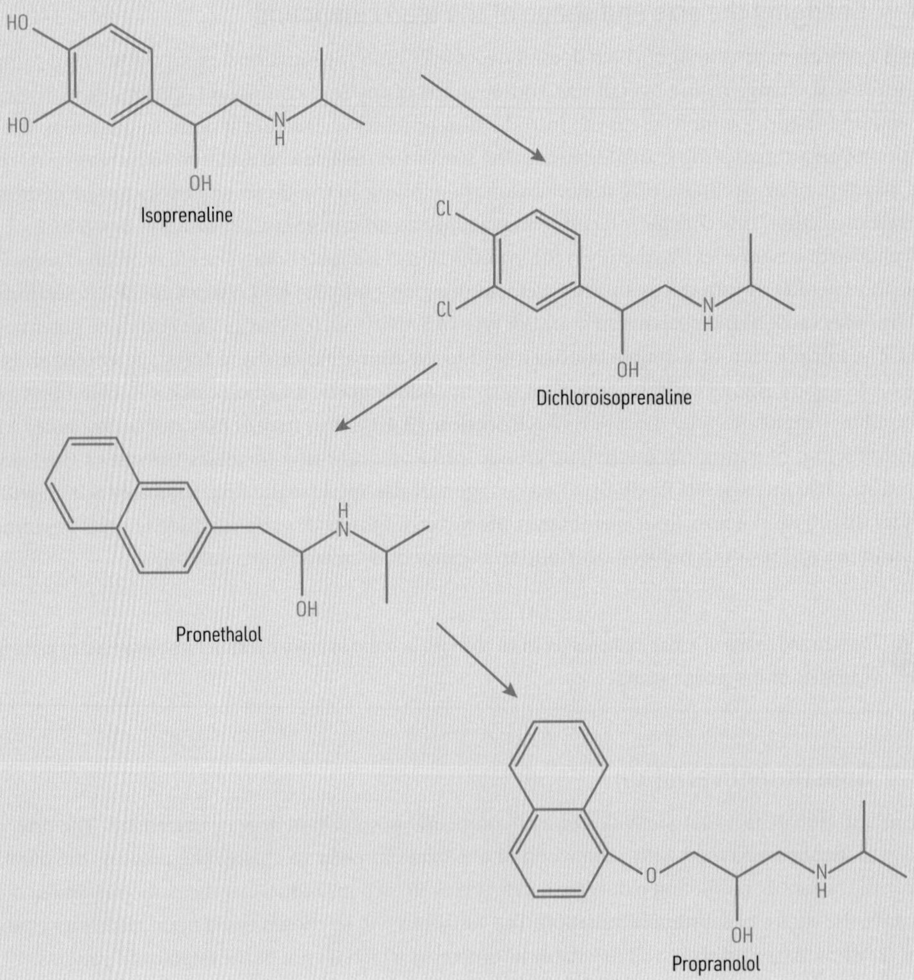

8.1.2.1 *Alkyl substituents*

The introduction of a new alkyl substituent will increase the lipophilicity of the lead compound which may improve the absorption and distribution profile of the molecule. However, introduction of a new alkyl group (particularly methyl) will very often increase the rate of metabolism of the molecule by oxidation or demethylation (▶ **XR Section 12.4.1**). Conversely the introduction of alkyl groups can be used to block the metabolism of a metabolically labile group such as an ester or amide (see Figure 8.10). If an alkyl group is already present in the lead compound, changing the size of that alkyl group may cause a change in selectivity. For example, when the N-methyl group of adrenaline, which acts as an agonist at both α and β adrenergic receptors, is converted to N-isopropyl (isoprenaline), this produces a selective β agonist (Figure 8.2).

 Alkyl substituents can be introduced into a lead compound to increase the lipophilicity and selectivity at the desired receptor. Alkyl groups will also affect metabolism of the lead compound.

8.1.2.2 *Halogen substituents*

Introduction of one or more halogen atoms into a lead compound will increase the lipophilicity of that molecule and this variation is usually carried out in order to improve transport properties in the body. However, care has to be exercised as polyhalogen molecules tend to accumulate in lipid tissues within the

Figure 8.2 Example of structural variation changing selectivity

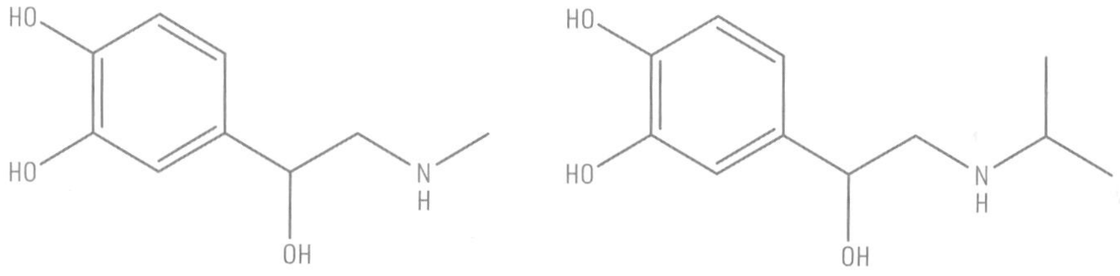

Adrenaline - an alpha and beta
adrenergic agonist

Isoprenaline - a selective beta agonist

Figure 8.3 Example of effect of introduction of an aromatic halogen atom

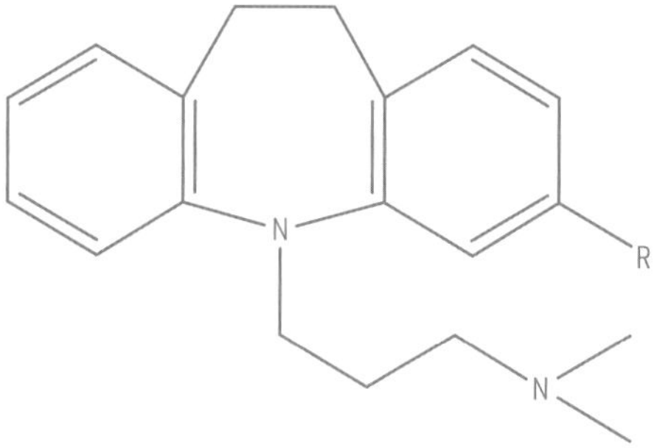

R = H Imipramine

R = Cl Clomipramine 50 times more active than
imipramine as an antidepressant

BOX 8.1   THE PROBLEM WITH DDT

Dichlorodiphenyltrichloroethane (DDT), when first introduced in 1939 as a highly effective insecticide, was regarded as a significant scientific breakthrough, particularly in the reduction of malaria by eradication of mosquito breeding areas. At that time, the advantage of DDT over other insecticides was its stability, thus it remains active for longer. Unfortunately, it was so stable that it began to accumulate in the food chain wherever it was heavily used. DDT is highly lipid soluble and accumulates in the lipid tissues of species at the top of the food chain (often humans) with serious toxic effects such as convulsions and respiratory paralysis. The use of DDT was subsequently banned worldwide, although some argue for its re-introduction for vector control in malaria is justified.

Figure 8.1.1 Dichlorodiphenyltrichloroethane (DDT)

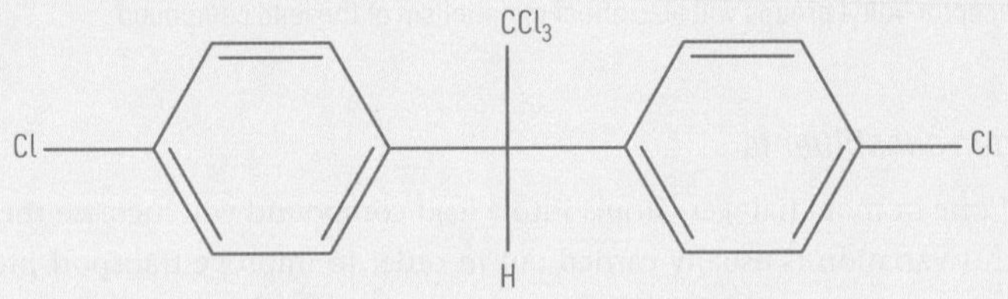

Dichlorodiphenyltrichloroethane - DDT

body (Box 8.1). Halogen atoms attached to aliphatic carbons are much more reactive than those attached to aromatic rings. Because of this, when halogen atoms are introduced as a substituent variation, they are usually attached to an aromatic ring (Figure 8.3). Aliphatic halogen atoms, because of their reactivity, are usually found in alkylating agents (➤ **XR Section 4.3.3**). One exception to this is the use of the trifluoromethyl group which is a similar size to a chlorine atom and increases the lipophilicity of a molecule without increasing its reactivity.

 Halogen substituents can be added, usually to aromatic rings, to increase the lipophilicity of a lead compound.

8.1.2.3 *Hydroxyl substituents*

The introduction of a hydroxyl group into a lead compound can potentially change the properties of that molecule significantly. It will introduce a potentially new hydrogen bonding interaction with the target—both as hydrogen bond donor and acceptor. It will also increase the hydrophilicity of the molecule, possibly aiding the **formulation** of the molecule. Because a hydroxyl group is easily oxidized (not tertiary alcohols) this can lead to increased metabolism.

 Introduction of hydroxyl groups will affect the capacity for hydrogen bonding and the hydrophilicity of the lead compound.

8.1.2.4 *Amine substituents*

Many drugs possess an amine group which will be protonated at physiological pH and often they are thought to be involved in ionic interaction with the target receptor site. The presence of an amine can also prove useful in formulation because of the ease of formation of a water-soluble salt. Amines are not the only basic group which can be used in this way and sometimes amidines, guanidines or a heterocyclic amine group is used (Figure 8.4).

8.1.2.5 *Acid substituents*

The introduction of an acidic group (carboxylic or sulphonic) will increase the water solubility of the lead compound and is sometimes used for improving formulation properties. However it has been found that the introduction of an acidic group often changes the type of biological activity exhibited by the molecule (Figure 8.5).

 The introduction of an amine or acidic group usually helps with formulation of the lead compound.

Figure 8.4 Examples of amine substituents

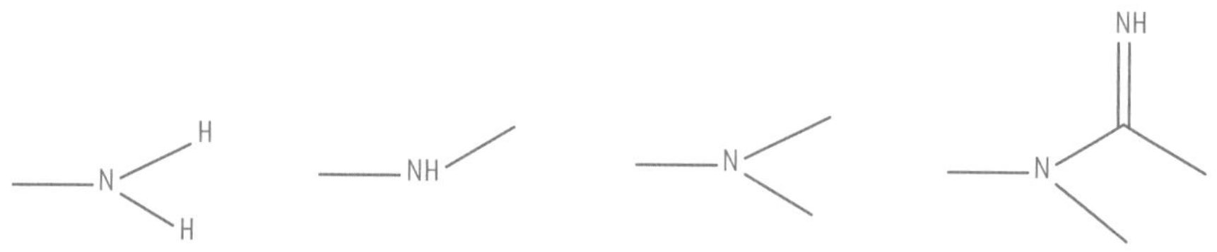

Primary amine   Secondary amine   Tertiary amine   Amidine

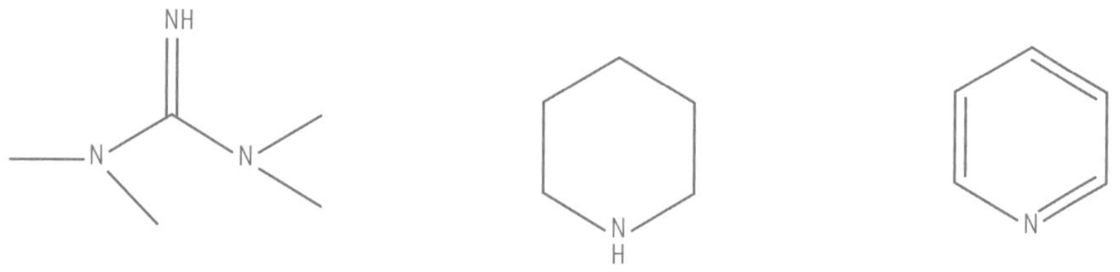

Guanidine   Aliphatic heterocyclic amine   Aromatic heterocyclic amine

Figure 8.5 Example of change of biological activity by insertion of carboxylic acid group

Phenol - antiseptic - toxic   Salicylic acid - anti-inflammatory - less toxic

8.1.2.6 *Aromatic substituents*

This variation in structure refers to changes in substitution of an aromatic ring which is already present in the lead compound. One approach often used is to vary the position of substituents on the aromatic ring. A change of position can have an important electronic effect on the aromatic ring, perhaps causing an increase or decrease in an electron-withdrawing effect and thus affecting binding to the target receptor. It should be noted that synthesis of such analogues is not always necessary, changes of this kind being conducive to the use of quantitative structure-activity relationship studies (QSAR) (**> XR Section 9.2**).

8.1.3 **Simplification of structure**

It is often the case that, when a lead compound is derived from a natural source, the molecular structure is quite complex. Such molecules are often difficult to extract and synthesize (**> XR Box 5.1**). In such cases, the strategy of simplification is used. The advantage of this strategy is that simpler molecules are

Figure 8.6 Examples of drugs produced by simplification of natural products

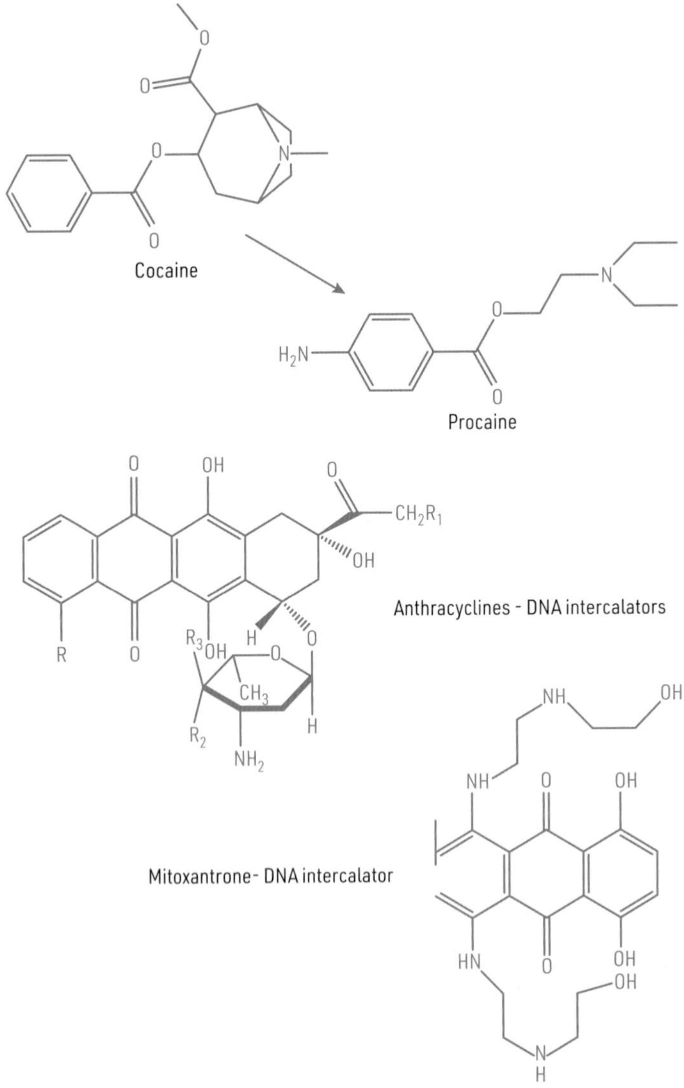

Cocaine

Procaine

Anthracyclines - DNA intercalators

Mitoxantrone - DNA intercalator

Tubocurarine - a neuromuscular blocker

Suxamethonium - a short-acting neuromuscular blocker

easier to synthesize. Usually the simplification process is carried out in a series of steps, gradually reducing the complexity of the lead compound, ensuring that the required biological activity is retained at each step. Figure 8.6 shows a number of drugs which have been developed by the simplification process (Figure 8.6). Care must be taken with the simplification process as simpler molecules will be more flexible, which may result in different binding to the target receptor, or binding to other receptors, leading to increased side effects.

 Simplification of the structure is often required when the lead compound is a complex natural product.

8.1.4 Rigidification of structure

A flexible molecule can, by virtue of rotation about carbon-carbon single bonds, adopt a number of different shapes (conformations). It is likely that only one of these will optimally fit the target receptor site. By making the lead compound more rigid it may be possible to fix the molecule in this optimal shape, potentially causing an increase in receptor selectivity. In flexible molecules key functionalities can interact with different receptors, leading to low selectivity. Fixing the spatial arrangement of these key functionalities increases the likelihood of interaction with only one receptor, leading to greater selectivity.

Rigidification may also result in greater affinity for the target receptor. When a flexible molecule binds to a receptor there is a restriction in its freedom of movement, causing a decrease in the entropy of the system—this is known as the adverse entropy effect. If a molecule is made more rigid (i.e. less initial free-dom of movement), when binding occurs there will be a lower adverse entropy effect, which is a more favourable thermodynamic situation, resulting in increased affinity for the target receptor.

In addition to possible increased selectivity and affinity, rigidification may also confer an improved stability to either chemical or metabolic degradation.

Rigidification can be achieved by the introduction of a group (usually methyl) which sterically hinders free rotation, one that allows the formation of an intramolecular hydrogen bond or by fixing of functionalities by cyclization. Restricted rotation can also be achieved by introduction of unsaturation (e.g. a carbon-carbon double bond) but this is used less frequently for reasons previously discussed (❯ XR Section 8.1.1).

Rigidification of the structure of a lead compound is usually carried out in order to increase the affinity and selectivity for the desired receptor.

8.1.5 Stereochemistry and drug design

Consideration of the stereochemistry of a lead compound and its analogues is something that is an important part of the drug design process. The existence of stereoisomerism in a lead compound and its analogues can potentially result in important differences between stereoisomers in terms of their types of biological activity, potency and side effects.

8.1.5.1 Geometrical isomerism

Geometrical isomerism (also referred to as Z/E isomerism) results from restricted rotation of groups at-tached to a double bond or cyclic system. Chemically speaking, geometrical isomers have always been regarded as different compounds because the isomers exhibit different physical and chemical properties. From the point of drug design it is almost always the case that one isomer will have the desired thera-peutic activity and the other isomer is an unwanted impurity with a reduced activity or even a different type of activity (Figure 8.7).

Figure 8.7 Different biological activities of geometrical isomers

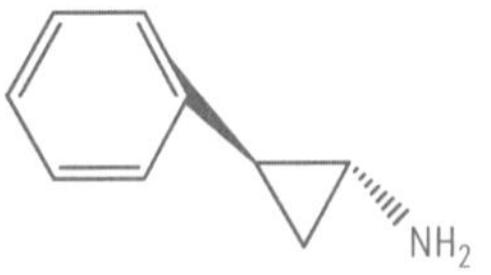

Tranylcypromine - only the trans isomer shown here is active as a monoamine oxidase inhibitor

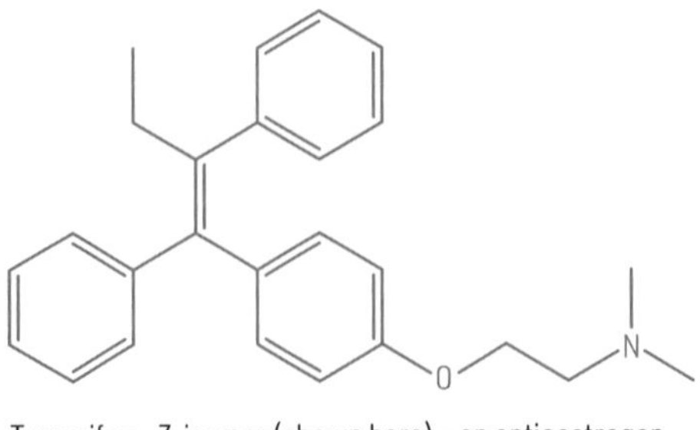

Tamoxifen - Z-isomer (shown here) - an antioestrogen
E-isomer - a weak oestrogen

Geometrical isomers often differ considerably in their biological activity.

8.1.5.2 *Optical isomerism*

Optical isomerism arises as a result of the presence of a chiral centre within a molecule. Optical isomers (**enantiomers**) have identical physical and chemical properties except when they are within a **chiral environment**. Because most receptors are protein in nature, and thus form a chiral environment, it is highly likely that optical isomers will exhibit different biological activities.

As optical isomers have identical solubilities, it would be expected that they have identical rates of absorption as this is usually by passive diffusion which relies solely on solubility profiles. Occasionally, differences will be observed when absorption involves active transport via a carrier system which will be a chiral environment. For example, the S-isomer of 3,4-dihydroxyphenylalanine (levodopa) is transported into the brain by the phenylalanine transporter protein whereas the R-isomer is not.

The distribution of a drug candidate around the body again, being based on solubility profile, ought not to exhibit any isomeric differences. However, binding to proteins (a chiral environment) within the plasma and also to certain tissues can lead to differences in circulating levels of free **enantiomeric** forms of the molecule. This situation may lead to different enantiomeric levels at the target receptor, resulting in apparent different pharmacodynamics for the two enantiomers. This differential protein binding may also result in different excretion rates as molecules bound to plasma protein cannot be removed by the kidney.

Enantiomeric differences would be expected in metabolism of drug molecules because xenobiotic-metabolizing enzymes are chiral environments. This situation is considered in detail in the later chapter on drug metabolism (❯ **XR Chapter 12**).

The interaction of a chiral drug candidate with a target receptor would be expected, in most cases, to exhibit enantiomeric differences. There are a number of possible consequences with respect to therapeutic activity which may arise due to the presence of one or more chiral centres in a drug candidate. Because of these potential consequences it is necessary, in drug design, to investigate fully the biological properties of both enantiomers (see Table 8.2). Indeed, drug regulatory authorities require a positive therapeutic benefit to be proven for the use of anything other than an individual enantiomer (❯ **XR Integration Box 6.6**).

Table 8.2 Variations in biological activity of isomers

Biological activity of enantiomers	Examples
Both isomers have activity of same type and potency	R and S isomers of chloroquine have equal antimalarial activity
	R and S isomers of promethazine have equal antihistamine activity
Both isomers have activity of same type but different potencies	S isomer of verapamil has 4 x the potency of the R isomer
One isomer is biologically active, the other isomer has no activity	S isomer of propranolol has β-blocking activity whereas the R isomer does not
	S isomer of methyldopa has antihypertensive activity whereas the R isomer does not
Both isomers are biologically active but have different types of activity	S isomer of ketamine has anaesthetic activity whereas the R isomer has psychotic activity
Both isomers have same type of activity but have different side effects	Both isomers of thalidomide have sedative activity, but S isomer is teratogenic whereas the R isomer is not

Many aspects of drug activity exhibit enantiomeric differences because they involve the drug being in a chiral environment.

8.2 OPTIMIZING ACCESS TO THE DRUG TARGET

As has been referred to in the previous section there are important aspects of drug design which do not relate directly to the interaction with a target receptor but are related to the ability of a potential drug to reach the target receptor. These aspects are often referred to as the absorption, distribution, metabolism, and excretion (ADME) profile of a drug candidate and are equally important to the drug design process. A drug candidate with an excellent activity at the target receptor is of no value if it cannot reach the target receptor.

8.2.1 Solubility properties

The solubility of a drug candidate is vital with respect to its absorption, distribution and excretion. If a molecule is too hydrophilic it will have difficulty being absorbed across the lipid cell membranes of the gastrointestinal tract. On the other hand, if a drug candidate is too lipophilic, it may be absorbed into the lipid cell membranes of the gastrointestinal tract but be unable to partition from there into the aqueous-based bloodstream for distribution around the body. Even if injected into the bloodstream, highly lipophilic drug molecules are likely to be taken up into lipid tissues, reducing the amount available to reach the target receptor. It is very important, therefore, to ensure the appropriate hydrophilic/lipophilic balance within a potential drug molecule (Integration Box 8.3).

It is unlikely that a lead compound will possess the ideal solubility properties, so a key part of the drug design process often requires changing functional groups to achieve the appropriate hydrophilic/lipophilic balance. One should always be aware, however, that modification of functional groups may affect the binding of the molecule to the target receptor. A molecule can be made more lipophilic by masking a polar group such as an alcohol, phenol or carboxylic acid by converting it to an ether or ester (Figure 8.8).An alternative approach is to add hydrophobic substituents such as alkyl groups (Figure 8.8).

If it is necessary to make a lead compound more hydrophilic (for example if it is too lipophilic to be easily distributed via the bloodstream) then polar groups such as hydroxyl, carboxyl or sulphonamide can be added (Figure 8.9). Care has to be taken that the hydrophilicity does not increase the excretion of the molecule so as to render it unusable.

INTEGRATION BOX 8.3   **LIPINSKI'S RULE OF FIVE**

Lipinski's rule of five has proved valuable in drug design. The rule was derived from examination of around 2,500 drug-like compounds with a view to identifying the structural features which determine an appropriate hydrophilic/lipophilic balance for oral activity. Features identified as being important in rendering a drug orally active were:

A molecular weight less than 500
A logP value of less than +5
No more than 5 hydrogen bond donor groups
No more than 10 hydrogen bond acceptor groups

It should be noted that there are not 5 rules, but that each of the numbers involves a multiple of 5, hence the name. It should also be noted that these are not strict rules but are useful guidelines. There are numerous exceptions to the rule (in particular, natural products used as drugs) but Lipinski himself said that this was to be expected.

Figure 8.8 Increasing lipophilicity

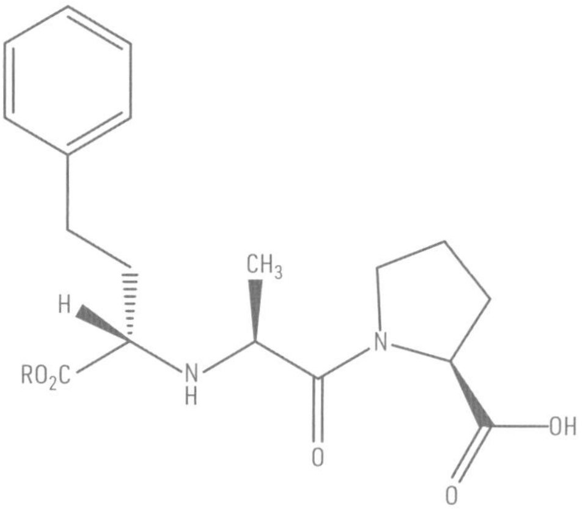

R = H Enalaprilat - not orally active as ACE inhibitor carboxylic acid too water-soluble to be absorbed
R = CH_2CH_3 Enalapril - orally active as ACE inhibitor prodrug- ester hydrolysed after absorption

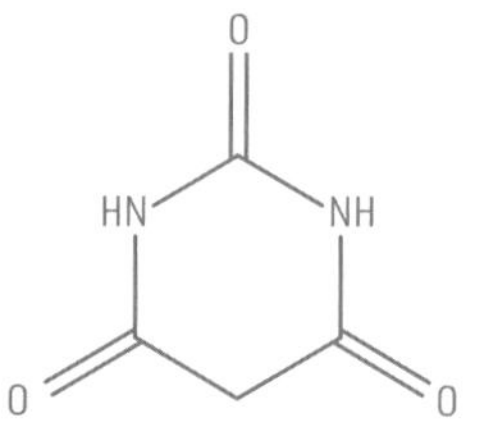

barbituric acid - no hypnotic activity
too water soluble

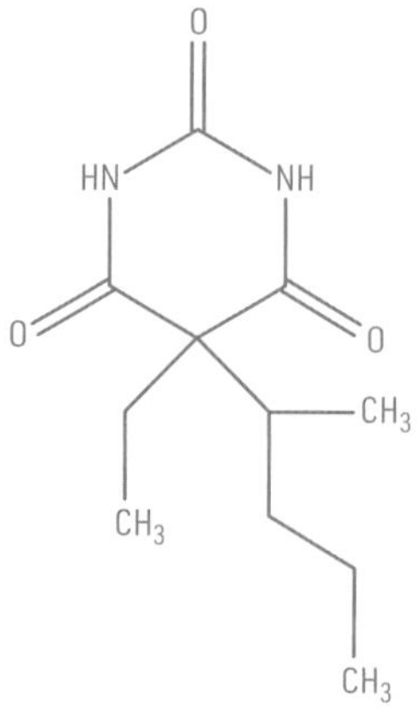

pentobarbital - hypnotic activity
more lipophilic due to added alkyl groups

It must not be forgotten that many drugs possess ionizable groups which will also influence solubility in the biological environment. Amines, being weak bases, have pKa values which result in a reasonable equilibrium between the ionized and non-ionized forms. The ionized form allows good solubility in the gastrointestinal tract and the blood and the non-ionized form readily crosses lipid cell membranes.

 It is important to ensure that a drug candidate has the appropriate hydrophilic/lipophilic balance in order to optimize absorption and distribution.

8.2.2 Increasing resistance to degradation

It may be the case that the presence of certain functional groups in a lead compound make it susceptible to chemical and/or enzymatic degradation. The most common functional groups which are susceptible in this way are those sensitive to hydrolysis (esters and amides), and oxidation (hydroxyls and thiols).

Figure 8.9 Increasing hydrophilicity

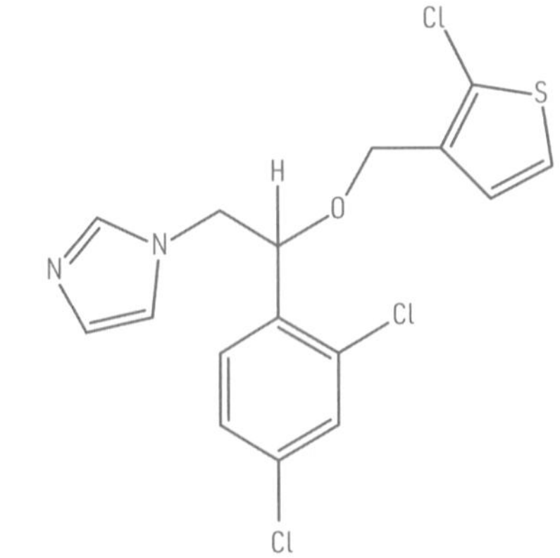

Tioconazole – only topical activity – poorly soluble in blood

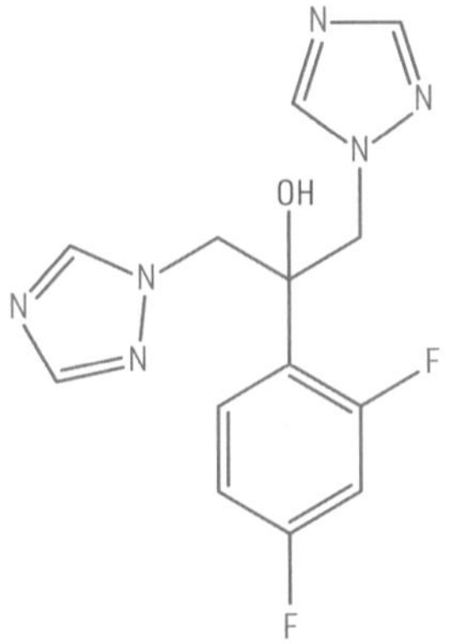

Fluconazole – orally active – improved water solubility

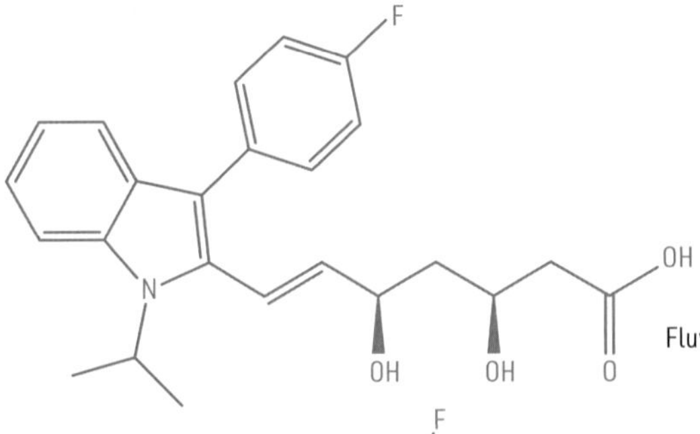

Fluvastatin – hydrophobic

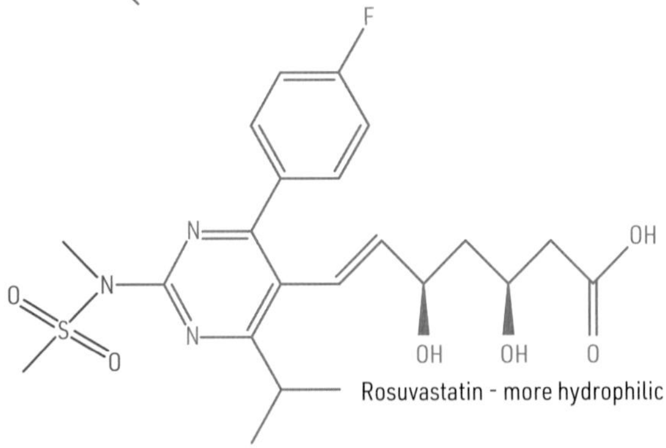

Rosuvastatin – more hydrophilic

Such groups can often be protected sterically by addition of groups which will hinder the approach of the attacking species, be it a nucleophile or an enzyme. Electronic effects can also be used by the involvement of bioisosteres (Figure 8.10) (❯ **XR Section 8.1**).

8.2.3 Increasing susceptibility to metabolism

It is not always desirable for a drug to have a prolonged duration of action and sometimes it is necessary to make changes which give rise to a more rapid metabolic inactivation of the drug candidate. Such situations can be addressed by introducing a functional group which is more susceptible to metabolic inactivation. Examples of such groups are hydroxyl or ester groups (Figure 8.11) (Integration Box 8.4). It is important that the groups that are introduced are rapidly metabolized by a predictable route and that the metabolites are pharmacologically inactive.

Figure 8.10 Increasing resistance to degradation

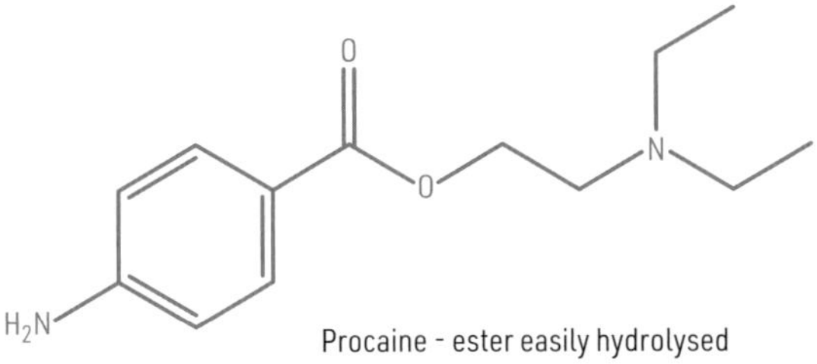

Procaine - ester easily hydrolysed

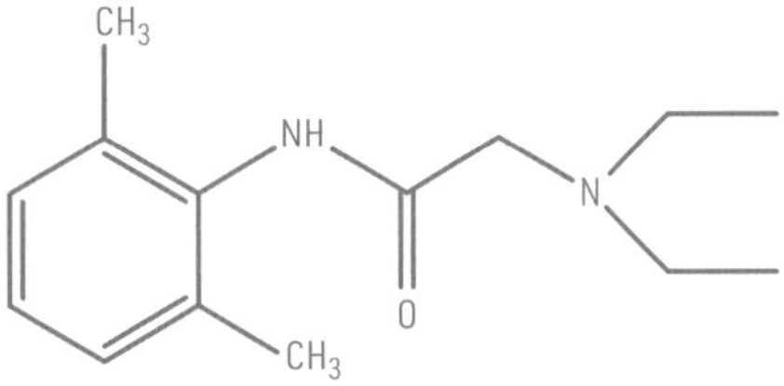

Lidocaine - amide less easily hydrolysed and
sterically protected by methyl groups

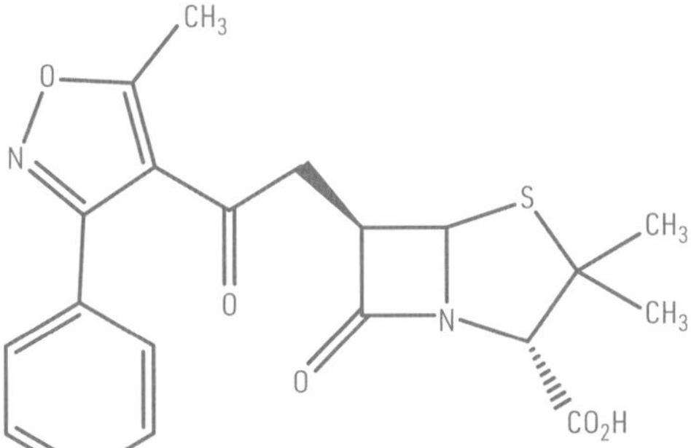

Oxacillin - isoxazoyl ring is bulky and electron-withdrawing
protects from beta-lactamase degradation

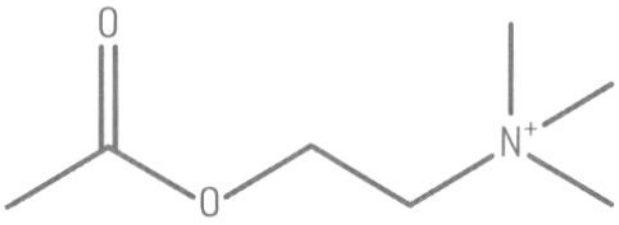

Acetylcholine - degraded by
acetylcholinesterase

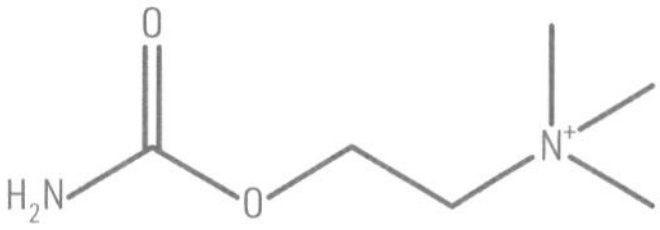

Carbachol - carbamate less susceptible to
degradation by acetylcholinesterase

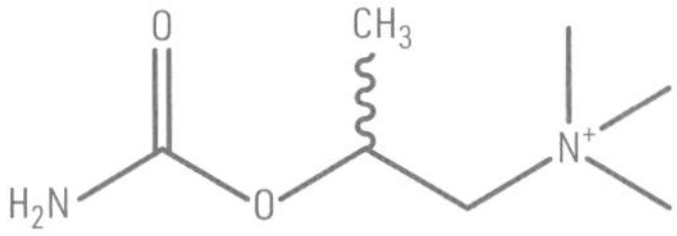

Bethanecol - additional protection from degradation
by acetylcholinesterase because of additional methyl

 Metabolically susceptible functional groups in a lead compound can be protected sterically or electronically.

8.2.4 Targeting drugs

The ideal situation in drug design would be the production of a drug which only reaches the exact target location necessary to produce the desired activity. This is extremely difficult to achieve in most cases and the majority of drugs still reach their desired target by a 'random walk' around the body. There have been a small number of instances where drugs have been designed to target specific areas of the body, e.g. the gastrointestinal tract, and the central nervous system. It is relatively easy to restrict the activity

Figure 8.11 Increasing susceptibility to metabolism

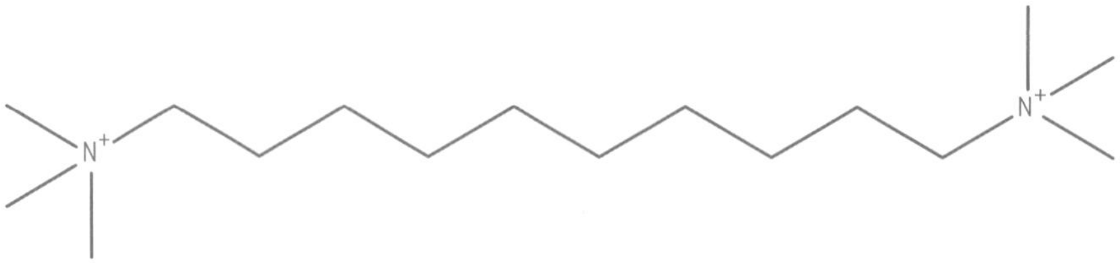

decamethonium - a long-acting neuromuscular blocker - not degraded by acetylcholinesterase

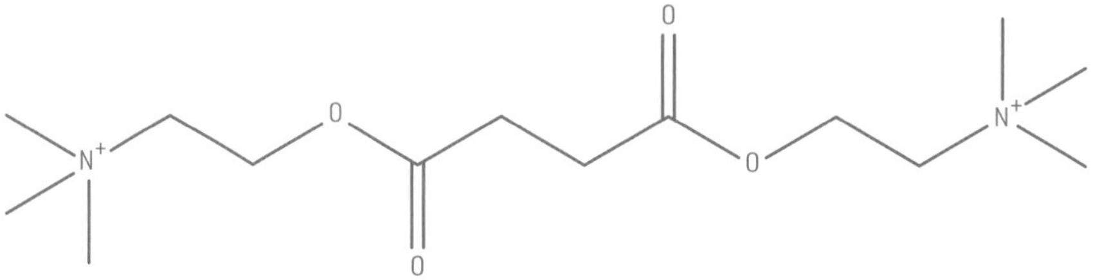

suxamethonium - a short-acting neuromuscular blocker - ester groups hydrolysed by plasma cholinesterase

of a drug to the gastrointestinal tract—if the drug is fully ionized it will not be able to cross the lipid cell membranes of the gut. Examples of this are the cholesterol-binding complexes and the antibacterial agent succinylsulfathiazole (Figure 8.12). Targeting the central nervous system is more difficult because the drug would have to be designed to cross the blood-brain barrier, which is reasonably effective at keeping foreign molecules out of the central nervous system. An example where this has been achieved is the drug levodopa (❭ XR 8.1.5.2) which uses the phenylalanine active transport system to penetrate the brain, although strictly speaking levodopa is a prodrug (❭ XR see Section 12.6.4). Preventing a drug from entering the central nervous system can be equally important. A good example of this is the statins (❭ XR see Case Study 6.1).

INTEGRATION BOX 8.4   SOFT DRUGS

Although widely used in society to refer to a particular type of recreational drug, soft drugs, scientifically speaking, are drugs designed to have a predictable and controllable metabolism to non-toxic and inactive products, after they have achieved their desired pharmacological effect. If the drug is deactivated and detoxified shortly after it has exerted its biological effect, the therapeutic index ought to be increased. A soft drug should have a close structural similarity to the lead compound but have a metabolically sensitive entity built into the lead structure. The metabolically sensitive entity should not affect the overall physicochemical properties of the lead compound. The advantages of soft drugs are the elimination of toxic metabolites, the avoidance of pharmacologically active metabolites, and the avoidance of pharmacokinetic problems caused by multiple active species. Endogenous ligands can be considered natural soft drugs as the body has fast and efficient metabolic pathways without the production of highly reactive metabolites. Examples of such drugs include suxamethonium (❭ XR Figure 8.6), esmolol and remifentanil.

→

→

Figure 2 Examples of soft drugs

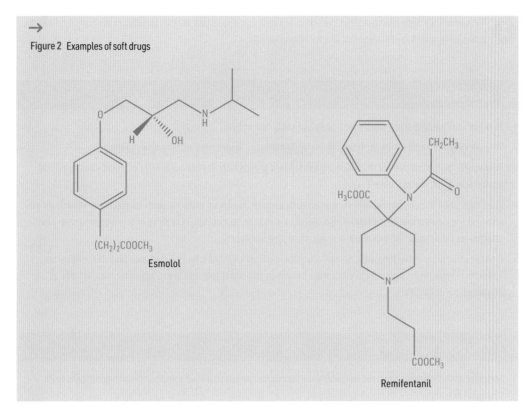

(CH$_2$)$_2$COOCH$_3$

Esmolol

H$_3$COOC

CH$_2$CH$_3$

COOCH$_3$

Remifentanil

If a candidate drug is required to have a short duration of action a metabolically sensitive group can be introduced to the lead compound.

Figure 8.12 Examples of drugs restricted to the gastrointestinal tract

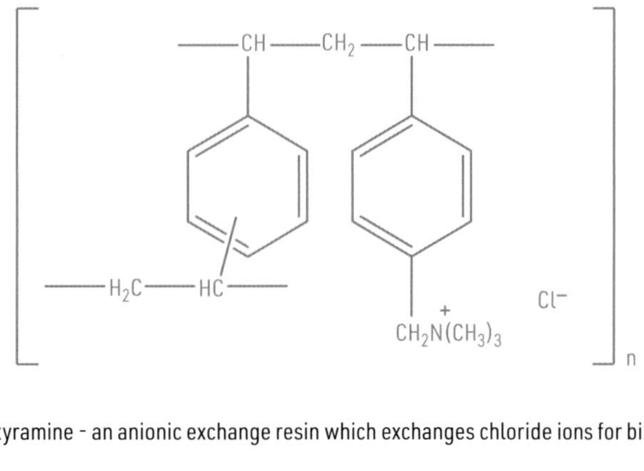

colestyramine – an anionic exchange resin which exchanges chloride ions for bile salts

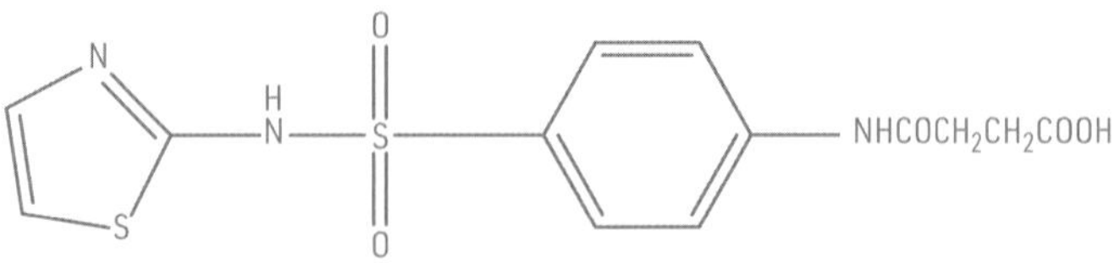

succinylsulfathiazole – the carboxylic acid ensures ionization in GIT so not absorbed into bloodstream

It is sometimes desirable to restrict the action of a lead compound to a specific location in the body. This can be achieved by addition of the appropriate functional groups.

Questions

1. Find five orally active drugs which don't obey Lipinski's rule of five.

2. Why are chlorine and fluorine preferred to the other halogens in structure activity investigations?

3. How would the introduction of the following substituent groups alter the bioavailability of a lead compound: sulphonic acid, thiol, methyl, ester?

4. The three-point attachment hypothesis was an early attempt to explain drug-receptor interactions. How could you interpret the interactions of the following molecules with their appropriate receptors in terms of the three-point attachment hypothesis: adrenaline, morphine, clozapine, captopril?

5. Find the structures of the following 'sartan' drugs (angiotensin II inhibitors: losartan, candesartan, irbesartan, valsartan). From their structures, try and work out which structural features are required for their activity as angiotensin II inhibitors.

Chapter summary

- Structure activity studies are used to identify the functional groups of a lead compound which contribute to its biological activity.

- Isosteric replacement is a process often used in the optimization of the interaction of a lead compound with the target receptor.

- Changing the size or shape of a lead compound can be achieved by addition of rings, alkene or alkyl groups.

- Variation of the substituent groups of a lead compound can potentially affect receptor affinity and selectivity, solubility properties, and metabolism.

- Simplification of the structure of a lead compound is carried out in order to identify any parts of the molecule which are not required for activity.

- Rigidification of the structure of a lead compound can be used in order to fix the molecule in its optimal shape for interaction with the target receptor.

- Geometrical isomers have different physical and chemical properties and often have very different biological effects.

- Optical isomers have identical physical and chemical properties except in a chiral environment. As many chiral environments exist within the body, optical isomers exhibit a variety of differences with respect to ADME and target receptor interactions.

- It is important to ensure that a drug candidate has the appropriate hydrophilic/lipophilic balance in order to optimize absorption and distribution.

- Increased resistance or increased sensitivity to metabolic degradation can be achieved by insertion of the appropriate functional groups into the lead compound.

- Targeting the lead compound to a specific location in the body is likely to lead to a reduction in unwanted side effects.

Further reading

Stocks, M. (2013) An introduction to biological and small molecule drug research and development. In Ganellin, R., Roberts, S.M., and Jeffries, R. (ed.) *The Small Molecule Drug Discovery Process.* Oxford: Elsevier, Chapter 3.

Contains key issues and a number of case studies regarding lead optimization.

Lipinski, C.A., Lombardo, F., Dominy, B.W., and Feeney, P.J. (1997) Experimental and computational approaches to estimate solubility and permeability in drug discovery and development settings, *Adv. Drug Discovery Rev.* 23: 3–25.

The original publication of Lipinski's rule of five.

Carson, R. (2000) *Silent Spring.* London: Penguin Modern Classics.

An account of environmental and human damage caused by indiscriminate use of pesticides, originally written in 1962.

CASE STUDY 8.1   A NEW ERA OF DRUG DESIGN—DEVELOPMENT OF RANITIDINE

For many years, the traditional design of a new drug depended on the discovery and extraction of a natural product that exhibited a particular desired pharmacological activity. The extracted natural product was then used as a lead compound, and numerous compounds with similar structures were synthesized and tested for their biological activity. At this stage, the researchers did not have any real understanding of the mechanism of this biological activity.

However, in the 1960s, a new era of drug development started to become the preferred method of drug design. This method commenced with the identification of the physiological cause of the condition to be treated, and it was from this starting point that a drug was logically designed, i.e. from first principles. Probably the best example of this was the development of the histamine H_2 receptor antagonists. The work was commenced at Smith, Kline and French (SKF) by James Black who, working for ICI, had been responsible for the development of β-blockers. He produced the β-blockers by leading the development of a molecule similar to the natural agonist (noradrenaline), which occupied the receptor but did not stimulate it—an antagonist. At SKF he was looking to repeat this approach but with histamine receptor antagonists.

Histamine (Figure CS8.1) is a neurotransmitter which is found throughout the body and, as such, has numerous roles, including allergic reactions and acid secretion in the stomach. The imidazole ring in histamine can exist in two tautomeric forms—the tele tautomer represented by τ and the pros tautomer represented by π. Previous work with antihistamine drugs, used to treat allergic reactions, indicated that they had no effect on gastric acid secretion.

Figure CS8.1 Histamine tautomers

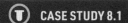

Histamine - tele
tautomer

Histamine - pros
tautomer

→

→

This suggested that there was more than one type of histamine receptor. If the receptor that controlled gastric acid secretion could be identified, this might lead to the production of an antagonist at that receptor—a potential anti-ulcer drug.

Thus, the lead compound in this case was histamine, and structural variations were produced in the search for an antagonist. Initially, none were found but an agonist, 5-methylhistamine (Figure CS8.2) was discovered, which stimulated gastric acid secretion without any of the other normal responses to histamine. This established the presence of a second type of histamine receptor, not involved in the allergic response, and it was labelled the histamine H_2 receptor. Many structural variations of 5-methylhistamine were made, but without any success.

As a result of advances in assay techniques, a more sensitive assay was developed, and re-testing of the compounds previously synthesized led to the identification of a partial antagonist. After a further 2 years, an active antagonist was produced, and named burimamide. However burimamide had only weak activity and was not orally active, and a new analogue was required. Burimamide had been produced from N^α-guanylhistamine (Figure CS8.3), which was a weak antagonist. The side-chain length was increased from two to four carbons and the strongly basic guanidine component was replaced by the neutral methylthiourea function shown in red in Figure CS8.4. The low activity of burimamide was thought to be due its non-basic electron-releasing sidechain which favours the N^π-imidazole tautomer (How?). Histamine itself has a basic electron-withdrawing sidechain which favours the high affinity N^τ-imidazole tautomer (How?). Inserting a thioether (shown in red in Figure CS8.5) function (which is electronegative) favours the N^τ tautomer (How?). Furthermore, introduction of the 5-methyl favours high H_2-receptor selectivity and oral bioavailability—this was metiamide (Figure CS8.5). Additionally, a methyl group was also introduced onto the thiourea sidechain.

Figure CS8.2 5-methylhistamine

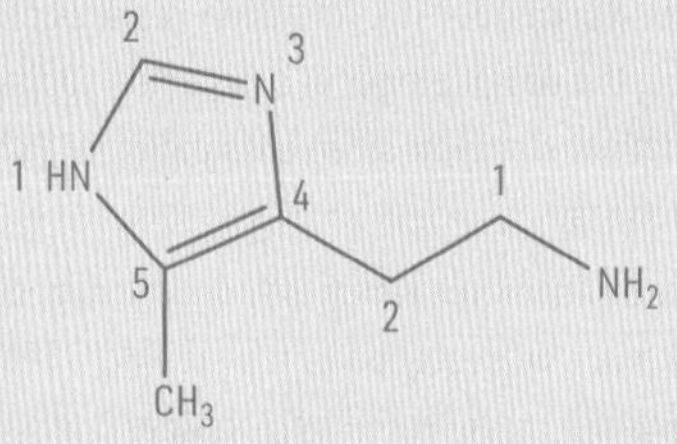

5-methylhistamine

Figure CS8.3 N^α-guanylhistamine

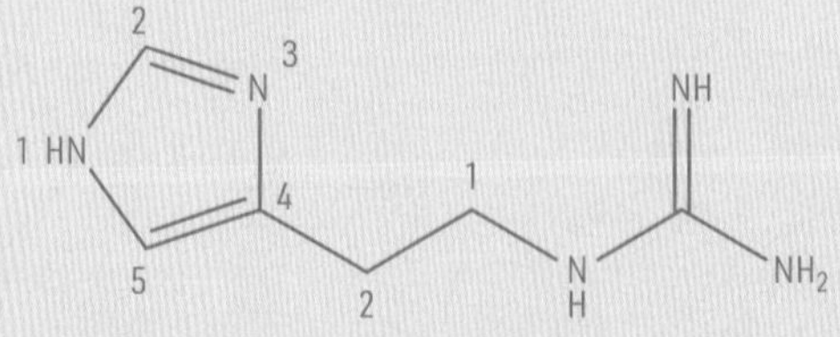

N^α-guanylhistamine

→

Figure CS8.4 Burimamide

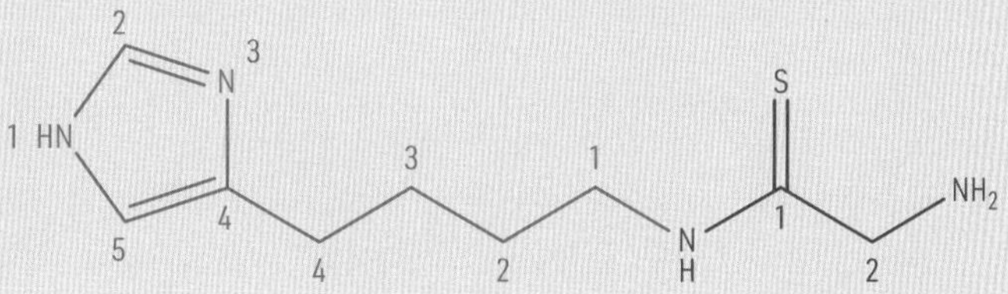

Burimamide

Figure CS8.5 Metiamide

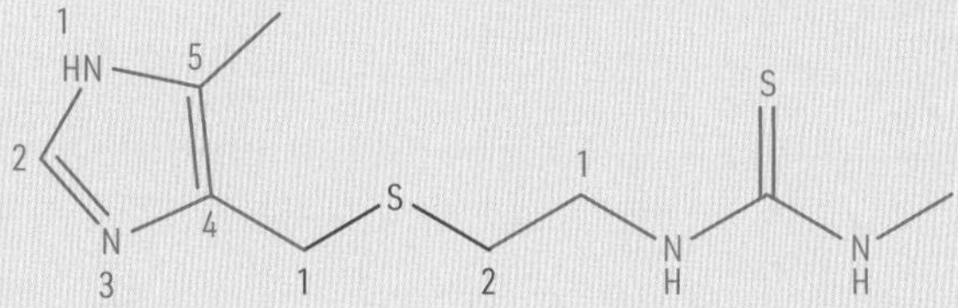

Metiamide

Figure CS8.6 Cimetidine

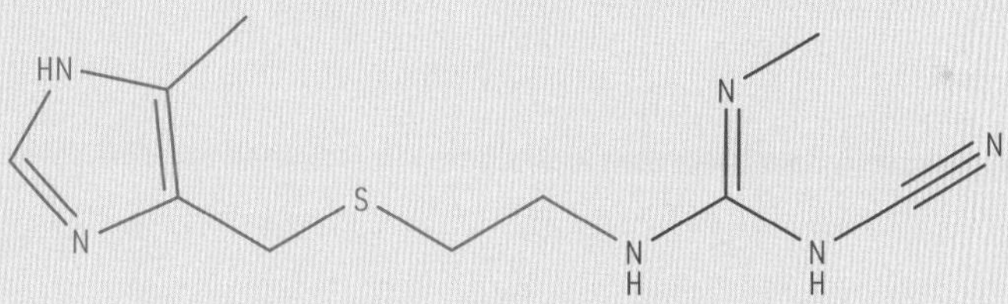

Cimetidine

Whilst initial clinical trial results were impressive, it soon became clear that metiamide gives rise to a blood disorder called agranulocytosis. It was thought that this was due to the thiourea group and it was replaced by a cyanoguanidine (shown in red)—this was cimetidine (Figure CS8.6). Despite its incredible success (it became the world's number one prescription drug), it was not without its problems. It is relatively short-acting (Why?) (leading to a frequent dosage regime), it interacts with the cytochrome P450 metabolizing system (leading to interaction with numerous other drugs), and it has anti-androgenic activity.

It was discovered that the imidazole ring was not required for antagonism at the H_2 receptor. Replacement of the imidazole ring by a variety of other heterocyclic rings led to the development of ranitidine, which in 1985, also became the world's number one prescription drug (Figure CS8.7).

→
Figure CS8.7 Ranitidine

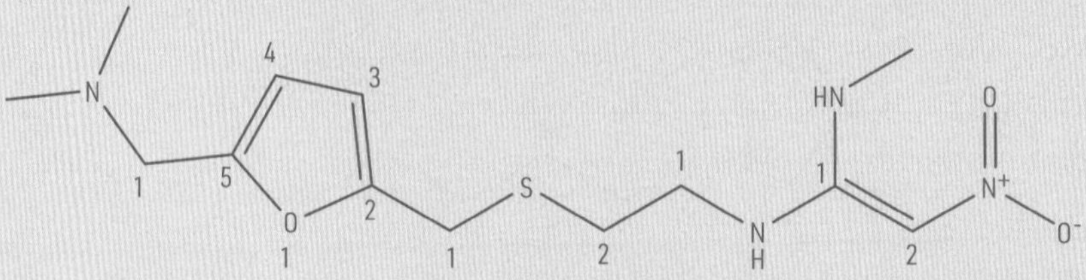

Ranitidine

Computer-aided Drug Design

9

Chapter 8 provides an overview of what a traditional drug design process would look like. The optimization of a lead compound can be brought about by making structural changes to the lead compound or by synthesizing new structures related to it, with a view to improving its pharmacodynamics and pharmacokinetic properties. In the early days of drug design, success often relied on a significant element of luck. As the drug design process developed, medicinal chemists were able to produce guidelines which made the process much less dependent on luck, allowing a more informed choice with respect to which molecules to synthesize. During the latter part of the twentieth century, the increase in the power of computers led to the realization that they could prove extremely useful in aiding the drug design process. This resulted in the development of a new tool to be used in drug design, namely computer-aided drug design. The use of computers in aiding drug design takes a number of forms, such as the storage and prediction of data (cheminformatics) (**▶ XR see Section 9.1**), quantitative structure-activity relationships (QSAR) (**▶ XR see Section 9.2**), and computer modelling of molecular properties, drug-receptor interactions, and receptor mapping (**▶ XR see Section 9.4**).

9.1 CHEMINFORMATICS

The use of computerized informational techniques to solve problems in drug design and elsewhere is known as cheminformatics. It includes the ability to store chemical structures, store information about chemical and physical properties, and to make predictions of biological activity (both desirable and undesirable) based on chemical and physical properties. Cheminformatics is useful in drug design and the production of new chemical entities (NCEs) by potentially decreasing the time and cost for a drug to reach the market and is widely used in the pharmaceutical industry today.

 Cheminformatics involves techniques for storage and retrieval of chemical structures and physicochemical properties.

9.1.1 Chemical information and its storage

Much of the information about a molecule is text-based and can be stored in traditional digital databases. A chemical structure, however, poses a different problem—how can this be represented in a digital format? The simplest way to do this is by use of a chemical code which represents the chemical structure and can be stored in a computer. These codes are known as 2D chemical codes and there are a variety of types in use. The most commonly used one is known as simplified molecular input line-entry specification (or SMILES). The SMILES code represents a chemical structure as a line of text. It has been in use since the 1980s and is relatively easy to understand, produce, and translate into a structure (Integration Box 9.1).

It must be remembered, however, that knowledge of the 3D structure of a drug candidate is absolutely vital and this cannot be represented by 2D coding. 3D representation is based around Cartesian x,y,z coordinates and requires more complex storage methods and there are a number of these that are used such as Chem3D, Alchemy, Sybyl, Hyperchem, Discovery Studio Pro, Spartan, and CACh (Figure 9.1). Computers can be used to construct large databases of these chemical structures which can be accessed at a later stage in order to identify potential new lead compounds.

9.1.2 Prediction of properties

These large databases (**▶ XR see Section 9.1.1**) can be used to predict physical and chemical properties. This predictive ability means that these properties do not necessarily have to be experimentally measured, thus saving vital resources such as time and money. It should be recognized, however, that

---

INTEGRATION BOX 9.1 | **HOW SMILES WORKS**

The use of SMILES to generate a 2D chemical code for a chemical structure involves following a set of straightforward rules. The first rule is that each atom in the structure is represented by the letter, or letters, which denotes the element in the periodic table (in upper case). Hydrogen atoms are ignored, and the presence of single bonds between atoms is implied. For example:

CH_4 becomes C, CH_3CH_3 becomes CC, CH_3CH_2OH becomes CCO.

Rule number 2 is that double bonds are represented by = and triple bonds by #. For example:

HCHO is C=O, carbon dioxide is O=C=O and ethyne is C#C.

Rule number 3 is that chain branches are represented by parentheses and they may be nested within one another. For example:

$$CH_3$$
$$|$$
$$H_3C \text{———} CH \text{———} CH_3$$

2-methylpropane

becomes CC(C)C and

$$O \qquad\qquad CH_3$$
$$\| \qquad\qquad |$$
$$H_3C \text{———} C \text{———} O \text{———} C \text{———} CH_3$$
$$|$$
$$CH_3$$

t-butyl ethanoate

→

becomes CC(=O)OC(C)(C)C.

Rule number 4 is about representing cyclic systems. Ring closures are represented by a pair of matching numbers. For example:

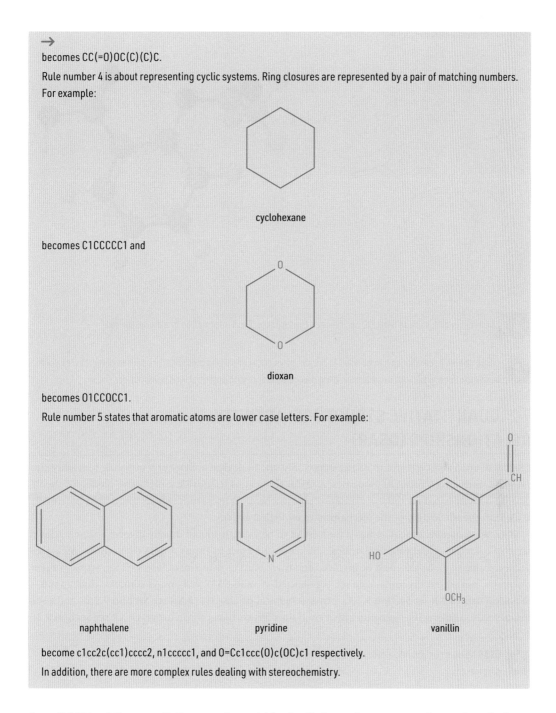

cyclohexane

becomes C1CCCCC1 and

dioxan

becomes O1CCOCC1.

Rule number 5 states that aromatic atoms are lower case letters. For example:

naphthalene   pyridine   vanillin

become c1cc2c(cc1)cccc2, n1ccccc1, and O=Cc1ccc(O)c(OC)c1 respectively.

In addition, there are more complex rules dealing with stereochemistry.

the reliability of these predictions can be variable. Predictions of some properties, such as logP, are usually reliable but prediction of others, such as pKa, are less reliable. Whilst the predictions are aimed primarily at identifying potential new lead compounds, they can be equally valuable at identifying molecules which are unlikely to be drug candidates because of, for example, poor oral availability, rapid metabolism, or toxicity. These databases can also be used to predict biological activities, both therapeutic and toxic, a process which is invaluable to drug design and development. By combining these capabilities, a quantitative relationship can be developed between structure and biological activity (▶ XR see Section 9.2).

Figure 9.1 3D representation of aspirin

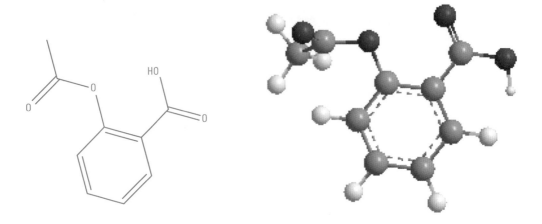

 Chemical codes, such as SMILES, can be used to store structural information in a digital format.

 Large chemical databases can be used to predict physicochemical and biological properties of molecules yet to be synthesized which can be helpful in drug design by identifying potential lead compounds.

9.2 QUANTITATIVE STRUCTURE-ACTIVITY RELATIONSHIPS (QSAR)

QSAR is defined as an attempt to relate, statistically, the biological activity of a molecule to its physico-chemical, including structural, properties. A QSAR study aims to provide a predictive model for the biological activity based on the calculation of physicochemical properties ,which could then potentially assist with the elucidation of the mechanism of biological activity.

There are a number of requirements for a QSAR to be valid. It should usually involve a closely related series of compounds and various statistical criteria must be met to ensure a valid relationship. An appropriate number of molecules must be involved and there must be evidence of how well the activity of new molecules, not within the initial data set, is predicted. A valid QSAR will always comprise three inputs—biological data (❯ XR see Section 9.2.1), physicochemical parameters (❯ XR see Section 9.2.2), and a statistical method linking the biological activity and the physicochemical parameters (❯ XR see Section 9.3).

 QSAR studies can provide a predictive model for biological activity based on calculated physicochemical parameters.

9.2.1 Biological data

In order to be used in QSAR studies, biological data must be as reliable as possible, always accepting that biological data is likely to contain errors because of biological variation. To make the data as reliable as possible, the information should involve the same biological test system carried out in the same laboratory by the same operator.

QSAR can use two different types of biological data, namely continuous data and categoric data. Continuous data utilizes a continuous numeric scale and is a quantitative measure of potency. In order to remove the effect of molecular weight, the data must be expressed in molar units of concentration.

The biological activity is normally expressed as $1/C$ where C is the molar concentration of a molecule required to achieve a defined level of biological activity. Thus an increase in activity will be represented by an increase in the value of $1/C$. Additionally in order to make the numbers easier to handle, $\log 1/C$ is usually used (Integration Box 9.2). Categoric data provides a qualitative measure of potency and utilizes a positive/negative (yes/no) response and is more useful in **pattern recognition**, for example in indicating what type of substituent group might confer biological activity on a molecule.

9.2.2 Physicochemical parameters

There have been many physicochemical properties used in QSAR but the most significant ones have been shown to be hydrophobicity, electronic distribution, and shape. The descriptors of these properties, also known as parameters, describe the physicochemical and structural aspects of molecules. QSAR relates one or more of these parameters to the biological activity of molecules. These parameters initially were measured but, ultimately, it is often possible to calculate the theoretical value of a parameter for an un-synthesized molecule and, from the QSAR equation, predict the possible biological activity. This allows the choice of which analogues of the lead compound to synthesize to be more informed, thus saving valuable resources.

9.2.2.1 Hydrophobic parameters

The hydrophobicity of a molecule governs, primarily, the ability to cross lipid membranes and so governs the ability of the molecule to be transported into and around the body. Additionally, the molecule may be involved in hydrophobic bonding at the target receptor. Two parameters have been used to represent hydrophobicity—partition coefficient (P) and the hydrophobicity substituent constant (π). The former relates to the whole molecule whilst the latter relates to substituent groups only.

The partition coefficient of a molecule is the measured relative distribution of that molecule between an octanol-water mixture. This relative distribution is represented by Equation 9.1.

P = concentration of molecule in octanol/concentration of molecule in water   Equation 9.1

From this equation it can be seen that a hydrophobic molecule will have a high P value (more soluble in octanol) whilst a hydrophilic molecule will have a low P value (more soluble in water). In order to produce linear relationships $\log P$ values are usually used in QSAR. Normally the aqueous phase used in measuring the partition coefficient is buffered to pH 7.4 to represent physiological pH.

Determination of the partition coefficients of a series of molecules is very time-consuming, as all the molecules have to be synthesized and their partition coefficients measured experimentally. It would be much more convenient if a value for P could be predicted. Hydrophobic substituent constant values can

---

INTEGRATION BOX 9.2   RATIONALE FOR THE FORM OF QSAR EQUATIONS

If we use an example of the development of a QSAR study of toxicity of a group of drugs relative to partition coefficient, it will help to explain why certain forms of data representation are used. The equation is,

$$\text{Log } 1/C\,(LD_{50}) = 1.517\log P + 4.4888$$

The reason why the biological response is expressed as a reciprocal is because this will produce a regression line with a positive slope. The logarithmic value of the biological response is used to produce a linear relationship plot and it makes the numbers easier to handle. If we take an example compound from the study to illustrate this last point, chlorpromazine has a value for C (LD_{50}) of 0.000006mmol. Expressed as 1/C this becomes 158489.32, which as log C is −5.2, but as log1/C is 5.2. In addition, the partition coefficient of chlorpromazine is 16595 but expressed as logP is 4.22. Thus, the reciprocal and logarithmic values are used to make the numbers easier to handle and easier to represent graphically.

In QSAR studies biological data is usually expressed as log 1/C where C is the molar concentration producing a specific biological response.

be used to calculate log P values. (π) is a measure of the hydrophobicity of a substituent relative to hydrogen (Equations 9.2 and 9.3).

$$\pi = \log P_X - \log P_H \qquad \text{Equation 9.2}$$

where P_X and P_H are the partition coefficients of the substituted molecule and the reference molecule respectively.

$$\pi_{Cl} = \log P_{(chlorobenzene)} - \log P_{(benzene)} \qquad \text{Equation 9.3}$$

If log P for chlorobenzene is 2.84 and log P for benzene is 2.13, then π_{Cl} is 0.71. In the octanol-water system a positive π value indicates a more hydrophobic substituent than hydrogen and a negative π indicates a less hydrophobic substituent than hydrogen. These π values can now be used to predict theoretical partition coefficients of a series of analogues simply by measuring the partition coefficient of the lead molecule and using π values to predict P values for all the other analogues (Integration Box 9.3).

INTEGRATION BOX 9.3   PREDICTION OF LOG*P* VALUES (CLOG*P*)

As an example of the prediction of log*P* we can look at the prediction of log*P* for *ortho*-toluic acid.

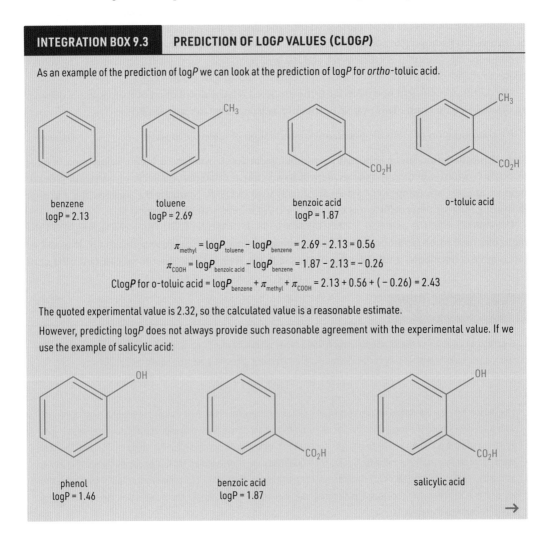

benzene	toluene	benzoic acid	o-toluic acid
logP = 2.13	logP = 2.69	logP = 1.87	

$$\pi_{methyl} = \log P_{toluene} - \log P_{benzene} = 2.69 - 2.13 = 0.56$$
$$\pi_{COOH} = \log P_{benzoic\ acid} - \log P_{benzene} = 1.87 - 2.13 = -0.26$$
$$\text{Clog}P \text{ for o-toluic acid} = \log P_{benzene} + \pi_{methyl} + \pi_{COOH} = 2.13 + 0.56 + (-0.26) = 2.43$$

The quoted experimental value is 2.32, so the calculated value is a reasonable estimate.

However, predicting log*P* does not always provide such reasonable agreement with the experimental value. If we use the example of salicylic acid:

phenol	benzoic acid	salicylic acid
logP = 1.46	logP = 1.87	

→

→

$$\pi_{OH} = \log P_{phenol} - \log P_{benzene} = 1.47 - 2.13 = -0.67$$

$$\pi_{COOH} = \log P_{benzoic\ acid} - \log P_{benzene} = 1.87 - 2.13 = -0.26$$

$$C\log P \text{ for salicylic acid} = \log P_{benzene} + \pi_{OH} + \pi_{COOH} = 2.13 + (-0.67) + (-0.26) = 1.20$$

The quoted experimental value is 2.26, so the predicted value varies considerably from the experimental value. This illustrates one of the dangers of relying too heavily on predicted values of logP. Here, the presence of intramolecular hydrogen bonds between the phenol group and the carboxylic acid group makes salicylic acid more hydrophobic than predicted by the use of hydrophobic substituent constants.

When constructing a QSAR, it should be remembered that logP and π do not represent the same hydrophobic influence within a molecule. LogP represents the overall hydrophobicity of a molecule and is related to the transport of a molecule to its target site. π represents the hydrophobicity of a particular region of the molecule and, more probably, is related to the hydrophobic bonding interaction of that region of the molecule with the target receptor site.

 The most commonly used hydrophobicity parameters in QSAR studies are partition coefficient, which relates to the whole molecule, and the hydrophobicity substituent constant, which relates to specific regions of the molecule.

9.2.2.2 Electronic parameters

The electronic distribution of a molecule can potentially have a considerable influence on a molecule's biological activity. The electronic distribution may affect its transport by influencing ionization. Electronic effects are also important to some types of drug-receptor binding such as ionic bonding, hydrogen bonding, and dipole-dipole attraction. The most widely used electronic parameter is the Hammett substituent constant (σ). This constant is a measure of the electron-donating or electron-withdrawing ability of a substituent. The values were originally determined using a series of substituted benzoic acids (Equation 9.4).

$$\sigma_X = \log K_X/K_H = \log K_X - \log K_H \qquad \text{Equation 9.4}$$

where K_H is the dissociation constant for benzoic acid itself, and K_X is the dissociation constant for the substituted benzoic acid. A negative value for σ indicates that the substituent exerts an electron-donating effect, whereas a positive value indicates an electron-withdrawing substituent.

The σ value varies with the position of the substituent because the Hammett constant reflects both the **inductive** and **mesomeric** contributions to the electronic distribution (Figure 9.2). Therefore the value of σ for a substituent will differ depending on whether the substituent is *meta* or *para*. There are two disadvantages associated with Hammett constants. Firstly, they only apply to substituents attached directly to an aromatic ring and, secondly, they cannot be used for *ortho* substituents because of interference from steric effects and, possibly, intramolecular hydrogen bonding. As a result a number of other electronic parameters such as dipole moment and **HOMO/LUMO** have been used in QSAR studies but Hammett constants are still the most widely used electronic parameter in QSAR.

9.2.2.3 Steric parameters

Steric parameters are used to describe the size and shape of a molecule which are important with respect to its ability to bind effectively to its target receptor site. Steric properties, particularly shape, are more difficult to quantify than hydrophobic or electronic properties. Several methods have been tried with varying degrees of success, however steric parameters are still used in many QSAR studies.

Figure 9.2 Hammett substituent constants

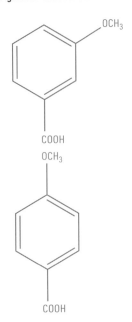

In m-methoxybenzoic acid the effect of the methoxy group is due to the electron-withdrawing inductive effect and σ value is 0.12

In p-methoxybenzoic acid the effect of the methoxy group is dominated by the electron-donating mesomeric effect and the σ value is -0.27

 The Hammett substituent constant, which reflect inductive and mesomeric contributions to electronic distribution within the substituents of a molecule, is the most widely electronic parameter in QSAR studies.

The simplest parameter to represent size is relative molecular mass (RMM) but this relates poorly to molecular shape. In order to better quantify molecular shape, parameters such as molecular surface area and molecular volume have been used. The Verloop steric parameter attempts to provide a representation of molecular shape based on a number of properties such as bond angles and lengths, van der Waals radii, and possible conformations. This parameter is very complex and is calculated using a computer program called Sterimol.

Molar refractivity (MR) is a measure of the volume of a molecule and its ease of polarization (Equation 9.5).

$$MR = (n^2 - 1)RMM/(n^2 + 1)\rho \hspace{2cm} \text{Equation 9.5}$$

where n = refractive index, MW = RMM and ρ = density.

MW/ρ is a measure of the molar volume and the refractive index term is a measure of polarizability.

The steric influence of substituent groups (similar to the Hammett substituent constants) can be represented by Taft's steric factor (E_s). Taft, in 1956, showed that the rates of hydrolysis of a series of aliphatic esters were almost entirely dependent on steric factors. Using methyl ethanoate as the standard ester he developed the following equation (Equation 9.6).

$$E_s = \log K_X - \log K_O \hspace{2cm} \text{Equation 9.6}$$

where K_X is the hydrolysis rate of the substituted ester and K_O is the hydrolysis rate for the standard ester. The main disadvantage of the Taft steric parameter is that it relates to an intramolecular steric effect, whereas interaction of a molecule at a target receptor site involves intermolecular effects.

 Steric parameters, relating to molecular size and shape, are more difficult to quantify than electronic or hydrophobic parameters.

9.2.2.4 *Topological parameters*

An alternative way of describing molecular structure is by topological parameters, which are based on graph theory, in which the bonds connecting the atoms are considered as a path that is traversed from one atom to another. Many such parameters exist, but the most commonly used is molecular connectivity. The details of how the values for these parameters are obtained is beyond the scope of this book, but more details can be found in the Further reading at the end of the chapter. Topological parameters are most often used in discriminant analysis, principal component analysis (PCA), and pattern recognition.

9.3 STATISTICAL METHODS

The point of a QSAR study is to attempt to establish a link between the desired biological activity and the physicochemical parameters used to describe the molecules in the study. This link can be established by a variety of methods, increasing in complexity as the number of parameters used increases. When the biological activity is related to only one parameter, then a simple plot of biological activity against that parameter can be used (Figure 9.3). Linear regression analysis can then be used

Figure 9.3a Example of QSAR plot

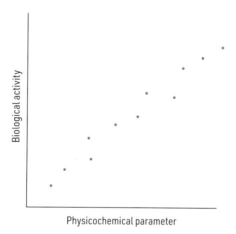

Figure 9.3b Example of linear regression analysis plot

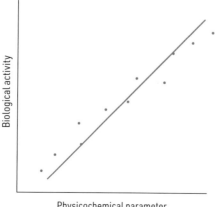

to produce an equation which represents the line of best fit—y = ax + c, where a is the slope of the line of best fit, and c is the intercept. There are many software programs available to carry out this type of analysis.

More often, however, two or more parameters are required to describe the biological activity and these situations require the use of multiple linear regression analyses, producing an equation of the form y = ax + bz + ...c. These equations are often referred to as Hansch equations (Box 9.1). Once established and verified, these equations can be used to provide information about the mechanism by which the molecules bring about their biological activity. They can also be used to predict the activity of molecules yet to be synthesized.

It may be the case that the QSAR has a large number of parameters. In this case, stepwise regression analysis can be used to identify the most relevant parameters. This process involves repeating linear regression analysis, including an additional parameter at each step to determine whether the additional parameter provides a better statistical relationship between the parameters and the biological activity.

Knowledge of just how meaningful the relationship is between the parameters and the biological activity requires the use of statistical measures of goodness of fit. The regression coefficient (r) is a measure of how well the parameters in the regression equation explain the observed biological activity. A regression coefficient of 1 indicates a perfect fit. It is impossible to obtain a perfect fit when working with biological data (which has inherent errors) and values of r above 0.9 are usually considered acceptable. The regression coefficient can also be quoted as r^2, in which case values above 0.8 are considered acceptable. Multiplication of the r^2 value by 100 gives an indication of the extent of variation in the biological activity data that is explained by the physicochemical parameters used, e.g. an r^2 value of 0.89 means that 89 per cent of the variation in the biological activity is explained by the parameters used in the regression equation. Another statistical value that should be used in the analysis is the standard error of the estimate (s). A value of zero for s would mean that there were no errors whatsoever in the biological data or the values of the parameters. Again, this situation is not feasible, but the value of s should be low. Finally, there are statistical tests which can be carried out in order to assess the significance of each parameter in the regression equation. These are the Fisher's (or F) tests. Application of these tests will yield p values which should be less than or equal to 0.05 if the parameter is significant (please see Integration Box 9.4 for an example of the interpretation of a QSAR regression equation). Chi square tests are procedures which test whether the observed distribution in the relationship is due to chance. Cross-validation methods (e.g. q^2 or r^2cv) are also used to evaluate the extent to which the relationship can predict the activity of compounds not in the original set.

BOX 9.1   CORWIN HANSCH

Corwin Hansch can be regarded as the pioneer of computer-assisted drug design. In the 1960s, he first proposed a multi-parameter approach to the problem of relating drug activity to measurable chemical properties. He realized that the biological activity of a molecule was dependent on its ability to reach and bind to its target site. He suggested that the transport of a drug to its site of action was dependent on its hydrophobicity and that this could be expressed numerically as a function of the drug's partition coefficient. The binding of the drug to the target site, however, would depend on the shape and electronic distribution of the groups involved in the binding, represented by, for example, the Taft steric factor and the Hammett electronic constant. The mathematical relationships between these physicochemical parameters and biological activity could be represented by equations which subsequently became known as Hansch equations. He produced over 300 publications as well as a number of books.

Linear regression analysis, simple or multiple, is used to find the equation which represents the best links of biological activity with one or more physicochemical parameters.

INTEGRATION BOX 9.4 **INTERPRETATION OF A QSAR EQUATION**

A study by Hansch of the adrenergic blocking activity of a series of β-haloarylamines in mice yielded the following equation.

$$\text{Log}1/\text{IC}_{50} = 1.22\pi - 1.59 + 7.89 \; n = 22, r^2 = 0.84, s = 0.238$$

IC_{50} represents the concentration which inhibits binding by 50%. The presence of π and σ in the equation tells us that the biological activity has a relationship with both hydrophobicity and electronic parameters and so both are important for the biological activity. The positive value for π shows that biological activity increases with increasing hydrophobicity and the negative value for σ shows that substituents should be electron-donating. The equation shows a good statistical fit (high r^2 value and low s value).

Figure 9.4 Linear regression plot with outliers

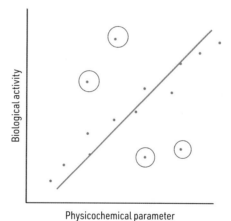

In a QSAR study sometimes molecules are identified that do not fit the QSAR equation. Such molecules are referred to as outliers (Figure 9.4). Their presence within the study will, of course, reduce the statistical fit of the QSAR regression equation and they need to be removed from the study. Normally, a reason for their removal should be identified such as they are atypical of the data set or may be bringing about their biological activity by a different mechanism to the other molecules in the data set.

9.4 MOLECULAR MODELLING

Advances in computer hardware and software have provided enormous advances in the design and development of drugs. Molecular modelling software is now readily available and there are numerous commercially available packages which allow the construction and visualization of 3D molecular structure (Figure 9.5). This text will not deal with the mechanisms by which the packages function and interested readers should consult the Further reading at the end of this chapter. Not only do these software packages allow the construction and 3D visualization of molecules but also have the ability to display a molecule

Figure 9.5 Examples of different 3D representations of morphine

a. 2D representation
b. 3D ball and stick representation
c. 3D space filling representation

d. 3D stick representation
e. Four 3D space filling representations identifying heteroatoms

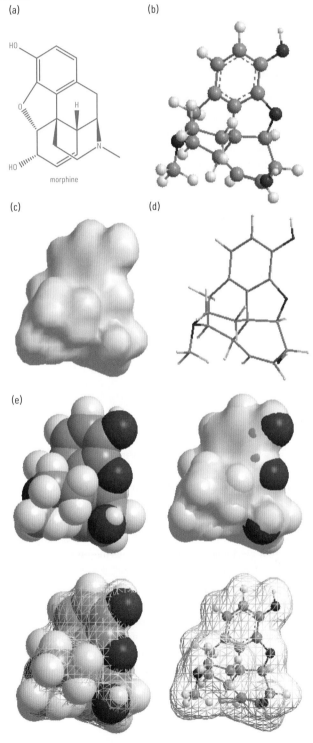

There are numerous computer software packages available to construct and display 3D molecular structures.

in different formats and calculate various properties such as dipole moment, charge density, and electrostatic potential (❯ XR see Section 9.4.1). Software packages are also available to model receptor sites (❯ XR see Section 9.4.2) and to model drug-receptor interactions (❯ XR see Section 9.4.3). All these possibilities make it easier to choose appropriate analogues of the lead compound to synthesize, thus reducing the cost of new drug development.

9.4.1 Molecular properties

Once a structure has been produced by a software modelling package, the process of energy minimization must be carried out. This involves manipulation of bond angles and lengths, torsion angles, and potential non-bonding interactions until the most stable conformation (i.e. the one with the minimum energy) is achieved. This energy-minimized structure can now be used to calculate and display various significant molecular parameters. All the bond lengths, bond angles, and torsion angles can now be accurately measured. Ionic charge is not usually fixed on a particular atom but can be distributed around other atoms in the molecule (Figure 9.5). This will have implications for any ionic bonding interaction with the target binding site. Charge distribution within a molecule can also be represented by molecular electrostatic potentials (MEPs) and this allows the identification of regions (rather than individual atoms) that possess an element of electrostatic charge, be it positive or negative (Figure 9.5).

The energy-minimized structure produced initially by the computer software will be a stable conformation. However, there is no certainty that the most stable conformation will be the biologically active conformation. It may be possible, using molecular mapping, to compare the conformations of biologically active compounds to identify those areas of 3D space occupied by potential binding groups.

 Molecular modelling software packages have the ability to calculate many molecular properties such as bond angles and lengths and use these values to produce the most stable conformation of a molecule.

9.4.2 Receptor mapping

Drug design ought to be made much simpler if the structure of the target receptor is known. As has been seen in earlier chapters (❯ XR Chapters 2, 3, and 4), most receptors are protein in nature. If the receptor protein can be crystallized, then the structure can be determined by X-ray crystallography. This method of structure determination is not always possible and, in these cases, molecular modelling can be used to create a model receptor. This model will be based on the primary amino acid sequence of the receptor protein (determined using standard techniques) and the X-ray determined structure of a related protein. For example, many G-protein coupled receptors (❯ XR see Section 2.2.4) were found to exhibit structural similarities to the protein bacteriorhodopsin because of possessing 7 transmembrane helices. The structure of this protein was used initially as a template to construct models of these receptors. Subsequently, the structure of bovine rhodopsin was determined by X-ray crystallography and this provided a better template because this protein actually is a G-protein coupled receptor and is remarkably similar to the β_2-adrenergic G-protein coupled receptor. Subsequently the crystal structures of a number of G-protein coupled receptors, with and without ligands, have been determined and have led to the awarding of several Nobel prizes.

9.4.3 Modelling drug-receptor interactions

The optimal use of molecular modelling would be the ability to model the interaction between potential drug molecules and their target receptor site. Computer programs have been used to create 3D models of the proposed drug molecules, and computer programs have been used to generate 3D images of the target receptor. Molecular modelling can now be used to fit the modelled molecules into the model receptor site (see Figure 9.6). This process is known as docking. The docking process can be under the control of parameters, such as bonding distance, determined by the operator. However, there are also programs which can automate the docking process and, by doing so, remove any bias that might arise from the operator. There is a wide variety of ways in which automatic docking can be carried out, and there are many modelling programs available for this process, e.g. DOCK, FLOG, Directed DOCK, FlexX, Hammerhead, SPROUT, LUDI, LEGEND. The method of operation of these programs is beyond the scope of this text but interested readers are directed to the Further reading at the end of this chapter.

9.4.4 3D QSAR

As the use of molecular modelling has become widespread, the original basis of QSAR, using physico-chemical parameters and 2D molecular representation has been adapted to 3D molecular properties. The theory of 3D QSAR assumes that the most important physicochemical properties of individual substituents, such as size, shape and electronic properties will apply to the molecules as a whole. A comparison of these molecular parameters with the biological activity for a large number of molecules (as in a normal QSAR study) will help to define the steric and electrostatic interactions which are favourable for the desired biological activity.

The outcome of a 3D QSAR study is often displayed in a lattice or on contour lines. These techniques are not without difficulty. For example, the active conformation of each molecule in the study has to be known, as has the pharmacophore and the molecules have to be aligned correctly. However, the advantages of 3D QSAR are that molecules of different structural classes can be compared and there is no

Figure 9.6 A view of atorvastatin bound to the active site of HMG-CoA reductase

(Credit: From Pharmaceutical Chemistry edited by Jill Barber and Chris Rostron (2013). Reproduced with permission of Oxford University Press through PLSclear).

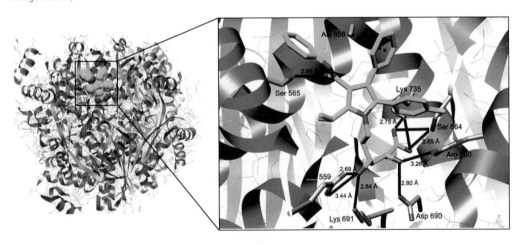

———— Hydrogen bond   ▪▪▪▪▪▪ Hydrophobic interaction

Molecular modelling packages can produce 3D models of both molecules and receptor sites and fit the modelled molecules to the modelled receptor in a process known as docking.

dependence on experimentally determined parameters. As with modelling drug-receptor interactions, a large number of 3D QSAR programmes have been developed such as COMFA, HINT, Quasar, and GRIND. Again, please refer to the Further reading at the end of the chapter for more information.

9.4.5 Virtual screening

Because of the potentially large number of structures arising from combinatorial chemistry (❯ **XR Section 10.2**), it is useful to evaluate their properties using computer programs (virtual screening). This filters impossibly large numbers of compounds to produce manageable numbers that are suitable for synthesis and testing. Essentially, virtual screening is an attempt to determine whether a compound is likely to interact with a known receptor and, equally importantly, which compounds will have appropriate pharmacokinetic properties.

❓ Questions

1. Derive the SMILES code for procaine.

2. Derive the structure from the following SMILES code:

   OC(=O)c1ccccc1OC(=O)C

3. Calculate the value of log$P$ for 4-hydroxybenzoic acid based on the values of log$P$ in Integration Box 9.3. Is the calculated value in reasonable agreement with the experimental value?

4. Using the ChemDraw package, draw the structure of a commonly used drug of your choice and display the 3D structure in as many ways as you can, using the ChemDraw package.

↻ Chapter summary

- The role of cheminformatics in drug design is to store information about chemical structure and properties by constructing large databases.

- Large databases of chemical structures are kept in order to assist in the search for potential new drug structures.

- These databases can be screened to predict desirable properties of potential lead compounds and also to screen compounds for undesirable properties such as toxicity.

- QSAR studies are used to predict biological activity based on molecular properties.

- QSAR studies use a predictive mathematical model based on physicochemical properties, measured experimentally or calculated.

- In order to be valid, a QSAR study must satisfy a number of statistical criteria.

- There are three components to a QSAR study—biological data, physicochemical parameters, and a statistical method linking the two.

- The main physicochemical parameters used in QSAR studies are hydrophobicity, electronic, and steric parameters.

- The link between biological activity and physicochemical parameters is achieved using linear regression analysis.

- QSAR studies are used in lead optimization to improve pharmacological activity, pharmacokinetic properties, and to reduce toxicity.
- 3D computing software packages are used to model molecular structures, receptor site structure and to visualize the interaction between molecules and model receptor sites.

📖 Further reading

Leach, A.R., Grillet, V. (2010) *An Introduction to Chemoinformatics.* Revised Edition, Dordrecht: Springer ISBN 978-1402062902.

A comprehensive review of all aspects of chemoinformatics.

Weininger, D. (1988) SMILES: A chemical language and information system 1 Introduction to methodology and encoding rules, *Journal of Chemical Information and Computer Science* 28: 31–6.

The original publication introducing SMILES.

Leach, A.R. (2001) *Molecular Modelling Principles and Application.* 2nd edn, London: Pearson Education.

Presents background theory and techniques of molecular modelling.

Hinchcliffe, A. (ed.) (2010) *Molecular Modelling for Beginners.* Weinheim: Wiley-VCH, ISBN 978-0-470-51313-2.

This book is written as an introduction to molecular modelling and is useful to readers new to this field.

Devilliers, J. and Balabon, A.T. (eds) (2002) *Topological Indices and Related Descriptors in QSAR and QSPR.* Amsterdam: Gordon and Breach. ISBN 90-5699-239-2.

An account of all topological descriptors.

Ⓣ CASE STUDY 9.1   DRUG-RECEPTOR INTERACTIONS—A QUESTION OF TIMING

In Chapter 2 we have dealt with the specific types of interactions between a drug and a receptor (❯ **XR Section 2.1**). The overall picture of drug-receptor interactions has tended to be governed by the affinity of a candidate drug for its target receptor. This is essentially the strength of the binding between the drug and the receptor.

Because only about 10 per cent of drug candidates that commence phase I clinical trials get approved by the regulatory authorities, pharmaceutical companies are constantly investigating ways by which this percentage can be increased. One such approach has been to commence investigation into the binding kinetics of drug-receptor interactions, i.e. the time a drug occupies a receptor–the so-called residence time. Much of the initial impetus in this case stemmed from the observation that candesartan was a more effective anti-hypertensive agent compared to others drugs in the same class–the sartans (for structures see ❯ **XR Case Study 3.1**). This may be because of the length of time candesartan spends attached to the receptor (several hours), as compared to, for example, losartan which only binds for minutes. Candesartan also has a much more rapid onset of action than, for example, losartan. Why might this be?

Binding kinetics is not a new science. It was first recognized in the 1960s by William Paton who suggested a rate theory of drug-receptor interaction. The accepted measure of affinity is the concentration of a drug at which 50 per cent of the target receptors are occupied and the time of occupation of the receptor has been somewhat ignored. By not considering receptor binding kinetics pharmaceutical companies could be missing out on potential drug candidates.

$\rightarrow$

A drug produces its clinical effect by stimulating (agonist) or blocking (antagonist) a target receptor. The binding of a drug to a receptor is often a dynamic process, although binding may be irreversible in some instances (covalent binding). Can you think of examples of drugs which act by covalent binding? The drug will associate with the receptor and, after a period of time, will dissociate from the receptor. As previously stated, much effort has been directed to the strength of the binding but, increasingly, attention is being directed to the time taken to bind and dissociate from the receptor—the binding kinetics. It is now recognized that clinical efficacy, duration of action, and incidence of side effects may all be influenced by binding kinetics.

In 2012, a 5 year project was commenced called Kinetics for Drug Discovery (K4DD). Its aim was to improve the efficacy and safety of a candidate drug in the clinic. In order to do this, it would be necessary to improve the understanding of drug-receptor binding kinetics and to develop appropriate software and assays that allow routine binding kinetic analysis. A significant effort has been with respect to G-protein coupled receptors because they are the target for at least 30 per cent of currently utilized drugs. The types of techniques that have been used to study the structure of receptors and their interaction with drugs include X-ray crystallography and radio-ligand binding. Kinetic data can be obtained by surface plasmon resonance, fluorescence spectroscopy, FTIR, and isothermal titration. Use of all of these techniques can provide more in-depth information about drug-receptor kinetics (how do these techniques provide this information?). This information can be added to existing knowledge about a drug's affinity for its target receptor and the mechanism by which it influences subsequent signalling processes. In this way, kinetics can be added to the factors that are useful in predicting good drug candidates. Part of the remit of K4DD was to construct a database of kinetic data in order generate computer tools to aid in the prediction of useful clinical drugs from preclinical data, in order to reduce the attrition rate from preclinical research to clinical trials.

Suggested reading

K4DD has a website containing lots of information about this project and its outcomes, https://www.k4dd.eu.

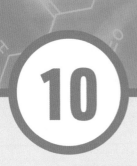

10

Combinatorial Chemistry and High Throughput Screening

Prior to the 1980s, the drug design process relied on the synthesis and biological testing of potential drug molecules in a serial manner. Each synthesized molecule was tested, and, depending upon the results, medicinal chemists used structure-activity relationships (SAR) and intuition to decide what other analogues should be synthesized. This process was very time consuming and, together with a success rate of production of a marketable drug of 1 in 10,000, resulted in drug design being a very expensive process. During the 1980s, a rapid increase in molecular biology techniques had resulted in the development of rapid, efficient drug testing systems, known as high throughput screening (HTS) (▶ **XR see Section 10.10**). These techniques were able to provide accurate results on extremely small quantities (µg) of test substances. However, in order to be used economically, HTS requires rapid production of very large numbers of test substances which could not be met by traditional synthesis. Combinatorial chemistry was developed to provide new test molecules in sufficient numbers to meet this need.

10.1 HISTORICAL DEVELOPMENT

The principle of combinatorial chemistry was first utilized in the 1960s for the synthesis of peptides. Merrifield, in 1963, introduced the first efficient solid state synthesis of peptides. This led to the development of rapid, automated synthesis of peptides for which Merrifield was awarded a Nobel Prize in Chemistry in 1984 (see Box 10.1). The application of solid state synthesis was not immediately applied to non-oligomeric substances because of the greater variety of reactants and reaction conditions required, unlike with peptides and other macromolecules. However, this changed in 1992, with the publication of the use of solid phase organic synthesis of 1,4-benzodiazepines, the first use of solid state synthesis for the production of drug-like molecules (Figure 10.1). The following few years saw an explosion in the use of combinatorial chemistry (as it was now called) in the synthesis of potential new drugs.

Figure 10.1 Solid phase organic synthesis of 1,4-benzodiazepines

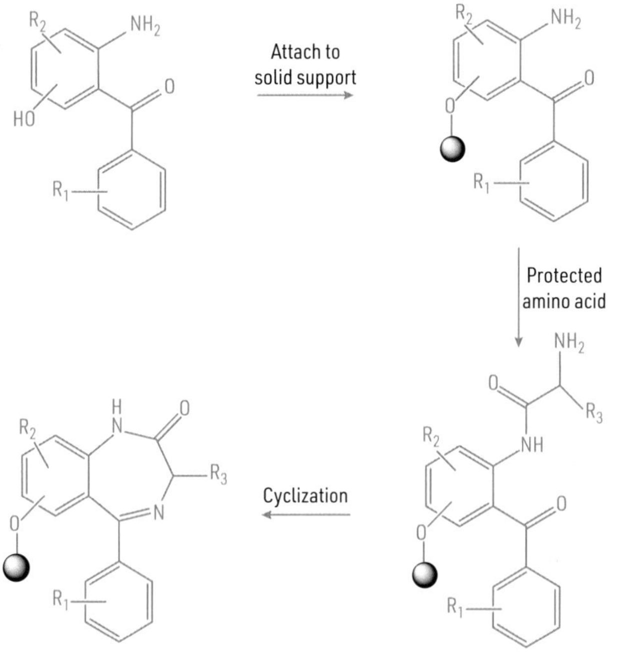

BOX 10.1 MERRIFIELD SOLID PHASE SUPPORT SYNTHESIS OF PEPTIDES

The initial process as used by Merrifield utilized a solid support of polystyrene-divinylbenzene resin beads functionalized with monochloromethyl sidechains. The initial amino acid in the peptide sequence reacted with the chloromethyl group at the C-terminus of the amino acid. In order for this to happen the N-terminus of the amino acid must be protected with a t-butyloxycarbonyl (Boc) group. After formation of the peptide bond, the protecting group can be removed by acid treatment and the now functionalized beads purified by washing. This cycle of reactions can now be repeated until the desired peptide is obtained (see Figure 10.1.1).

Figure 10.1.1 Merrifield solid phase support synthesis

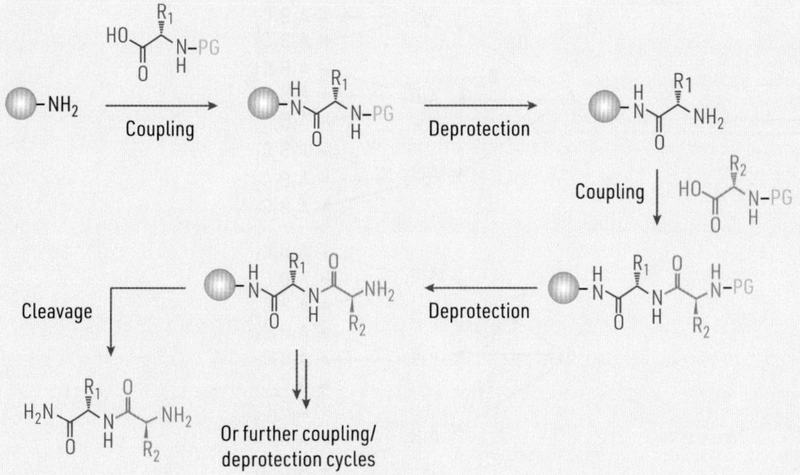

10.2 WHAT IS COMBINATORIAL CHEMISTRY?

Traditional drug synthesis involves the joining together of individual molecular building blocks in a linear fashion (Figure 10.2a). This is, by necessity, a slow process and can only yield relatively small numbers of new chemical entities (NCEs). Combinatorial chemistry involves the simultaneous reaction of a set of molecules (A) with a second set of molecules (B) to form what is known as a combinatorial library of new compounds (Figure 10.2b). The products of the initial reactions may be used in further iterations of reactions with a third set of molecules (C). This process has been described as 'a method of increasing the size of the haystack in which to find your needle'. Combinatorial libraries can vary in size, quantities and purity of compounds produced and molecular complexity. The number of molecules produced in a combinatorial library can easily be huge.

 Combinatorial chemistry involves the simultaneous reaction of a set of molecules with a number of sets of molecules to form a combinatorial library.

Two types of combinatorial library exist—the unbiased (or random) library and the directed library (**❯ XR see also Section 10.9**). An unbiased library typically has a common chemical core known as the

Figure 10.2a Traditional drug synthesis

$$A \ + \ B \longrightarrow A \!-\! B \xrightarrow{\ C\ } A \!-\! B \!-\! C$$

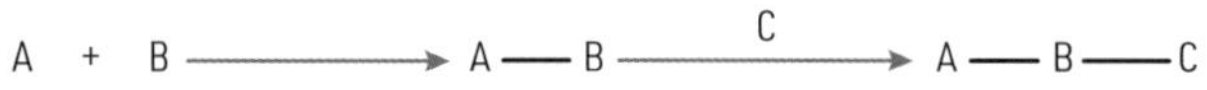

Figure 10.2b Combinatorial synthesis

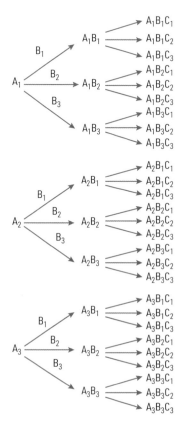

Figure 10.3 Spider scaffold for combinatorial synthesis

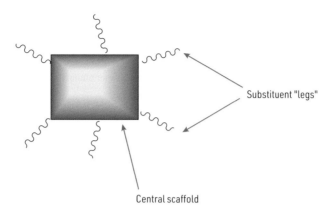

Substituent "legs"

Central scaffold

starting scaffold. In drug design the most useful scaffolds are spider scaffolds because various substituents ('legs') radiate from the centre. It is better for the legs to be spaced evenly around the scaffold as this allows a more effective probing of the 3D space around the scaffold (Figure 10.3). This type of library utilizes a large number of diverse building blocks and is aimed at generating lead molecules with the possibility of biological activity at numerous target sites. Directed libraries also have a common chemical scaffold but utilize a limited number of building blocks and are usually directed towards a specific target site, building on what is referred to as a 'privileged' structure, often based on modelling ligand-receptor interactions. It is estimated that between 1991 and 2003 about 2,500 combinatorial libraries were constructed, producing between 1 million and 2 million compounds.

 There are two types of combinatorial library—unbiased and directed.

There are two possible strategies for combinatorial synthesis—oligomer production and template production. Oligomer production proceeds by building blocks being added to the preceding structure and so the molecule grows in one direction only. In template production, synthesis proceeds in different directions from the initial scaffold (Figure 10.4). Both methods may require the use of protecting groups to ensure selectivity of reactions. Reactions in combinatorial chemistry must form a covalent bond between the

Figure 10.4 Oligomer and template production

$$W \xrightarrow{X} W - X \xrightarrow{Y} W - X - Y \xrightarrow{Z} W - X - Y - Z$$

Oligomer production

Template production

$$W \xrightarrow{X} W - X \xrightarrow{Y} W - X - Y \xrightarrow{Z} W - X - Y - Z$$

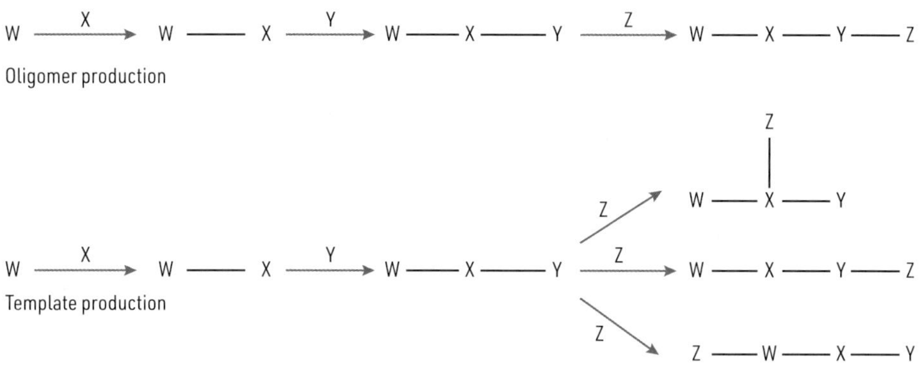

building blocks, they should provide predictable products, give a high yield, and be suitable for use in automated equipment. The building blocks should be readily available and be as diverse as possible in order to provide as wide a range of structures as possible in the final products.

 The two main strategies used in combinatorial synthesis are oligomer production and template production.

10.3 SOLID PHASE SYNTHESIS

The solid phase support synthetic method was pioneered by Merrifield in 1963 for peptide synthesis. The starting material is attached to an insoluble solid support—Merrifield used polystyrene-resin beads. These have now been replaced by resins which are more suitable for non-peptide synthesis, such as TentaGel resin, to which polyethylene glycol is attached, and polyacrylamide resins. The starting material is usually attached to the polymeric support material via a link molecule which is covalently attached to the polymeric chain. The link molecule possesses a functional group which can react with the starting material. Once this attachment is achieved, an excess of the next reactant is added, mixed and the excess reactant removed by filtration, the solid support is washed, and the next reactant added and so on. Once all the reactions are complete, the link to the solid support is cleaved to yield the target compound (Figure 10.5).

The advantages of using a solid support are that excess reagents can be used to drive the reactions to completion and can be easily removed by washing when the reaction is complete. Intermediates in the synthesis remain attached to the support and so do not need to be purified. In addition to beads, pins and chips and polyethylene bags (the 'tea bag method') have been used (Figure 10.6). In the bead, pin, and chip support methods, the synthesized molecules are attached to the support in an appropriate way. For bead supports the starting material is attached, via a linker, to the beads which are then immersed in a set of wells. For pins, the compounds are attached to 'crowns' placed on top of the pins, which are then suspended in a set of wells. The chip support is analogous to integrated circuit chips where films of starting materials are attached to silicon chips which are then immersed in solutions of reagents. The 'tea bag' consists of a number of mesh pockets with μm size pores filled with resin beads, each of which contains a compound attached to the beads. This method has the advantage of being able to label the bags, allowing for ease of identification of the product. Additionally, the method allows for the production of greater quantities (multi-mg) of each product, enabling easier structural identification. Just like a teabag, where the mesh size is too small to allow the tea to escape but water can penetrate, so the compounds attached to the resin beads cannot escape but reagents and solvent can penetrate.

Figure 10.5 Solid phase support synthesis

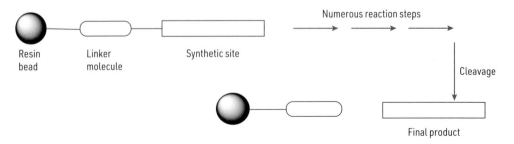

Figure 10.6 'Tea bag' method

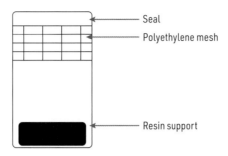

- Seal
- Polyethylene mesh
- Resin support

In solid phase support synthesis the starting material is linked to insoluble support material such as beads, pins, chips, or bags.

Solid phase support synthesis was initially used to produce libraries of separate compounds and this is referred to as parallel synthesis. The compounds are prepared in separate reaction vessels at the same time, i.e. in parallel. The process involves the use of an array of reaction vessels such as a 96 well plate or a pin and tray arrangement (Figure 10.7). Such equipment is suitable for automated control of the reactions and it is easy to keep track of each compound produced. Parallel synthesis is, however, only applicable to producing libraries of relatively small numbers of compounds (of the order of hundreds).

However other approaches have been made to generate libraries by pooling reactants and intermediates. The pool and split synthetic method is useful for producing both small and large combinatorial libraries. The compounds are still synthesized on solid supports such as beads. Each bead can contain a large number of molecules but all the molecules are the same. Different beads have different structures attached but are then mixed together in a single reaction vessel so that all the molecules undergo the same reaction. The resulting structures are not separated and purified but are tested for biological activity as a mixture (Figure 10.8). As this process is not a 'one vessel one product' process, unlike parallel synthesis, it is not possible to identify the history of a bead by a grid reference. Other methods must be used such as tagging (❯ **XR Section 10.6**) or deconvolution (❯ **XR Section 10.7**).

Figure 10.7 Examples of reaction vessels

a. 96 well plate

b. Pin and tray

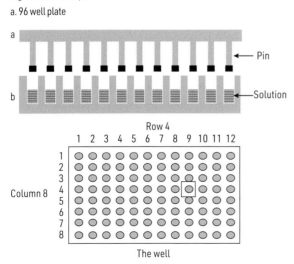

- Pin
- Solution

Row 4

Column 8

The well

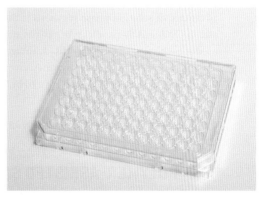

Figure 10.8 Pool and split synthetic method

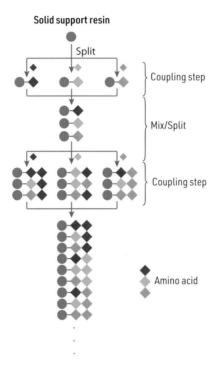

 Solid phase support can be used for parallel or pool and split synthesis.

10.4 SOLUTION PHASE SYNTHESIS

Most organic reactions take place in solution so it would appear to make sense to utilize solution phase synthesis. In its simplest form this is a number of solution phase reactions carried out simultaneously, i.e. parallel synthesis. Libraries of mixtures can be prepared by reacting each of the members of a set of similar compounds (Y1–8) in a 96 well plate with the mixture of all the members of a second set of compounds (X1–12) (Figure 10.9). This will yield, at this stage, ninety-six different compounds. The primary advantage of solution phase synthesis is the ease of characterization of products, as well as intermediates, if produced by parallel synthesis as standard characterization methods (such as HPLC-MS) can be used at each step. The primary disadvantage of this method is the purification that has to be carried out at each step. If solution phase synthesis were used to prepare mixtures of compounds then deconvolution (❯ XR Section 10.7) would have to be used to identify the biologically active compounds.

 Solution phase synthesis is used mainly for parallel synthesis.

10.5 POLYMER-ASSISTED SOLUTION PHASE SYNTHESIS

This method is essentially a hybrid between solid and solution phase synthesis. Some of the disadvantages of solution phase synthesis can be avoided by this method. The reagents are added to each step on a solid support, but with an excess of one of the reactants present in solution in order to drive the reaction

Figure 10.9 Solution phase parallel synthesis

A. Placement of first set of building blocks in ninety-six well plate

	A	B	C	D	E	F	G	H
1	Y1	Y2	Y3	Y4	Y5	Y6	Y7	Y8
2	Y1	Y2	Y3	Y4	Y5	Y6	Y7	Y8
3	Y1	Y2	Y3	Y4	Y5	Y6	Y7	Y8
4	Y1	Y2	Y3	Y4	Y5	Y6	Y7	Y8
5	Y1	Y2	Y3	Y4	Y5	Y6	Y7	Y8
6	Y1	Y2	Y3	Y4	Y5	Y6	Y7	Y8
7	Y1	Y2	Y3	Y4	Y5	Y6	Y7	Y8
8	Y1	Y2	Y3	Y4	Y5	Y6	Y7	Y8
9	Y1	Y2	Y3	Y4	Y5	Y6	Y7	Y8
10	Y1	Y2	Y3	Y4	Y5	Y6	Y7	Y8
11	Y1	Y2	Y3	Y4	Y5	Y6	Y7	Y8
12	Y1	Y2	Y3	Y4	Y5	Y6	Y7	Y8

B. Addition of second set of building blocks

	A	B	C	D	E	F	G	H
1	Y1-X1	Y2-X1	Y3-X1	Y4-X1	Y5-X1	Y6-X1	Y7-X1	Y8-X1
2	Y1-X2	Y2-X2	Y3-X2	Y4-X2	Y5-X2	Y6-X2	Y7-X2	Y8-X2
3	Y1-X3	Y2-X3	Y3-X3	Y4-X3	Y5-X3	Y6-X3	Y7-X3	Y8-X3
4	Y1-X4	Y2-X4	Y3-X4	Y4-X4	Y5-X4	Y6-X4	Y7-X4	Y8-X4
5	Y1-X5	Y2-X5	Y3-X5	Y4-X5	Y5-X5	Y6-X5	Y7-X5	Y8-X5
6	Y1-X6	Y2-X6	Y3-X6	Y4-X6	Y5-X6	Y6-X6	Y7-X6	Y8-X6
7	Y1-X7	Y2-X7	Y3-X7	Y4-X7	Y5-X7	Y6-X7	Y7-X7	Y8-X7
8	Y1-X8	Y2-X8	Y3-X8	Y4-X8	Y5-X8	Y6-X8	Y7-X8	Y8-X8
9	Y1-X9	Y2-X9	Y3-X9	Y4-X9	Y5-X9	Y6-X9	Y7-X9	Y8-X9
10	Y1-X10	Y2-X10	Y3-X10	Y4-X10	Y5-X10	Y6-X10	Y7-X10	Y8-X10
11	Y1-X11	Y2-X11	Y3-X11	Y4-X11	Y5-X11	Y6-X11	Y7-X11	Y8-X11
12	Y1-X12	Y2-X12	Y3-X12	Y4-X12	Y5-X12	Y6-X12	Y7-X12	Y8-X12

to completion. At the end of the reaction, the reaction mixture will comprise AB (the product) and excess reactant (B). Excess (B) can now be removed by use of a scavenger attached to a solid support designed to react with the reactant (B). This can now be removed by filtration. Excess reagent can be also removed in the same way. The solution now contains only the product (AB) and this can be isolated by removal of the solvent (see Figure 10.10).

 Polymer-assisted solution phase synthesis, as the name suggests, is a hybrid of solid phase and solution phase synthesis.

Figure 10.10 Polymer-assisted solution phase synthesis

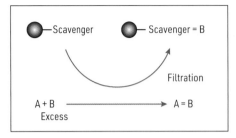
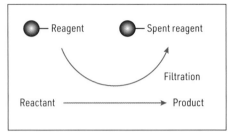

10.6 TAGGING

In pool and split techniques specialized tagging (also referred to as encoding) methods have to be used so that the reaction history of each bead can be known. There is a variety of methods used, including placing an identifiable tag compound onto the bead at each synthetic step (❯ XR Section 10.6.1), using a radiofrequency transponder chip (❯ XR Section 10.6.2) and barcoding methods (❯ XR Section 10.6.3).

 Tagging is a way of ensuring that the reaction history can be determined when using pool and split synthetic techniques.

10.6.1 Chemical tagging

In this method specific compounds (or tags) are added as a code for each step of the synthesis. The tags are attached to the same bead as the library compound at each step of the synthesis. When the synthesis is complete both the tag compound and the library compound are released from the bead. The tag can then be decoded to provide the history and the possible structure of the library compound (Figure 10.11). Tag compounds should satisfy several criteria. The tagging reaction must utilize reaction conditions compatible with those used in the library synthesis and the tag must be easily removed and separated from the library compound at the end of the synthesis. The analysis of the tag should be rapid, accurate and sensitive enough so that only a small amount of the tag is required, i.e. it should only occupy a small

Figure 10.11 Chemical tagging

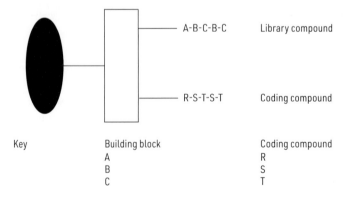

proportion of the linkers to the bead. The types of molecules used as tags are usually amino acids or oligonucleotides. The drawback of the tagging process is that it makes the whole combinatorial synthetic process more time-consuming and complicated. Tagging requires extra protection steps and may limit the type of reactions that can be used—oligonucleotides are particularly unstable.

 Chemical tagging involves attaching a chemical tag to the same beads as the library compounds.

10.6.2 **Radiofrequency transponder chips**

This method involves the use of silicon chips which can be coded to receive and store radio signals in the form of a binary code which is used as a code for the individual building blocks of the synthesis. The silicon chip and the beads are placed in a container which is porous to the reagents, essentially the 'tea bag' method of combinatorial synthesis. Each container is reacted with its required building blocks and the chip is irradiated with the appropriate radio signal for that building block. The pool and mix process is then carried out with the chips being appropriately irradiated at each step. At the end of the synthesis, the library compounds are separated from the chip and the radio signals from the chips decoded to reveal the history of the compounds.

 In the tea bag method of combinatorial synthesis a radiofrequency-labelled silicon chip is used to follow the reaction history.

10.6.3 **Barcoding**

This method of encoding involves assigning each building block its own chemical equivalent of a binary code for each stage of the synthesis. Often aryl halides are used because they are relatively inert, can be linked to the bead by a photo-labile bond (easily removed by irradiation) and can be detected in very small amounts by gas chromatography, in which the retention times can be equally spaced by appropriate choice of halide (Figure 10.12A). The gas chromatograph trace resembles a barcode (Figure 10.12B).

 Aryl halides are used as a chemical means of barcoding reactions in combinatorial synthesis.

Figure 10.12 **A.** Barcoding; **B.** GLC trace of released aryl halide tags

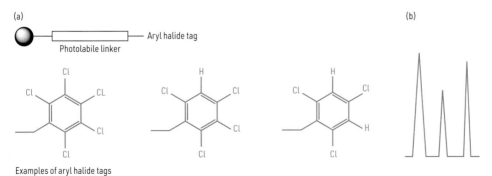

10.7 **DECONVOLUTION**

The success of combinatorial synthesis depends not only on the library containing the biologically active compounds, but also on the efficiency of the screening process for the biological activity. Very large combinatorial libraries require a very large amount of work to screen. Deconvolution is an important process in this respect and is the process of reducing the number of screening tests required to identify the most active member of a library. There are two types of deconvolution—iterative and subtractive.

 Deconvolution is the process used to identify the biologically active members of a combinatorial library.

Iterative deconvolution is the oldest type of deconvolution and was first used in the early days of combinatorial synthesis. Assume the combinatorial synthesis has produced the twenty-seven compounds in Figure 10.2b. Any given structure only appears in one of the groups (check this for yourself). If the biological activity is found only when C_3 is present (nine compounds), we know that C_3 is required for activity. Now, the smaller library is synthesized and these mixtures are screened and biological activity is found only when B_2 is present (three compounds), meaning that B_2 is also required for activity. Finally, $A_1B_2C_3$, $A_2B_2C_3$ and $A_3B_2C_3$ are synthesized separately and screened, revealing $A_2B_2C_3$ as the active structure.

 In iterative deconvolution the size of the combinatorial library is gradually reduced until the active structure is identified.

Subtractive deconvolution uses negative logic to reveal the biologically active member. Having carried out the original screen and identified biological activity, the same assay is carried out on a secondary library which has one building block missing. If the secondary library still shows the same activity as the original library, the missing building block is not part of the active structure. The process is repeated, each secondary library missing one building block. In this way the most important functional groups required for biological activity can be identified. Subsequently, a reduced library containing only these functional groups is prepared and the most active compounds identified by iterative deconvolution and one compound synthesis. This is the simplest case scenario and the situation may be more complicated if, for example, there is more than one active compound in the initial library. There may also be a number of poorly active compounds which show additive activity (false positive) or partial binding of inactive structures may prevent the binding of an active compound (false negative).

 In subtractive deconvolution combinatorial libraries with building blocks removed are screened to identify the functionalities required for biological activity.

10.8 **PURIFICATION AND ANALYSIS**

Combinatorial synthesis places significant demands on purification and analytical techniques. In many cases purification requires an extraction process. Liquid-liquid extraction is extensively used in solution phase combinatorial synthesis but can be problematical if emulsions are formed or if any of the impurities present have the same solubility properties as the desired products. Solid phase extraction can be used for acidic or basic impurities. An acidic chromatography column will remove basic impurities whilst a basic column will remove acidic impurities, the impurities remaining on the column as the product solution passes through the column.

Purification is important in solution phase combinatorial synthesis.

Analysis in combinatorial synthesis can be challenging because the methods used must be rapid, able to analyse very small quantities of material (nanomoles or picomoles of product) and, because the products then have to be biologically tested, non-destructive. Very few single analytical techniques can satisfy all these requirements and this leads to the use of 'hyphenated' analytical techniques such as HPLC-MS, FT-IR and certain NMR techniques (see Integration Box 10.1 Hyphenated analytical techniques).

INTEGRATION BOX 10.1   **HYPHENATED ANALYTICAL TECHNIQUES**

These techniques combine separation techniques with an appropriate analytical detection technique, thus exploiting the advantages of both of these techniques. The separation technique is usually some form of chromatography, e.g. GC, HPLC, **capillary electrophoresis**. These separation methods can produce pure fractions of the chemical components of a mixture, obtained, for example, by combinatorial chemistry. The linked analytical method can then provide information, both qualitative and quantitative, about the individual components. The most commonly used analytical method is mass spectrometry because of its sensitivity and the ability, from the fragmentation pattern, to determine the identity of the component being analysed. More recently, as a result of increasing sophistication of all of these techniques, so-called double hybrid techniques have become more common, e.g. LC-MS-MS, SE (solid phase extraction)-LC-MS.

 Mainly hyphenated analytical techniques are required in combinatorial synthesis because of the minute quantities produced.

10.9 ESTABLISHMENT AND FORMAT OF COMBINATORIAL LIBRARIES

The design of a combinatorial library will be dependent on the specific purpose of the production of that library. Essentially, there are two basic types of combinatorial library. The first of these is an unbiased or random library. This is typically based on a common chemical scaffold and will involve a large number of highly diverse building blocks. This type of library is looking to generate lead molecules directed, probably, towards a number of biological targets, will generate in excess of 5,000 compounds and usually employs solid phase synthesis (one bead one compound if possible). The second type is a directed library which is used to optimize lead structures and is directed towards a specific biological target. Such a library usually contains less than 5,000 compounds and can be produced by solid phase or solution synthesis.

The format of combinatorial libraries can be divided into three groups—one bead one compound, pre-encoded, and spatially addressable. One bead one compound format is used for very large libraries and utilizes the pool and split solid phase synthesis. The size of the library varies between 10,000 and 2,000,000 compounds and produces approximately 0.1–1nmole of product. Because of the size of the library and the fact that it produces a mixture of compounds, deconvolution is necessary, and the purity of selected members only is assessed.

Pre-encoded (i.e. tagged) libraries are used to produce individual compounds in mg quantities. These employ pool and split solid phase synthesis with radiofrequency or other labelling. The size of these

Figure 10.13 Automated combinatorial synthesis workstation

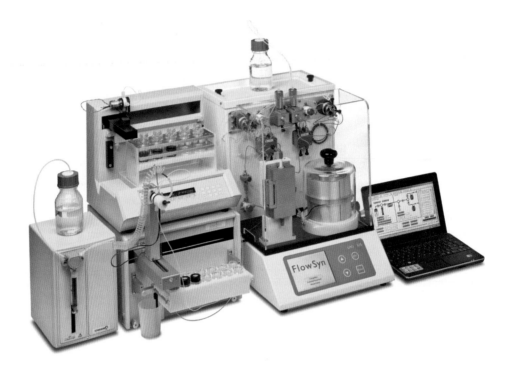

libraries is between 1000 and 100,000 compounds and yields 5—100µmole of product. Because of the quantity of product produced, the purity of smaller libraries can be assessed prior to screening.

Spatially addressed libraries (the structure of a compound can be inferred from its position in the library) utilize parallel solid phase or solution phase synthesis in arrayed reaction vessels. The solid phase method is used to produce libraries of 100–20,000 compounds in 10–100µmole quantities, whereas the solution phase method is used to produce libraries of 100–5000 compounds in 10–250µmole quantities. Because these are both parallel syntheses, purity can be determined prior to screening. Spatially addressed libraries tend to utilize fully automated workstations such as in Figure 10.13.

 The format of a combinatorial library will depend on the purpose of the production of that library and can vary in the number and amounts of compounds produced.

10.10 HIGH THROUGHPUT SCREENING (HTS)

Advances in biotechnology have allowed the automation and miniaturization of *in vitro* tests using genetically modified cells. Now large numbers of compounds (typically several thousands) can be tested simultaneously in a range of biochemical tests (up to fifty). This is known as high throughput screening (HTS).

As stated in the introduction to this chapter, the development of HTS was responsible for the development of combinatorial synthesis, in order to meet the demands for the very large numbers of compounds required to operate HTS efficiently. Indeed, the increase in efficiency of combinatorial synthesis has meant that attempts are being made to make HTS more efficient. Originally, HTS involved automated tests on 96 well plates of capacity 0.1ml. These days the test plates used contain 1,536 wells with volumes of 1—10μl. Further miniaturization to allow use of volumes below 1μl requires closed systems and the use of microfluidics. There are now analytical instruments that can support 10^5 separate bioassays on a nanolitre scale on a 10×10 cm silicon wafer.

 HTS is designed to screen large numbers of compounds, present in minute quantities, in a variety of biological assays.

Any HTS assay must be accurate, reproducible and have a high signal-to-noise ratio because of the minute quantities of the test compounds. Often the outcome of HTS is a qualitative (yes/no) or semi-quantitative (high/medium/low) one, rather than a precise numerical value such as ED_{50} or LD_{50}. The enzymic methods used for detection are either radiometric or non-radiometric. The radiometric methods involve the use of radioisotopes, such as the filtration radiometric assays. In this type of assay the radioactive substrate which is bound to a **capture group** is cleaved by its enzyme, thus removing the radioactivity from the capture group. The mixture is filtered and the capture group remains on the filter. A **scintillation fluid** is added to the product on the filter and the radioactivity is measured. The degree to which the radioactivity is retained measures the strength of the inhibition of the enzyme (Figure 10.14).

 Many HTS assays tend to have a qualitative or semi-quantitative endpoint.

Non-radiometric methods include UV absorbance, fluorescence, and luminescence spectroscopy. Other HTS assay methods include the use of bacteria and yeast cells, cloned mammalian receptors in micro-organisms, protein-protein interactions, and DNA and protein array assays. For further details of these types of assays please refer to the Further reading at the end of this chapter.

Figure 10.14 Filtration radiometric enzymic assay

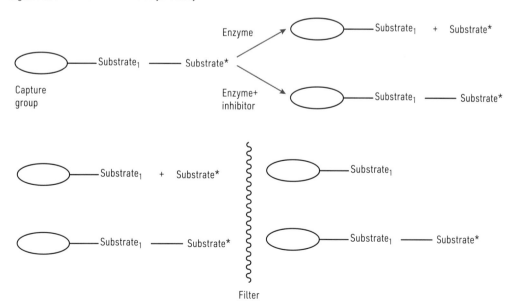

10.11 CHEMOGENOMICS

In theory, chemogenomics can be defined as the screening of all possible chemical compounds against all potential drug targets. In reality, it is the study of the genomic response of a biological system to a selection of chemical compounds. It involves systematic screening of targeted chemical libraries of small molecules against individual drug target families (e.g. GPCRs, kinases etc.) to identify novel drugs and drug targets and utilizes known active compounds which function as ligands as probes of genomic function. Chemogenomics can be investigated in the forward (classical) or reverse manner. Forward chemogenomics is an attempt to identify drug targets by searching for molecules which give a particular **phenotypic** effect thus allowing an investigation of the mechanism of action of that effect. In reverse chemogenomics gene sequences of interest are expressed as target proteins and screened against compound libraries in order to learn more about the role of the protein in the phenotypic response.

? Questions

1. What are the desirable properties for the building blocks in a combinatorial synthesis?

2. What are the desirable properties for a linker molecule to be used in solid phase support synthesis?

3. In the solid phase synthesis of a range of dipeptides what precautions are necessary when including the following amino acids: methionine, tyrosine, serine, and lysine?

↻ Chapter summary

- Combinatorial synthesis was first used in the 1960s for production of peptides but it was not until the 1990s that it was used for synthesis of drug-like molecules.

- Combinatorial synthesis involves the simultaneous reaction of a set of structurally similar molecules with one or more sets of different molecules to yield a combinatorial library.

- Combinatorial chemistry can involve solid phase support or solution phase methods.

- Combinatorial chemistry can involve parallel synthesis or pool and split synthesis.

- Pool and split synthetic methods require the use of tagging to identify the history of each synthetic step.

- Reactions can be tagged by using specific tag compounds at each reaction step, by using radiofrequency labelled chips at each step, or by using chemical barcoding.

- Deconvolution is the process used to identify the biologically active members of a combinatorial library and is necessary because of the large numbers of compounds in combinatorial libraries.

- Deconvolution involves reducing the number of screening tests required to identify the most biologically active member of a combinatorial library and may be an iterative process or a subtractive process.

- Purification steps are more often required in solution phase synthesis.

- Analytical methods must be rapid and able to work effectively with very small amounts of material.

- The design of a combinatorial library will depend on the purpose for the production of that library and may be random or directed.

- HTS is designed to screen large numbers of compounds, present in minute quantities, in a variety of biological assays and tend to have a qualitative or semi-quantitative output.

📖 Further reading

Merrifield, R.B. (1963) Solid phase peptide synthesis 1. The synthesis of tetrapeptides, *Journal of the American Chemical Society* 85: 2149–53.

The original publication on combinatorial synthesis.

Furka, A. (2002) Combinatorial chemistry: 20 years . . ., *Drug Discovery Today* 7: 1–4.

A review of the first 20 years of combinatorial chemistry.

Combinatorial Chemistry (2012) http:/youtube.com/watch?v=MVgsX7PM4F4.

A Youtube video from the Royal Society of Chemistry.

Dittrich, P.S. and Manz, A. (2006) Lab-on-a-chip: Microfluidics in drug discovery, *Nature Reviews Drug Discovery* 5: 210–18.

An account of the role of microfluidics in drug discovery.

Landro, J.A. et al. (2000) HTS in the new millennium—the role of pharmacology and flexibility, *Journal of Pharmacological and Toxicological* 44: 273–89.

A review of HTS from a biological viewpoint.

Venton, D.L. and Woodbury, C.P. (1999) Screening combinatorial libraries, *Chemometrics and Intelligent Laboratory Systems* 48: 131–50.

A thorough review of high throughput screening.

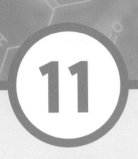

11

Biotechnology and Biopharmaceuticals

The rapid developments in biotechnology over the last 30 years have not only impacted on the biological assays of potential drug molecules (▶ **XR Section 10.10**) but also have changed the nature of drug design and development. Whereas small molecules dominated the search for new drugs for many years and have been the focus of previous chapters, biopharmaceuticals (also known as biologicals) now tend to dominate the search for and design of potential new drugs. These biopharmaceuticals are being produced by recombinant DNA (rDNA) technology (▶ **XR Section 11.2**). rDNA largely gives rises to molecules that are protein in nature (▶ **XR Section 11.3**) with all the difficulties associated with the production, delivery and use of such molecules as drugs (▶ **XR Section 11.3.1**). The protein molecules, currently used or being investigated as drugs, include hormones (▶ **XR Section 11.4**), cytokines (▶ **XR Section 11.5**), antibodies (▶ **XR Section 11.6**). In addition, advances in genomics has led to the development of gene therapy (▶ **XR Section 11.8**) and antisense therapy (▶ **XR Section 11.7**), involving recombinant genes and oligonucleotides respectively as therapeutic agents.

11.1 BIOTECHNOLOGY AND DRUG DESIGN

The Oxford Dictionary definition of biotechnology is 'the exploitation of biological processes for industrial and other purposes, especially the genetic manipulation of microorganisms for the production of antibodies, hormones etc.'. Within this definition, biotechnology can be said to include proteomics, design and development of biopharmaceuticals, genomics and gene therapy, possibly with a view towards the generation of personalized medicines, i.e. the elimination of the 'one drug fits all' basis of pharmaceutical care (see Integration Box 11.1).

INTEGRATION BOX 11.1	PERSONALIZED MEDICINE

Every individual is genetically unique and individual variations in their genes can influence an individual's health and responses to disease. Until recently a lack of knowledge of these genetic variations has meant that medication has relied on the 'one size fits all' approach, although it was often apparent that not all drugs worked equally well for all patients, e.g. antidepressants only work for about 60 per cent of patients. Advances in biotechnology such as genome sequencing has led towards the ability to diagnose which therapies would be appropriate based on the patient's genetic makeup, now termed **pharmacogenomics**. Pharmacogenomics could be used to determine appropriate doses of drugs and to help prevent adverse effects or, indeed, whether a drug will be of any value to a particular patient. There are, however, many ethical issues to be resolved regarding personalized medicine before it becomes more widely accepted (see Questions at end of the chapter).

In the past, drug therapy has been based on so-called 'small molecule' drugs and these still comprise the major proportion of therapeutic agents used today. These small drugs have been developed by partial or complete chemical synthesis and are generally small organic compounds with a molecular weight of less than 500. Mostly they have been developed for oral administration and are absorbed into the bloodstream from the gastrointestinal tract. However, since the 1990s, there has been an increasing emphasis on the development of what are now known as biopharmaceuticals. These are usually chemically similar to endogenous biomolecules which are more effective at interacting with their target receptors. The use of biopharmaceuticals does, however, present some challenges. Being chemically similar to endogenous molecules, they are easily metabolized by endogenous catabolic routes and thus are not stable *in vivo*. Because they are mostly protein in nature oral administration is usually not possible due to degradation in, and poor absorption from, the gastrointestinal tract. In addition, by comparison with most small organic molecules, they are more difficult and costly to manufacture. Nevertheless the use of biopharmaceuticals has led to the introduction of therapeutic agents for conditions which were previously considered difficult or impossible to treat by conventional drug therapy such as cancers and some autoimmune diseases (see Table 11.1).

Initially biotechnology was used to produce pharmaceutical products such as antibiotics like β-lactams, tetracyclines and macrolides. More recently, biotechnology has been used to produce biological therapeutic products such as blood products, hormones, vaccines etc. The more recent focus has been on protein or nucleic acid based therapeutic agents such as monoclonal antibodies, cytokines, and oligonucleotides produced in genetically engineered organisms by recombinant DNA technology.

Table 11.1 Examples of therapeutic uses of biopharmaceuticals

Types of biopharmaceutical product	Therapeutic area
Hormones	Diabetes, neurology
Interferons	Oncology, hepatitis
Interleukins	Oncology, blood disorders
Blood products	Blood disorders
Tumour necrosis factor	Rheumatoid arthritis
Monoclonal antibodies	Diagnostic testing, oncology
Antisense nucleotides	Oncology, AIDS
Gene therapy	Inherited genetic diseases, oncology

Biotechnology processes are used to produce existing drugs like antibiotics but are increasingly being used to produce biologically based therapeutic agents.

11.2 RECOMBINANT DNA (rDNA) TECHNOLOGY

The key development which led to the increase in the use of biotechnology was that of rDNA which allows the extraction of genetic material from one organism and the insertion of it into another organism, allowing it to produce protein. In order to understand the processes involved in rDNA technology it would be very useful to read the material relating to the normal transcription of DNA into RNA, and the translation of RNA into protein in an earlier chapter (❯ (**XR Sections 4.1.2 and 4.1.3**).

rDNA technology involves a number of steps—retrieving or isolating a gene of interest, fusing the gene with a vector, introducing the vector into a host, selecting the transgenic host, propagating the gene and expressing the protein. In order for rDNA techniques to be successful there are a number of requirements which must be satisfied. There must be an efficient method for cleaving and re-joining fragments of DNA (genes) derived from a variety of sources. There must be suitable vectors capable of replicating the foreign DNA placed in them (and capable of replicating themselves). Finally, there must be a means of introducing the rDNA into a host organism and the ability to select the population of that organism which possesses the rDNA molecule.

 Recombinant DNA technology allows the insertion of genetic material from one organism into another organism.

11.2.1 Obtaining the gene of interest

There are three sources which can be used in the production of rDNA—these are genomic DNA, DNA libraries and synthesized DNA. The use of genomic DNA involves the isolation of the mRNA that encodes for the protein of specific interest. This mRNA is then treated with reverse transcriptase in the presence of nucleotide triphosphates. This causes a strand of DNA to be produced which is complementary to the mRNA, producing an RNA-DNA hybrid (Figure 11.1). The RNA strand is then degraded in alkaline conditions to yield a single strand of DNA. Use of DNA polymerase produces a complementary strand of DNA, (cDNA), which can be fused with a vector.

The use of DNA libraries involves the creation of a library of DNA fragments from a cell's genome (which represents all the genes present). This library is then screened using special DNA probes. The genomic contents are lysed to generate a variety of DNA fragments, some of which will contain the DNA sequence which encodes the specific protein required. Using DNA probes (which have been synthesized to specifically hybridize with the required fragments) labelled with fluorescent or radioactive tags, double-stranded DNA can be identified and isolated. This DNA is subsequently amplified by a polymerase chain reaction (PCR) and fused with a vector.

The final method of obtaining DNA is by automated synthesis using combinatorial chemistry (❯ **XR Section 10.2**), although this method is only suitable for the production of DNA encoding for small proteins. The synthetic DNA is then fused with a vector.

 There are three sources used in the production of rDNA—genomic DNA, library DNA, and synthetic DNA.

Figure 11.1 Retrieving the gene of interest

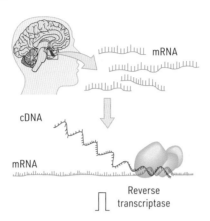

11.2.2 Inserting the gene into a vector

Vectors (or carriers) are the most widely used methods for inserting foreign (or passenger) DNA into a host cell. The types of vectors most commonly used are bacterial **plasmids**, **bacteriophages** or viruses which have been genetically engineered to accept fragments of foreign DNA (see Integration Box 11.2).

Initially, the DNA fragment of interest must be excised from the larger DNA molecule. This is achieved by the use of restriction endonucleases, which can be regarded as a set of 'molecular scissors'. Restriction endonucleases are enzymes which cleave phosphodiester bonds within a DNA molecule. This cleavage occurs at specific sites of nucleotide sequences of six to eight base pairs. There are a large number of restriction endonucleases (> 500) and they operate at more than a hundred cleavage sites. The same restriction endonuclease is also used to cleave the vector DNA, and then the two DNA fragments are joined together by a process called annealing. Initially, the vector DNA is heated, and this causes unwinding of the double helix. The DNA to be inserted (passenger DNA) is added, and the mixture cooled causing pairing of complementary strands. The phosphodiester bonds are regenerated by enzymes called DNA ligases. This process is known as ligation and results in the linking of the vector and the passenger DNA molecules. The vector is then effectively a rDNA molecule which can be inserted into a host cell (Figure 11.2). In many cases an antibiotic resistance gene is inserted linked to the required gene, in order to aid subsequent selection of the transgenic host.

INTEGRATION BOX 11.2   PLASMIDS AND BACTERIOPHAGES

Plasmids are the most commonly used vectors to introduce passenger DNA into host cells such as bacterial or yeast cells. A plasmid is a small circular double-stranded DNA molecule. For example, the *E.coli* bacterial plasmid contains 4,361 base pairs and can transport relatively small amounts of DNA. Plasmids are normally transported between bacterial cells via their **pili** to allow the 'sharing' of genetic information and are a means of generating antibiotic resistance by transferring mutated genes that have coded for improved antibiotic resistance.

Bacteriophages are much larger than plasmids and are, in fact, bacterial viruses. They contain up to 500,000 base pairs and can accommodate much larger amounts of passenger DNA. They can also be responsible for the development of bacterial antibiotic resistance.

Figure 11.2   Fusing the gene with a vector

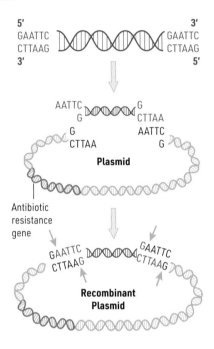

 Plasmids, bacteriophages and viruses are used as vectors for insertion of foreign DNA into a host cell.

11.2.3 Inserting the vector into a host

Host cells are most often bacterial cells (e.g. *E.coli*), yeast cells (e.g. *Saccharomyces* spp.), or mammalian cell lines (Figure 11.3). From a production point of view it is more appropriate to use bacterial or yeast cells as these are able to produce high protein yields by the use of fermentation. Mammalian cell lines, although they produce lower protein yields, are used when the product requires post-translation modifications because these cannot occur in bacteria (see Integration Box 11.3).

INTEGRATION BOX 11.3   **POST-TRANSLATION MODIFICATION**

Following translation, many proteins are modified in some way. They can be made more resistant to degradation by proteases by N-acetylation at the N-terminal. Hydroxyl groups in serine, threonine, and tyrosine may be phosphorylated, which takes place in certain cell signalling pathways (➤ **XR e.g. Section 2.2.5**). Often proteins, particularly those at the cell surface, are linked to carbohydrates and are vital in cell-cell recognition and disease processes. A number of proteins are broken down into smaller proteins, or even peptides, following translation. For example, insulin, a two-chain protein, was initially produced as two separate single polypeptide chains in separate bacterial strains, the chains isolated and attached to each other by disulphide linkages. It has now been found to be more efficient to produce recombinant proinsulin which is then converted to insulin by proteolytic cleavage (➤ **XR Section 11.4.1**).

Figure 11.3   Introducing the vector into a host

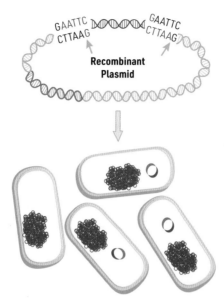

The two main methods for introducing the vector into the host cells are electroporation and gene guns. Electroporation is a technique which uses an electric field to increase the permeability of cell membranes, allowing the entry of the vector to the cell. The application of an electrostatic field causes the formation of water-filled pores in the cell membrane through which the vector can pass.

A gene gun is, as the name suggests, a delivery system that injects the vector into a cell and the 'bullet' is a heavy metal particle coated with the vector DNA. Originally, the heavy metal used was tungsten, but gold is used more often now as it is more uniform in nature and less toxic to cells. The propellant used to 'fire' the particle is pressurized helium.

 Bacterial cells, yeast cells or mammalian cells can be used as host cells for the foreign DNA which is introduced into these cells by electroporation or use of a gene gun.

11.2.4 Selecting the transgenic host

Host cells containing the vector are grown in small-scale cultures and screened for the required gene using selective growth media. For example, if the host cell is a bacterial cell, the antibiotic resistance gene (❯ XR Section 11.2.2) will enable the bacteria to grow on a medium containing the antibiotic, whereas bacteria not containing the resistance gene will not grow, thus allowing selection of the host cells possessing the required gene.

 Host cells are grown on selective media to allow the selection of those host cells containing the foreign DNA.

11.2.5 Propagating the gene and expressing the protein

Once the clone providing the correct protein and the best protein yield has been isolated, the selected organism is grown under carefully controlled conditions. The production conditions, which need to be investigated for optimization, are the pH and composition of the growth medium, the control of temperature, and the extent of agitation and aeration. Under the optimum conditions the host cells divide, the DNA within them replicates and the required protein is expressed. This process will, initially, be carried out on a pilot scale and, once successful, is scaled up for large-scale production. The host cells will, of course, produce their own proteins, as well as the recombinant protein, and thus some purification will be necessary before the recombinant protein can be developed as a new pharmaceutical product.

The purification of recombinant proteins was originally based on standard chromatographic methods. More recently, however, the process involves centrifugation, column chromatography and, finally, sodium dodecyl sulphate-polyacrylamide gel electrophoresis (SDS-PAGE). Differential centrifugation isolates the various cellular fragments. The appropriate fractions are further separated by column chromatography, during which molecules can be separated by size (gel filtration), charge (ion exchange chromatography), and specific binding characteristics (affinity chromatography). Finally, individual proteins can be separated and visualized by SDS-PAGE (see Box 11.1 Separation techniques).

BOX 11.1   SEPARATION TECHNIQUES

In gel filtration a column is filled with beads of different pore sizes. As a protein mixture passes down the column, large proteins which cannot fit into the pores pass through the column rapidly, whereas smaller proteins can enter the pores and, therefore, flow more slowly. Different fractions can be collected from the column by eluting with buffer solutions. Ion exchange chromatographic columns have beads which possess charged groups at their surface. Positive charges bind acidic amino acids and negative charges bind basic amino acids. Different proteins bind with differing affinities depending on their amino acid composition. The eluent used is one of increasing salt concentration (either NaCl or KCl), and different proteins elute at different salt concentrations. In affinity chromatography columns, beads are tagged with a specific compound, e.g. glutathione. Proteins also tagged with glutathione will bind to the beads, by disulphide linkages, and so are retained. Non-tagged proteins will be washed through the column. The glutathione-tagged proteins can then be eluted from the column with glutathione which competes with the protein for the glutathione on the beads. SDS-PAGE involves heating the protein sample with sodium dodecyl sulphate (SDS) and β-mercaptoethanol. The acidic surfactant SDS coats the proteins and masks the proteins' surface charge, thus giving each protein a similar mass/charge ratio. The proteins are then loaded onto the polyacrylamide gel (PAG) and an electric field applied. Because the charges on the proteins are similar, the proteins move through the gel at different speeds according to their mass.

 Once selected, the host cells containing the foreign DNA are grown under appropriate conditions to allow optimum division of the cells and expression of the recombinant protein.

11.3 RECOMBINANT PROTEINS AS DRUGS

Before dealing with the classes of recombinant proteins that are being used or researched as drugs, the various pharmaceutical problems which they pose must be highlighted. By their very nature, proteins give rise to significant deviations from the general pharmacokinetic and pharmacodynamics principles which apply to small drug molecules. They are structurally similar to endogenous molecules and are involved in normal physiological processes leading to difficulty in detection and analysis in the body. Additionally they are relatively large in size (❯ **XR Integration Box 8.3**). The consequences of all these factors have significant effects on the absorption, distribution, and metabolism of such molecules.

The use of proteins as drugs poses a number of significant pharmaceutical problems.

11.3.1 Pharmacokinetic challenges of protein drugs

From an absorption point of view, recombinant protein molecules are generally not active by oral administration because they are unstable to gastrointestinal enzymes and exhibit poor absorption through the intestinal mucosa. Parenteral administration is most often used (SC, IM, IV), as this provides a higher bioavailability but has the disadvantage of requiring a sterile product and is not particularly suitable for patient self-administration. Inhalational administration is a good route for biopharmaceuticals as it avoids first pass metabolism, and the respiratory passages and lungs provide rapid access to the bloodstream because they are highly vascularized. Transdermal delivery is being progressively used as a route of administration, particularly for recombinant insulin.

Recombinant proteins can bind significantly to endogenous proteins, particularly plasma proteins such as serum albumin. This binding will add another biodistribution compartment to the pharmacokinetic profile and will increase the half-life, affecting the dose required to achieve a steady state.

Recombinant proteins are particularly susceptible to breakdown by proteolytic enzymes. These enzymes are not only present in the gastrointestinal tract (as previously mentioned), but also in the liver, kidneys, blood, and, to some extent, in most other body fluids and tissues.

In addition to the pharmacokinetic issues, recombinant proteins are associated with the issue of immunogenicity. Therapeutic proteins can be recognized as foreign protein and may trigger an immune response with varying clinical consequences. The cause of the immune response may be structural, in that modifications may have been made deliberately to the protein (such as amino acid substitution) or may have happened as part of the production process such as incorrect protein folding or oxidation of a sulphur amino acid. In addition to these structural factors, if the production process has involved the use of a bacterial vector, there may be some residual bacterial protein in the final product. All of these factors will contribute to the antigenicity of the final product which, when administered to a patient, will cause the immune system to react against it. However, if the protein has been engineered to a 100 per cent complementarity to the human form, most of these immunogenicity issues should be avoided and so current research is aimed at producing 100 per cent human protein drugs, such as has been achieved with insulin (**>** XR Section 11.4.1).

 Recombinant proteins exhibit difficult pharmacokinetic profiles in that they are poorly absorbed, susceptible to degradation by proteolytic enzymes and bind to endogenous proteins such as serum albumin. They can also trigger an immune response when administered to patients.

11.4 HORMONES

Many hormones are used clinically as therapeutic or diagnostic agents and this use has increased due to the use of biotechnologically produced products. It should always be remembered that most hormones have a number of biological actions, and may, therefore, give rise to clinically significant side effects.

11.4.1 Insulin

Insulin is produced by the β-cells of the pancreas in response to high levels of glucose in the blood and induces cellular uptake of glucose as well as stimulating glycolysis and fatty acid synthesis. It is composed of two polypeptide chains (A and B) linked by disulphide bridges, comprising of a total of fifty-one

Figure 11.4 Insulin

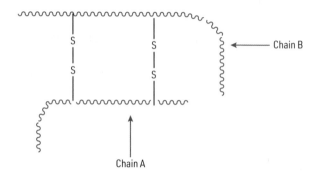

amino acids (Figure 11.4). Insulin has been used as the first line treatment for insulin-dependent (type 1) diabetes for many years. Originally the insulin used was obtained from porcine and bovine pancreatic sources. The use of insulin from both of these sources, which differ slightly from human insulin, caused immunological reactions in some patients.

These difficulties were overcome by the approval, in 1982, of genetically engineered human insulin. This was the first biopharmaceutically engineered product to be introduced. The recombinant insulin is chemically and physically indistinguishable from the human pancreatic hormone and the immunological problem has been eliminated. Originally, the recombinant insulin was produced using different vectors for the two peptide chains and joining them together after expression (Figure 11.5). Now, recombinant DNA technology is used to produce proinsulin from a proinsulin gene, and the connecting peptide is cleaved enzymatically just as happens in the pancreas.

11.4.2 Glucagon

Glucagon is also produced in the pancreas in response to low levels of glucose, resulting in a breakdown of glycogen and gluconeogenesis, both of which will raise blood glucose levels. Glucagon is a single chain peptide comprised of twenty-nine amino acids and has two clinical uses. It is used to treat insulin-induced hypoglycaemia in insulin-dependent diabetics and is also used diagnostically to relax smooth muscles of the gastrointestinal tract in order to reduce gastric motility during radiological examination. Unlike insulin, glucagon from bovine and porcine sources is identical to human glucagon so there ought to be no need for recombinant glucagon. However, the anxiety about the acquiring of bovine spongiform encephalopathy (mad cow disease) (see Box 11.2), from bovine sources has led to the use of recombinant glucagon produced using *Saccharomyces cerevisiae*.

Figure 11.5 Production of recombinant insulin

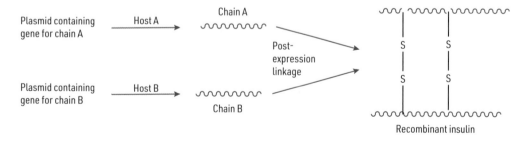

11.4.3 Human growth hormone (hGH)

Produced by the anterior pituitary gland, hGH promotes normal body growth and development and has been used since the 1950s for successful treatment of growth hormone deficiency (pituitary dwarfism), Turner's syndrome (lack of one X chromosome), chronic renal insufficiency, and failure to lactate in women. hGH used to be extracted from deceased humans as it is highly species specific. However this was stopped as it was a suspected cause of Creutzfeldt–Jakob disease (see Box 11.2).

BOX 11.2   PRIONS

Prion diseases are characterized by degenerative changes in the central nervous system, usually developing over several years. These conditions are characterized by impairment of brain function, dementia, and difficulty with coordinating movement (ataxia). They have been shown to be responsible for bovine spongiform encephalopathy (BSE), also known as mad cow disease and Creutzfeldt–Jakob disease (CJD) and its variant (vCJD). These conditions were originally thought to be caused by viruses but are now known to be caused by prions which have been inadvertently ingested or injected. A prion consists of protease resistant protein without any detectable DNA or RNA and this protein (PrP) is found in healthy people on the membranes of cells and is termed PrP^c (where c = cellular). In infected tissue, PrP has a different physical structure known as an isoform. This isoform of PrP replicates by triggering the conversion of normal PrP into the infected form by changing the normal protein into its own abnormal conformation via a protein-protein interaction. Once the initial conversion has occurred a chain reaction takes place whereby large amounts of the abnormal prion protein are formed, producing protein aggregates which are highly stable and accumulate in infected tissue. The resistance of prion protein to degradation poses a problem with respect to containment and makes destruction of prions difficult.

The first recombinant hGH was introduced in 1985 and was produced using *E.coli*. This preparation contained 192 amino acids with a terminal methionine, whereas the natural hGH contains only 191 amino acids. Natural sequence hGH has now been produced in mammalian (mouse) cell cultures.

Because hGH promotes lipolysis (in order to increase body lean mass/fat ratio) it has been tried as an anti-obesity treatment but without any appreciable success. hGH is currently undergoing clinical trials as a treatment for severe burns on the basis that it reduces protein catabolism which is a response to severe burns.

 The human hormones insulin, glucagon and human growth hormone are now produced by recombinant technology.

11.5 CYTOKINES

Cytokines are a group of regulatory proteins that act as intercellular chemical messengers. They are produced mainly by leucocytes and other cells of the immune system and are involved in haemopoiesis and the immune response. Cytokines include interferons, interleukins, haematopoietic growth factors, and tumour necrosis factor.

11.5.1 Interferons

The interferons are a family of proteins first discovered in the 1950s, and their name is derived from the property of interfering with the viral infection of eukaryotic cells (Figure 11.6). Interferons have two effects: initially they cause the recruitment of natural killer cells to kill the virally infected host cells and then they induce antiviral resistance in neighbouring cells, thus preventing the spread of the virus. There are three classes of interferons which have been characterized (Table 11.2), currently totalling more than eighteen distinct interferons. Interferons are all glycoproteins with α-interferons, derived from human leucocytes, β-interferons from fibroblasts, and macrophages and γ-interferons from human T lymphocytes, and natural killer cells. Although there are a number in clinical usage, it must always be borne in mind that most interferons inhibit cytochrome P450, raising the likelihood of interactions with drugs metabolized by this system.

11.5.2 Interleukins (IL)

The interleukins are a large group of proteins (currently about 30) with roles in immune cell growth and differentiation (see Table 11.3 for examples). The interleukins which have found most clinical usage are IL-2 and IL-11.

Figure 11.6 Activity of interferons

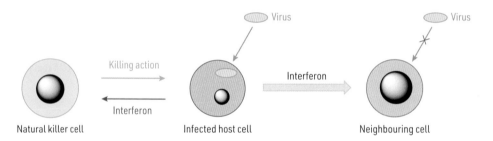

Table 11.2 Examples of clinically used interferons

Interferon	Source	Clinical use
Interferon alfa-2a	E. coli	Hairy cell leukaemia, chronic hepatitis C, AIDS-related Kaposi's sarcoma
Peginterferon alfa-2a	E. coli	Chronic hepatitis C
Interferon alfa-2b	E. coli	Hairy cell leukaemia, chronic hepatitis C, AIDS-related Kaposi's sarcoma, genital warts
Interferon alfa-n1	Human lymphoblastoid cell line	Chronic hepatitis C
Interferon Alpha-n3	Human leucocytes	Genital warts
Interferon Alfacon-1	E. coli	Chronic hepatitis C
Interferon Beta-1a	CHO cells	Multiple sclerosis
Interferon Beta-1b	E. coli	Multiple sclerosis
Interferon Gamma-1b	E. coli	Infections in chronic granulomatous disease

Table 11.3 Examples of interleukins

Interleukin	Source	Trade name	Clinical use
IL-1	*E. coli*		Rheumatoid arthritis
IL-2	*E. coli*		Renal cell carcinoma
IL-2	*E. coli*		T-cell lymphoma
IL-11	*E. coli*		Severe thrombocytopenia

Recombinant IL-2 has been used to treat renal cell carcinoma and, in combination with diphtheria toxin, to treat T cell leukaemia. Natural IL-2 is secreted by T-helper cells and its role is to convert T cells into natural killer cells. In addition it activates the division of B cells and the production of antibodies (❯ **XR Section 11.6**). rIL-2 is produced using *E.coli* and it is similar but not identical to natural IL-2.

Recombinant denileukin diftitox is a fusion protein and is expressed by *E.coli* and is a combination of the diphtheria toxin and IL-2. The IL-2 component acts as a recognition component which binds selectively to diseased cells, and then the diphtheria toxin inhibits cellular protein synthesis, causing cell death. The IL-2 targets certain leukaemia cells, and thus, denileukin diftitox is used to treat T-cell leukaemia.

IL-11 is secreted by a number of tissues and stimulates the proliferation of haematopoietic cells leading to increased production of platelets. rIL-11 (oprelvekin) is expressed via *E.coli* and, again, differs slightly from natural IL-11. It is used to treat severe **thrombocytopenia**, particularly that induced by chemotherapy for acute **myelogenous** leukaemia.

11.5.3 Haematopoietic growth factor

Haematopoietic growth factors are the cytokines which regulate the production and differentiation of blood cells (Table 11.4). The haematopoietic growth factors which have been genetically engineered are erythropoietin (EPO), granulocyte colony stimulating factor (GCSF), and granulocyte-macrophage colony stimulating factor (GMCSF).

EPO stimulates red blood cell production and rEPO (epoetin) is expressed in mammalian cells and is identical to the natural protein. It is used to treat various types of anaemia but, perhaps, is more recognizable from its use in blood doping in sport (❯ **XR Box 2.2**). Both GCSF (filgrastim), and GMCSF

Table 11.4 Examples of haematopoietic growth factors (HGF)

HGF	Source	Trade name	Clinical use
Epoetin alfa (EPO)	Mammalian cells	Epogen	Anaemia associated with chronic renal failure, antiviral HIV treatment and cancer chemotherapy
Granulocyte colony-stimulating factor (filgrastim)	*E. coli*	Neupoge	Chemotherapy-induced neutropenia, support haematopoiesis in bone marrow transplants and acute myelogenous leukaemia, prevention of infection in AIDS patients
Granulocyte-macrophage colony-stimulating factor (sargramostim)	*S. cerevisiae*	Leukine	Support haematopoiesis in bone marrow transplants, acute myelogenous leukaemia
Platelet-derived growth factor (becaplermin)	*S. cerevisiae*		Skin ulcerations

(molgramostim) are used to aid haematopoiesis in acute myelogenous leukaemia and to prevent bone marrow transplant or graft failure.

11.5.4 Tumour necrosis factor (TNF)

TNF is a cytokine produced at the initial site of an infection and causes cytotoxicity and inflammation and is also a trigger to the immune response. rTNF (etanercept) is a fusion protein (Figure 11.7) consisting of the extracellular binding domain of the human TNF receptor linked to the Fc protein of human IgG_1. Etanercept is expressed in Chinese Hamster Ovary (CHO) cell cultures. Its mode of action is to bind to TNF and prevent its interaction with cell surface receptor sites. Clinically, it is used to reduce symptoms of severe rheumatoid arthritis.

 A number of cytokines, which are regulatory proteins, such as interferons, interleukins, haematopoietic growth factor, and tumour necrosis factor are now being produced by recombinant technology for the treatment of a variety of disease states.

11.6 MONOCLONAL ANTIBODIES

All cells possess, on their cell surface, cell recognition molecules which act as antigens. Different species have different antigens, but the human body does not (usually) react to its own antigens. However, the body does react to antigens from other individuals or species ('foreign' cells) and responds by producing antibodies. The antibodies bind to the foreign antigens producing an immune response intended to destroy the foreign cell.

Antibodies are Y-shaped proteins made up of four peptide chains linked by disulphide bridges (Figure 11.8). The tip of the Fab region is the antigen-binding region. As there are two branches to the Y-shape, this means an antibody can bind two antigen molecules. The peptide sequence of most antibodies is similar, except in the hypervariable region, and the amino acid sequence in this region determines the nature of the antibody.

The cloning of antibody-producing cells produces more than one type of antibody known as polyclonal antibodies. However the cloning of specifically prepared B lymphocytes produces highly homogenous and focused antibodies known as monoclonal antibodies.

Figure 11.7 Diagrammatic representation of etanercept

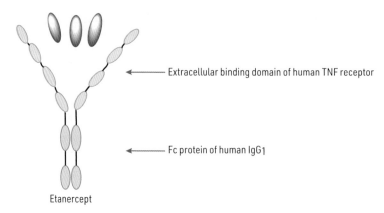

Extracellular binding domain of human TNF receptor

Fc protein of human IgG1

Etanercept

Figure 11.8 Structure of an antibody

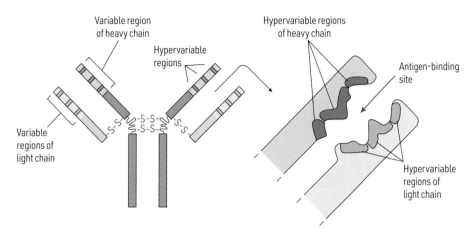

 Antibodies bind to foreign antigens to produce an immune response. Monoclonal antibodies are produced by cloning specifically prepared B lymphocytes to produce homogenous and focused antibodies.

11.6.1 Hybridoma production on monoclonal antibodies

The biotechnology techniques which allowed the production of long-lived antibody-producing cells were first introduced in 1976, when antibody-producing cells were fused with an immortal cell line to produce hybridomas—long-lived antibody-producing cells. In this technique (Figure 11.9) a mouse is made sensitive to an antigen. When the mouse is highly sensitized it is sacrificed, and the spleen cells isolated and fused (hybridized) with **immortal** myeloma cells in order to prolong the life of the spleen cells, which are B lymphocytes. Selection of the correctly fused cells is achieved by growth on a special medium (using ninety-six well plates), and the selected cells are cultured and purified. At this stage, the monoclonal antibodies will be immunogenic in humans because the antibodies have been produced in mice. In order to make the antibodies more useful to humans the mouse immunogenic properties must be removed, i.e. the monoclonal antibodies must be humanized. In this process, the constant regions of the antibody are human, and the variable regions are from the mouse antibody, producing what are known as **chimeric** antibodies. More recently, methods have been developed, using transgenic mice, for the production of antibodies which are 95–100 per cent human.

 Long-lived antibody producing cells are produced by fusing them with an immortal cell line to produce hybridomas.

11.6.2 Clinical uses of monoclonal antibodies

Increasingly monoclonal antibodies are being used both for diagnostic testing and therapeutic purposes (Table 11.5). Passive immunotherapy aims to provide assistance to the patient in combating a disease or infection without stimulating the patient's immune system. Active immunotherapy aims to trigger the patient's immune system and is used particularly against cancer cells. Monoclonal antibody therapy is the most widely used example of cancer immunotherapy and it is a form of passive immunotherapy. This can also be classed as targeted therapy because the monoclonal antibodies have a single target,

Figure 11.9 Hybridoma production of monoclonal antibodies

Step 1—sensitization of mouse to antigen, Step 2—spleen cells containing antibodies removed, Step 3—myeloma cells harvested, Step 4—fusion of antibodies with myeloma cells, Step 5—growth of selected hybridoma, Step 6—selection of correctly fused cells, Step 7 growth of selected cells in host, Step 8—harvesting of monoclonal antibodies.

(Credit: Martin Brändli / Wikimedia Commons (CC BY-SA 2.5))

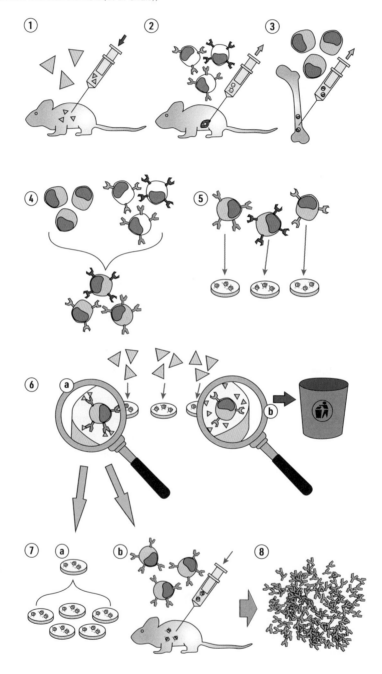

Table 11.5 Examples of clinical use of monoclonal antibodies

Diagnostic use	Therapeutic use
Pregnancy testing	Passive immunotherapy
Elisa (antigen analysis)	Active immunotherapy
Western blotting (analysis of proteins)	Targeting of drugs
Flow cytometry	
Radio-imaging	

Table 11.6 Examples of monoclonal antibodies used for cancer immunotherapy

Antibody	Target	Clinical use
Rituximab	B-cells	Non-Hodgkin's lymphoma
Gemtuzumab	CD33 cells	Acute myeloid leukaemia
Alemtuzumab	CD52 cells	B-cell chronic lymphocytic leukaemia
Basiliximab	CD25/IL-2 receptor	Prophylaxis in renal transplantation
Daclizumab	IL-2 receptor	Prophylaxis in renal transplantation
Muromonab-CD3	CD3 cells	Treatment of acute graft rejection in heart and liver transplants
Trastuzumab	HER2 receptor	Metastatic breast cancer
Infliximab	TNFα	Crohn's disease

i.e. a cancer cell surface antigen. Examples of such therapies are shown in Table 11.6 (❯ **XR see also Case Study 11.1**). The type of hybridoma, used to produce the monoclonal antibodies, is reflected in their names. The ending –omab (little used these days) is from a mouse hybridoma. A chimeric mouse hybridoma monoclonal antibody ends in –ximab and a humanized mouse hybridoma one ends in –zumab. Transgenic mouse human hybridoma antibodies end in –mumab.

In terms of cancer treatment, monoclonal antibodies have not proved to be the 'magic bullet' originally proposed. There may be a number of reasons for this. They are not as targeted as first thought, cancers being extremely diverse, meaning that they express numerous antigens. Tumour cells mutate and thus the antigen that the monoclonal antibodies are targeting changes. Finally, the toxicities are generally higher than predicted, perhaps due to lack of specificity or ineffective purification. At present positive responses to monoclonal antibody cancer therapy is between 20–30 per cent.

 Monoclonal antibodies have been mainly used in the treatment of various cancers but have only achieved moderate success.

11.7 OLIGONUCLEOTIDES

The emphasis in the previous sections on recombinant technology has been on the expression and manipulation of proteins via mRNA. A more recent development has been the use of oligonucleotides to block the message of coded mRNA, known as antisense therapy. If the sequence of a mRNA molecule is known, an oligonucleotide is produced by combinatorial synthesis (➤ **XR Section 10.2**), which is complementary to part of the mRNA molecule—this is the antisense nucleotide (Figure 11.10). This antisense nucleotide will bind to the mRNA and block any translation into protein. The antisense nucleotide-mRNA complex also is recognized by ribonuclease H which destroys the mRNA.

Antisense nucleotides, however, are very susceptible to degradation by endonucleases and are not readily transported through cell membranes. As a result, modifications have been made (Figure 11.11) in order to improve their stability to endonucleases, and to make them less polar to improve absorption. A number of these antisense nucleotides are being developed and are in clinical trials (Table 11.7); however, to date, only one, fomivirsen (Figure 11.12), has been approved for clinical usage.

 Antisense nucleotides block mRNA translation into protein, but they are easily degraded and poorly absorbed. Drug design efforts have focused on modifications to address these problems.

Figure 11.10 Antisense therapy

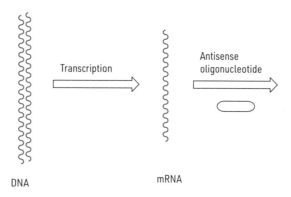

Figure 11.11 Example of structural modification to increase stability of antisense oligonucleotides

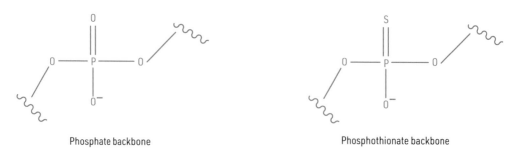

Phosphate backbone

Phosphothionate backbone

Figure 11.12 Fomivirsen

d(P-thio) (G-C-G-T-T-T-G-C-T-C-T-T-C-T-T-C-T-T-G-C-G)

(P-thio) = phosphothionate backbone

Table 11.7 Examples of antisense therapy

Name	Target gene	Clinical indication	Status
Fomivirsen	Cytomegalovirus (CMV) IE2	CMV retinitis in HIV patients	Approved
Alicaforsen	ICAM-1	Ulcerative colitis	Phase II
Affinitak	Protein kinase C-alpha	Small cell lung cancer	Phase III
Genasense	B-cell lymphoma (Bcl-2)	Chronic lymphocytic leukaemia, B-cell lymphoma, breast cancer	Phase III
ISIS 2503	H-ras	Solid tumours	Phase I
GEM 231	Protein kinase A	Solid tumours	Phase I

11.8 GENE THERAPY

Whereas oligonucleotide therapy modulates the translation and transcription of an abnormal gene, gene therapy, in the true sense, replaces an abnormal gene and, therefore, only works for those diseases where there is a correlation with one particular gene. Obvious candidates are monogenetic inherited diseases such as cystic fibrosis, sickle cell anaemia, and haemophilia. Gene therapy is also a possibility in some cancers where a genetic mutation is contributing to the malignancy such as prostate, lung, and pancreatic cancers.

Gene therapy operates via a number of stages. The initial stage is identification and isolation of the gene responsible for the condition. This gene must then be cloned and amplified using recombinant DNA technology or polymerase chain reaction (PCR) and then expressed in a suitable host. Finally, and this is probably the most difficult stage, the gene must be delivered to the appropriate cellular target. Genes are large molecules and not easily delivered into cells. Additionally, they are inherently unstable in the body. Therefore, suitable vectors need to be used to ensure efficient delivery. To date, mainly viral vectors have been used because viruses introduce genetic material into the host cell as part of their normal replication cycle (❯ **XR Section 4.4**). This mechanism has been exploited to introduce therapeutic genes into human cells (Integration Box 11.4), albeit with limited success to date.

INTEGRATION BOX 11.4   GENE THERAPY FOR CYSTIC FIBROSIS

Cystic fibrosis is a monogenetic inherited condition caused by a mutated gene known as CFTR. This mutation causes the build-up of thick sticky mucus in the lungs, which leads to pulmonary obstruction and infection. The aim of gene therapy, in this instance, is to replace the defective gene with a healthy non-mutated gene. Previous attempts to use a virus as a means of delivering the normal gene were unsuccessful because the normal defence mechanisms of the lung against infection prevented the virus from entering the cells. Recently, however, a measure of success has been achieved by encasing the normal gene in liposomes which are delivered to the lungs by nebulizer. In a clinical trial in 2015, this gene therapy produced a modest but significant improvement in lung function.

 Gene therapy involves the replacement of a faulty gene, which is causing a particular condition, by a genetically engineered normal gene.

? Questions

1. By what means might the pharmacokinetic profile of recombinant protein drugs be improved?

2. What could be the potential effects of interferon therapy on co-administration of the following drugs: warfarin, morphine, diazepam, azathioprine?

3. Explain why the therapeutic use of monoclonal antibodies has not yet been as successful as was first hoped.

4. The gene therapy described in Section 11.8 is known as somatic gene therapy. There is an alternative type of gene therapy known as germline gene therapy. What are the differences between these two types of gene therapy?

↻ Chapter summary

- Advances in biotechnology have changed the emphasis in drug design from small organic molecules to biopharmaceuticals.

- Initially, biotechnology was used simply to produce existing drug molecules, but is now increasingly used to produce biologically based therapeutic agents.

- Recombinant DNA technology allows the transfer of genetic material from one organism to another, allowing it to produce recombinant protein.

- The formation of recombinant protein involves several steps: identifying and isolating the gene of interest, inserting the gene into a vector, inserting the vector into a host, selecting the transgenic host, propagating the gene, and expressing the protein.

- The therapeutic use of recombinant proteins poses several pharmacokinetic challenges.

- There are now a number of therapeutically useful hormones which are produced by recombinant DNA technology such as insulin, glucagon, and human growth hormone.

- A number of cytokines, which are regulatory proteins, such as interferons, interleukins, haematopoietic growth factor, and tumour necrosis factor are now being produced by recombinant technology for the treatment of a variety of disease states.

- Monoclonal antibodies are being increasingly used for a variety of diagnostic and therapeutic purposes.

- Oligonucleotides, produced by combinatorial synthesis, can be used to block the translation of mRNA into protein—this is known as antisense therapy.

- Gene therapy involves the insertion of a genetically engineered healthy gene into a human cell to replace a gene identified as faulty.

📖 Further reading

Lindpaintner, K. (2002) The impact of pharmacogenetics and pharmacogenomics on drug discovery, *Nature Reviews Drug Discovery* 1: 463–9.

A view of the way in which advances in genetic science are affecting traditional drug discovery processes.

Crommelin, D.J.A., Sindelar, R.D., and Meibohm (eds) (2019) *Pharmaceutical Biotechnology: Fundamentals and Applications*. New York: Springer, ISBN 978-1-4614-6486-3.

The basic science and applications of biotechnology-derived pharmaceuticals.

Deweerdt, S., (2014) Gene therapy: A treatment coming of age, *Pharmaceutical Journal* 293: 366–8.

A review of the progress of gene therapy.

ⓣ CASE STUDY 11.1   DEVELOPMENT OF TRASTUZUMAB–A BIOPHARMACEUTICAL PRODUCT

The development of this drug, used to treat certain types of breast cancer, demonstrates the journey of drug development from the identification of a target through to clinical usage and involves the use of a biopharmaceutical product.

The story begins in 1976 with the discovery that cancer-causing genes (oncogenes) were present in human cells. One particular type of these genes, HER2, instructs cells to form receptors on their surface that send signals instructing them to grow and divide. This is part of the body's mechanism that regulates the growth, division, and replication of healthy cells. HER2 is an abbreviation of human epidermal growth factor receptor 2 and is a member of the human epidermal growth factor receptor family. They are a family of receptor tyrosine kinases and they promote cell proliferation and must be tightly regulated in order to prevent uncontrolled cell growth. In some individuals (about 15–30 per cent of breast cancer patients) this particular gene is over-expressed and is associated with increased disease re-occurrence. So this was the target, but how was a drug to attack this target gene to be produced?

The initial approach was to use monoclonal antibodies–man-made copies of proteins that are produced naturally by the body's immune system to ward off bacteria and viruses. This approach was originally identified in the 1970s but clinical trials utilizing such an approach had been very disappointing. The problem with these initial antibodies was that they were being produced in mice and the human body recognized them as foreign protein and rejected them. Eventually, in the 1990s, scientists at Genetech took sections of the mouse antibodies known to bind to HER2 and grafted them onto a human antibody, producing a humanized antibody that wouldn't be rejected by the human immune system. However, at this stage, the large-scale clinical trials required for FDA approval were considered too risky and the company stopped the programme's development. It was at this point that serendipity played a role. The mother of a senior manager at Genetech was diagnosed with breast cancer and he convinced his colleagues that the HER2 project was worthy of support.

Clinical trials with what was now called trastuzumab were conducted by Dennis Sloan, a director of research at a cancer centre in Los Angeles. Once the initial trial had commenced, Genetech were inundated with requests for the drug from patients who thought that it might help them. However, the problems of large-scale manufacture of such a complex biopharmaceutical product had still to be overcome. These clinical trials continued for 6 years and, in 1998, the FDA approved trastuzumab therapy for treatment of HER2-positive metastatic breast cancer. At the same time, a diagnostic test for HER2-positive breast cancer was developed, allowing the drug to be given to those patients who would be most likely to benefit from the treatment–one of the first examples of personalized medicine.

In 2006 Roche, who now owned Genetech, started a clinical trial where trastuzumab was combined with docetaxel and in 2012 the FDA approved this combination therapy as first-line treatment for HER2-positive metastatic breast cancer. This approval of such trastuzumab-chemotherapeutic combination therapies has led to the introduction of therapies which include a number of other chemotherapy drugs linked to trastuzumab.

Of course there are still potentially serious side effects associated with this therapy. One of the main problems with cancer chemotherapy is that drugs which are designed to kill rapidly-dividing cancer cells will also kill healthy cells which rapidly divide such as cells of the bone marrow, bowel, stomach and hair follicles, giving rise to many of the side effects associated with cancer chemotherapy. After approval of trastuzumab, scientists began to speculate whether the ability of targeted medicine would reduce these side effects. Could a chemotherapeutic agent be attached to an antibody designed to target specific cells (an antibody-drug conjugate) and delivered directly to the cancer cells? In order to produce such a conjugate there would have to be an appropriate linker between the chemotherapeutic agent and the antibody. This linkage would need to be stable so that the chemotherapeutic agent wouldn't be released into the general circulation. Additionally, the linkage would need to break down in the cancer

→

→

cell. What are the most common linkages used and why? In 2013, Kadcycla, which is ado-trastuzumab emtansine, was given FDA approval. The side effect problem has still not been solved—patients still suffered significant side effects but development work still continues, 40 years after the initial discovery of the target.

As has been stated previously, the first monoclonal antibody to target HER2 was produced in mice. The cells that produce the antibodies are extracted from the mouse's spleen. These are then fused with human myeloma cells to produce hybridomas which are screened for the cells that produce only the required antibodies. Trastuzumab is made by DNA that is 95 per cent human and 5 per cent mouse. These genes are grown in Chinese hamster ovary cells. Originally trastuzumab was formulated as an intravenous injection which has to be administered under the control of a healthcare professional in hospital and administration takes around 2–3 hours. Additionally, for a prolonged course of treatment, an indwelling catheter is often required, with all the potential problems that may cause such as thrombosis and/or infection. A subcutaneous formulation has now been introduced which only takes about 5 minutes for administration and, potentially, offers the possibility of administration at home. The additional component that allows subcutaneous administration is a recombinant hyaluronidase enzyme. This enzyme breaks down subcutaneous hyaluronic acid and, therefore, improves delivery by subcutaneous injection. Additionally, the time taken for administration is, as previously stated, a matter of minutes and requires the patient to spend less time in the oncology unit and involves less healthcare professional time. This produces significant advantages in terms of a better patient experience, cost saving, reduction in healthcare professional time, and could increase capacity in an oncology unit.

Suggested reading

R. Brazell (1998) HER-2: *The Making of Herceptin, a Revolutionary Treatment for Breast Cancer*, New York, USA, Random House Inc., p. 234, ISBN 0-679-45702-X.

A detailed account, written by a science correspondent of NBC, of the development of Herceptin, including personal stories of the women who participated in the initial trials.

PART 3

Biological Aspects of Drug Development

Part 3 deals with the biologically based studies which take place between the identification of a potential drug candidate and the entry of such a candidate into clinical trials. This phase of drug development is often referred to as preclinical testing. The studies involved are usually pharmacodynamic studies (*in vitro* or in animals), pharmacokinetic studies, the influence of genetics, and toxicity testing. Pharmacodynamic studies are beyond the scope of this text but the significance of drug metabolism is described in Chapter 12 (XR Chapter 12), the increasing importance of genetics on drug activity in Chapter 13 (XR Chapter 13), and toxicity testing in Chapter 14 (XR Chapter 14).

Drug Metabolism

12

Part 1 of this book was largely concerned with what is known as the pharmacodynamic phase of drug action, i.e. the relationship between a drug and its site of action. Traditional drug design involves the investigation of the nature of the active site (**> XR Part 1**) and the discovery of molecules which interact with that site and subsequent molecular modification to attempt to improve that interaction (**> XR Part 2**). This chapter will deal with one of the significant aspects of the pharmacokinetic phase of drug action, i.e. those factors which control the journey of a drug from initial delivery to its site of action.

12.1 PHARMACOKINETICS AND DRUG DESIGN

An increasingly important aspect of drug design involves designing a drug with an appropriate pharmacokinetic profile. A drug will be of little use if it cannot reach its site of action at a sufficient concentration to elicit a response. The factors controlling the pharmacokinetics of a drug are absorption, distribution, metabolism, and excretion (ADME). Absorption, distribution, and excretion are largely controlled by drug solubility and ionization. In the drug design process, these aspects are most often dealt within the **preformulation** stage of drug development and will be considered in detail in Part 4 of this book (**> XR Part 4**).

Drug metabolism can be defined as the chemical alteration of a drug by a biological system, with the principal objective of eliminating the drug from that system. Metabolism is a protective mechanism by which the body can remove potentially toxic foreign molecules from the body and is often called **xenobiotic** metabolism. As most drugs are molecules which are foreign to the body, they are subjected to these metabolic processes. A significant factor controlling the concentration of a drug reaching its site of action will be how much of it will be metabolized before it reaches its site of action. The design of a new drug, therefore, demands an understanding of the metabolic processes for that drug and, equally importantly, the biological activity of any products of that metabolism.

 Knowledge of how a potential new drug is metabolized is a vital aspect of drug design.

12.2 DRUG METABOLISM—WHAT IS IT?

Excretion by the kidneys (renal excretion) is enhanced by increased water solubility. As most drugs are quite lipid soluble, metabolism is designed to increase the water solubility of drugs and so increase their rate of removal from the body by renal excretion. The majority of metabolic reactions are enzyme controlled and, as such, exhibit many of the features of enzyme controlled reactions such as substrate specificity, control by substrate concentration and stereoselectivity. Often metabolism of a drug will involve different reaction routes, giving rise to a number of different products (metabolites). These metabolites may have no biological activity, reduced activity, increased activity, or even a different biological activity, potentially leading to unwanted side effects or toxicity (❯ **XR Section 12.6**).

 Metabolism is a process within the body which aims to increase the water solubility of a drug (or any xenobiotic) in order to facilitate its excretion via the kidney.

12.3 DRUG METABOLISM—WHERE DOES IT HAPPEN?

As xenobiotic metabolism is a process designed to protect the body from ingested molecules which might be toxic, it makes sense for it to take place as soon after absorption as possible. Consequently, the majority of drug metabolism occurs in the liver, although drug metabolism can take place in a number of other body tissues (see Table 12.1).

The majority of drugs are delivered orally and immediately after ingestion drug absorption can take place via the gastro-intestinal mucosa. However, not all drugs absorbed into the gastro-intestinal mucosa reach the general blood circulation. P-glycoprotein, which is an ATP-dependent efflux pump for xenobiotics, can secrete drugs such as digoxin from the intestinal mucosa back into the lumen of the gastro-intestinal tract thus being responsible for decreased drug accumulation in the blood. Additionally certain esterases present in the intestine can hydrolyse esters and amides (❯ **XR Section 12.4.3**). However, most drugs are absorbed relatively unchanged through the intestinal wall into the bloodstream. The gastro-intestinal blood supply (portal blood supply) passes through the liver before distribution to the rest of the body and it is in the liver that the vast majority of drug metabolism occurs, and this is often referred to as first pass metabolism. This process can greatly affect the **bioavailability** of a drug and, in extreme cases, may require an alternative route of administration to avoid the initial hepatic metabolism (see Integration Box 12.1 and Figure 12.1).

Although the liver is the major site of drug metabolism, other sites in the body may be involved (see Table 12.1). The metabolic processes which occur in these alternative tissues tend to be rather more

---

INTEGRATION BOX 12.1   **LIDOCAINE METABOLISM**

Lidocaine was originally designed as a local anaesthetic but is also a very useful antiarrhythmic drug. It is the drug of choice for the emergency treatment of ventricular arrhythmia. It is very useful in this regard because of its rapid metabolism, because the therapy can be rapidly modified in response to changes in the patient's status. Lidocaine can only be used as an antiarrhythmic when administered parenterally. Activity is not seen after oral administration because of the rapid first pass metabolism. Knowledge of the metabolism of lidocaine has also led to the production of tocainide which also has antiarrhythmic activity but is orally active. The plasma half-life of tocainide is about 12 hours compared with about 15 minutes for lidocaine.

Figure 12.1 Lidocaine and tocainide

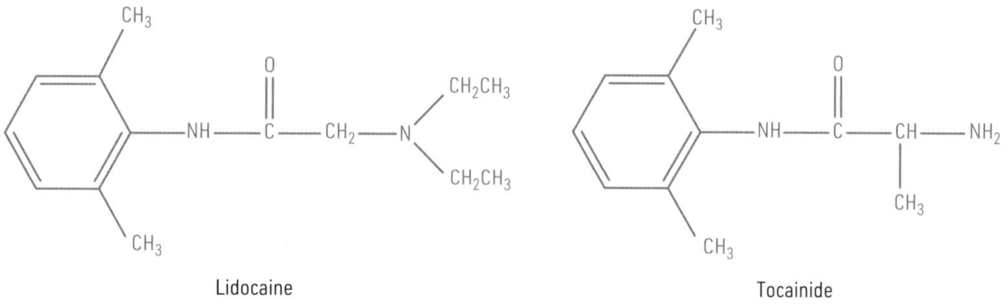

Lidocaine

Tocainide

Table 12.1 Types of metabolism and where they take place

Body tissue	Principal type of metabolism
Liver	Most types
Gastro-intestinal tract	Hydrolysis, reduction, conjugation
Lungs	Oxidation
Blood	Hydrolysis
Skin	Oxidation
Kidneys	Oxidation, hydrolysis
Brain	Oxidation
Placenta	Oxidation

substrate-specific than those which take place in the liver. For example, ester and amide hydrolysis takes place via esterases and related enzymes in the plasma (❯ XR Table 12.1 and Section 12.4.3).

 Drug metabolism can take place in a number of body tissues, but the liver is the primary site of metabolism.

The metabolic processes taking place in the liver can occur in various cell tissues, such as the mito-chondria and the cytosol. However, the vast majority of metabolic reactions involve cytochrome P450 enzymes (❯ XR Section 12.4.1 and Integration Box 12.2) which are associated with the endoplasmic reticulum of the liver cells.

 Drug metabolism takes place in a number of locations within liver cells, but the main site is the endoplasmic reticulum.

12.4 DRUG METABOLISM–HOW DOES IT HAPPEN?

Drug metabolic reactions are conveniently classified into Phase I and Phase II reactions. Phase I metab-olism involves the conversion of a drug to a more water-soluble molecule. Improved water solubility re-quires a functional group with a good hydrogen bonding capacity and involves the introduction of such a group or the unmasking of such a group (for example, the conversion of an ester to a carboxylic acid).

If the metabolites are now sufficiently water-soluble renal excretion can occur. Phase I metabolic re-actions are classified as oxidation, reduction and hydrolysis. The Phase I metabolites may still not be sufficiently water soluble to be readily excreted. In this situation Phase II metabolism may take place (**❯ XR Section 12.4.4**).

 Drug metabolism takes place in two steps—Phases I and II. Phase I introduces or unmasks a group with increased water solubility. Phase II involves a reaction to further increase water solubility if necessary.

12.4.1 Oxidation reactions

Oxidative reactions are the most important reactions of Phase I metabolism. They generally involve the introduction of a hydroxyl (OH) group (hydroxylation), the oxidation of a sulphur or nitrogen atom (S- or N- oxidation), or the removal of an alkyl group from nitrogen or oxygen (N- or O-dealkylation) (see Figure 12.2).

Figure 12.2 Examples of oxidative metabolic reactions: (a) Hydroxylation, (b) S-oxidation, (c) N-oxidation, (d) N-dealkylation, (e) O-dealkylation

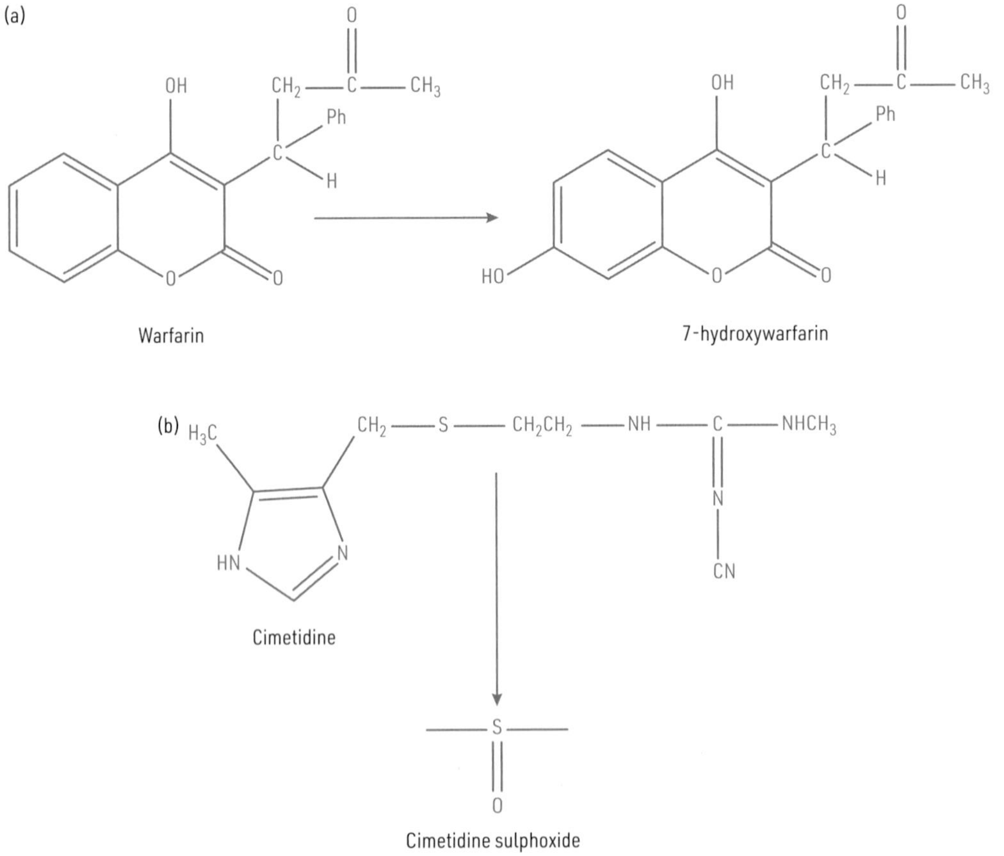

Figure 12.2 (*Cont.*)

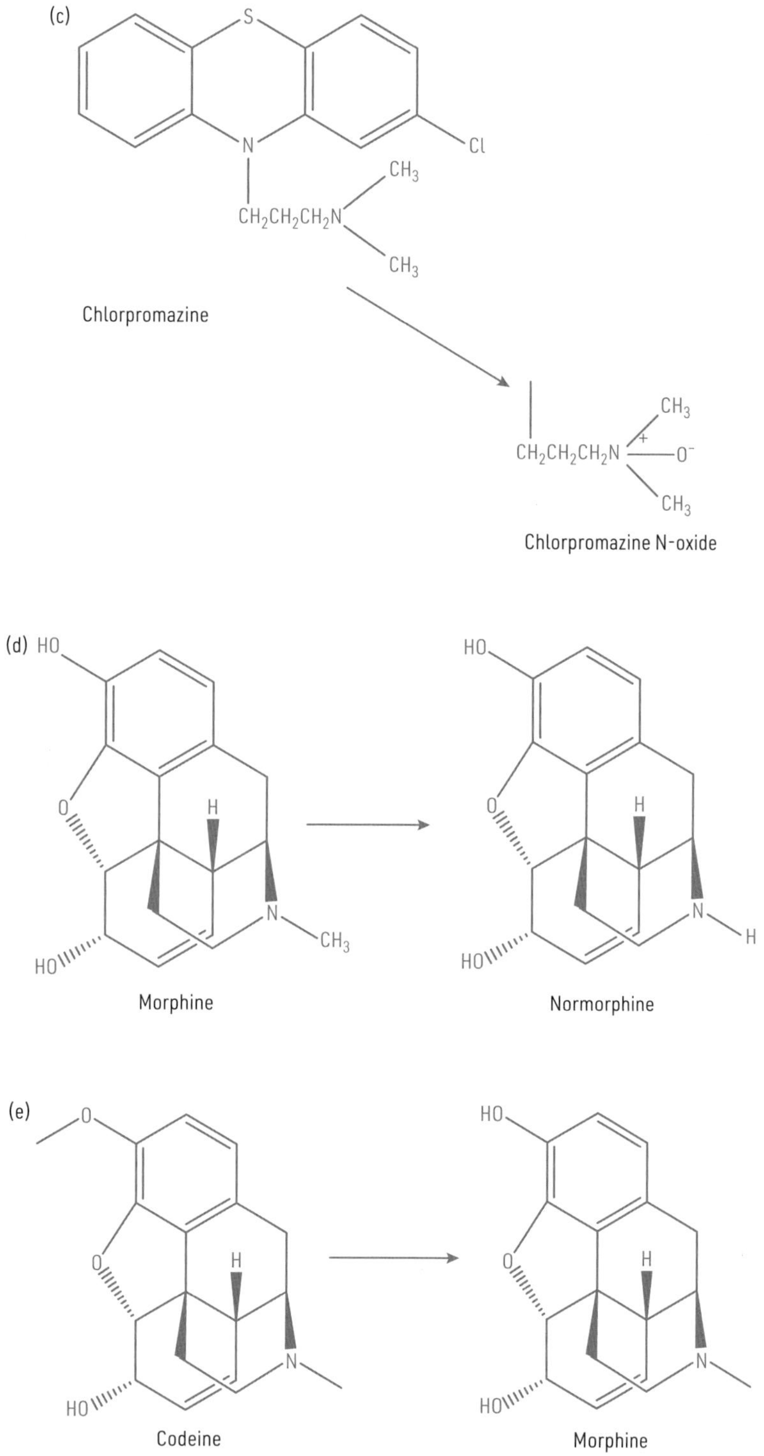
(c)
S
N
Cl
CH2CH2CH2N
CH3
CH3
Chlorpromazine
CH2CH2CH2N
+
O−
CH3
CH3
Chlorpromazine N-oxide
(d) HO
O
H
N
CH3
HO
Morphine
HO
O
H
N
H
HO
Normorphine
(e)
O
O
H
N
HO
Codeine
HO
O
H
N
HO
Morphine

INTEGRATION BOX 12.2 | **CYTOCHROME P450s**

Cytochrome P450s are a family of enzymes that have an important role in metabolism of xenobiotics. The title P450 arises from the fact that they complex with carbon monoxide and the complexes absorb light of about 450 nm. They all have a similar structure, having an iron atom (Fe^{2+}) which forms coordinate bonds with four nitrogen atoms of haem and the thiol group of a cysteine residue in a globin protein (see Figure 12.3). The final coordination position is occupied by water or other ligands, which are easily exchanged. The nomenclature of cytochromes can appear quite complex but is actually relatively straightforward. The letters CYP represents the cytochrome system. This is followed by the cytochrome family number (CYP1, CYP2 etc.). This is then followed by an upper-case letter representing the sub-family (CYP1A, CYP2B etc.). Specific enzymes which catalyse a specific reaction are indicated by a final number (CYP1A1).

Figure 12.3 The structure of haem and cytochrome

(Credit: From Pharmaceutical Chemistry edited by Jill Barber and Chris Rostron (2013). Reproduced with permission of Oxford University Press through PLSclear).

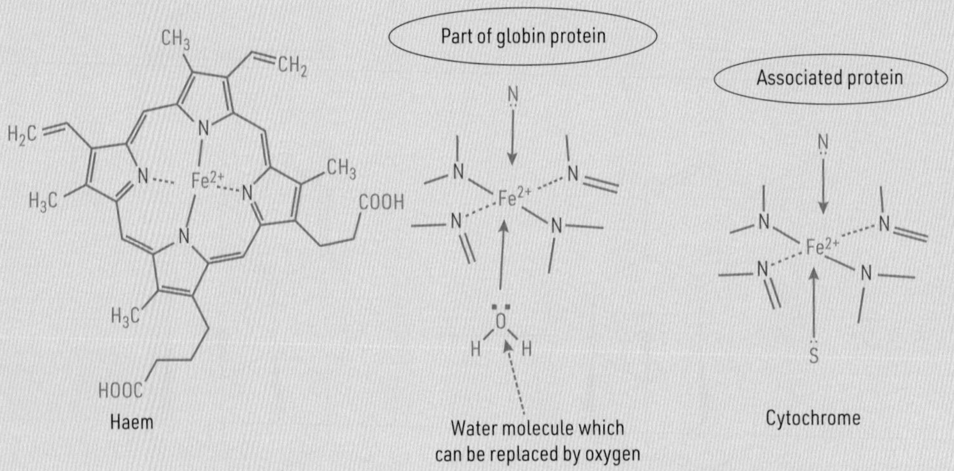

Haem · Water molecule which can be replaced by oxygen · Cytochrome

These oxidation reactions are catalysed by mixed-function oxidases or monooxygenases (oxidation at carbon atoms and N- or O-dealkylation), flavin monooxygenases (oxidation of atoms other than carbon, e.g. nitrogen, sulphur, or phosphorus) and monoamine oxidases (oxidative deamination). The mixed-function oxidases are mainly present in the endoplasmic reticulum of liver cells. These oxidative reactions occur in a series of steps and cytochrome P450s are involved in one or more of these steps (see Integration Box 12.2).

Cytochrome P450s are actually a whole family of **isozymes** which have different substrate specificity and spectral characteristics. Some are them are capable of being induced by specific substrates, e.g. CYP2B by phenobarbitone and CYP1A1 by polyaromatic hydrocarbons (▶ **XR Section 12.5.4** and **Box 12.1**).

Oxidation by flavin monooxygenases involves the oxidation of nucleophilic atoms such as nitrogen and sulphur and requires nicotinamide adenine dinucleotide (NAD^+) or nicotinamide adenine dinucleotide phosphate ($NADP^+$) as coenzymes. The reaction occurs by the attack of the nucleophilic atom on a hydroperoxide found on the flavin prosthetic group of the enzymes.

Monoamine oxidases belong to a group of substrate-specific enzymes. Their usual role is in the deamination of catecholamines, such as noradrenaline, but they can also oxidize some drugs,

---

BOX 12.1   THE DANGERS OF SMOKING

The statistics linking smoking and lung cancer were first published in 1950. However, the proof of the connection was not published until 25 years later, when the polyaromatic hydrocarbon benzo-[a]-pyrene was shown to be responsible (see Figure 12.4). Or rather, it was an oxidative metabolic product which contains an epoxide and a diol that is mostly responsible for the carcinogenicity. The reactive metabolite reacts with a guanine moiety in DNA, causing DNA damage, which can result in carcinogenesis. The situation is made even more dangerous because benzo-[a]-pyrene from cigarette smoke induces the production of cytochrome CYP1A1, which leads to the production of the toxic reactive metabolite.

Figure 12.4 Benzo-[a]-pyrene

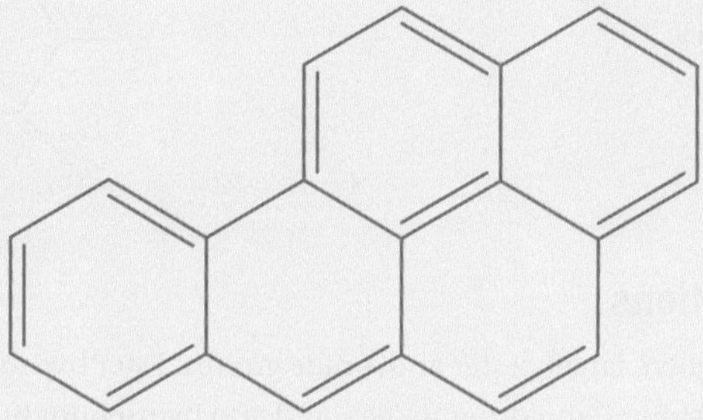

Benzo-[a]-pyrene

---

e.g. amphetamine. Also included in the substrate-specific category of metabolic enzymes are alcohol dehydrogenase and xanthine oxidase, which can also oxidize drugs structurally related to the natural substrate.

 Many oxidative metabolic reactions involve cytochrome P450 enzyme systems, although flavin monooxygenases and monoamine oxidases can also be involved.

12.4.2 Reduction reactions

Reductive metabolic reactions usually involve specific reductase enzymes. Although reductive reactions are less common than oxidative ones, they involve some alcohols, aldehydes, and ketones and, less commonly, the reduction of nitro groups to amines. Aldehydes are relatively easily oxidized and so reduction is less often involved. Ketones, however, are resistant to oxidation and so are often reduced to secondary alcohols. Reductive drug metabolic reactions, such as reduction of aldehydes and ketones to alcohols, often lead to the formation of a new asymmetric carbon atom and, therefore, two stereoisomers (see Figure 12.5). This situation can have significant consequences for biological activity (**› XR Section 12.5.7**) and is often a consideration in drug design and development.

 Reductive metabolic reactions usually involve drugs with ketone or nitro groups.

Figure 12.5 Example of metabolic reduction of ketone producing stereoisomers

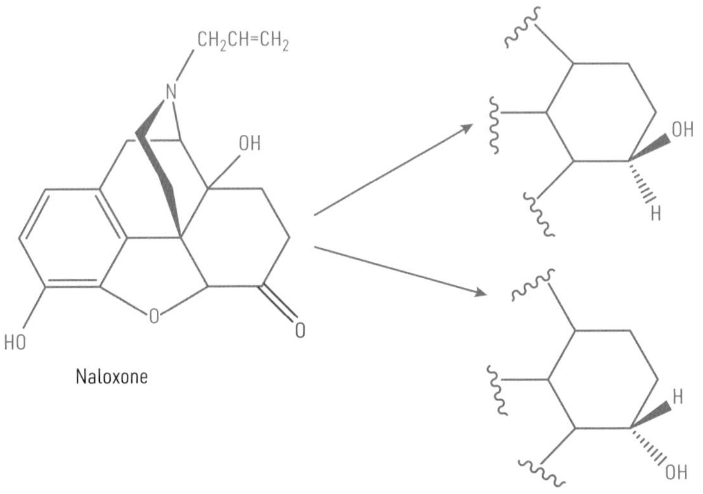

Naloxone

12.4.3 Hydrolysis reactions

These metabolic reactions involve largely ester and amide groups. Ester hydrolysis can take place by non-specific esterases in the liver, kidney, and other tissues, and also by **pseudocholinesterases** in the plasma. Amide hydrolysis usually involves nonspecific amidases, carboxypeptidases and aminopeptidases. Ester hydrolysis is usually more rapid than amide hydrolysis and is widely used in the design of prodrugs (❯ **XR Section 12.6.4**).

Hydrolytic metabolic processes mainly involve drugs containing an ester or amide group.

12.4.4 Phase II metabolism

In this process a functional group present in the drug, or its metabolites, reacts with an endogenous substance and forms a highly polar (water-soluble) conjugate. Phase II metabolism is also known as conjugation. The endogenous substances include glucuronic acid, sulphate, acetic acid and a number of amino acids. Phase II metabolism is often the final step in drug metabolism, and the conjugates are excreted in the urine and/or the bile. Conjugates are usually biologically inactive, with few exceptions, whereas Phase I metabolites can retain some biological activity (❯ **XR Section 12.6**).

Reaction with glucuronic acid is the most important of the Phase II reactions. The body has plenty of available glucuronic acid and reaction (glucuronidation) can take place with alcohols, phenols, thiols, amines and carboxylic acids within drugs or their metabolites (see Figure 12.6a). The drug, or its Phase I metabolite, reacts with an activated form of glucuronic acid, uridine diphosphate glucuronic acid (UDP-GA), and the reaction is catalysed by UDPG transferase.

Sulphate formation is a metabolic route for phenols and, occasionally, alcohols and amines (see Figure 12.6b).The sulphate is obtained from the body's sulphate pool (see Integration Box 12.3), is activated by reaction with ATP, and the process is catalysed by magnesium ions. The sulphates are normally excreted in the urine, except steroid sulphates which are excreted in the bile. Sulphate formation can also take place in the gastro-intestinal tract, leading to reduced absorption.

Figure 12.6 Examples of Phase II metabolic reactions: (a) Glucuronidation, (b) Sulphation, (c) Acetylation, (d) Amino acid conjugation, (e) Glutathione conjugation

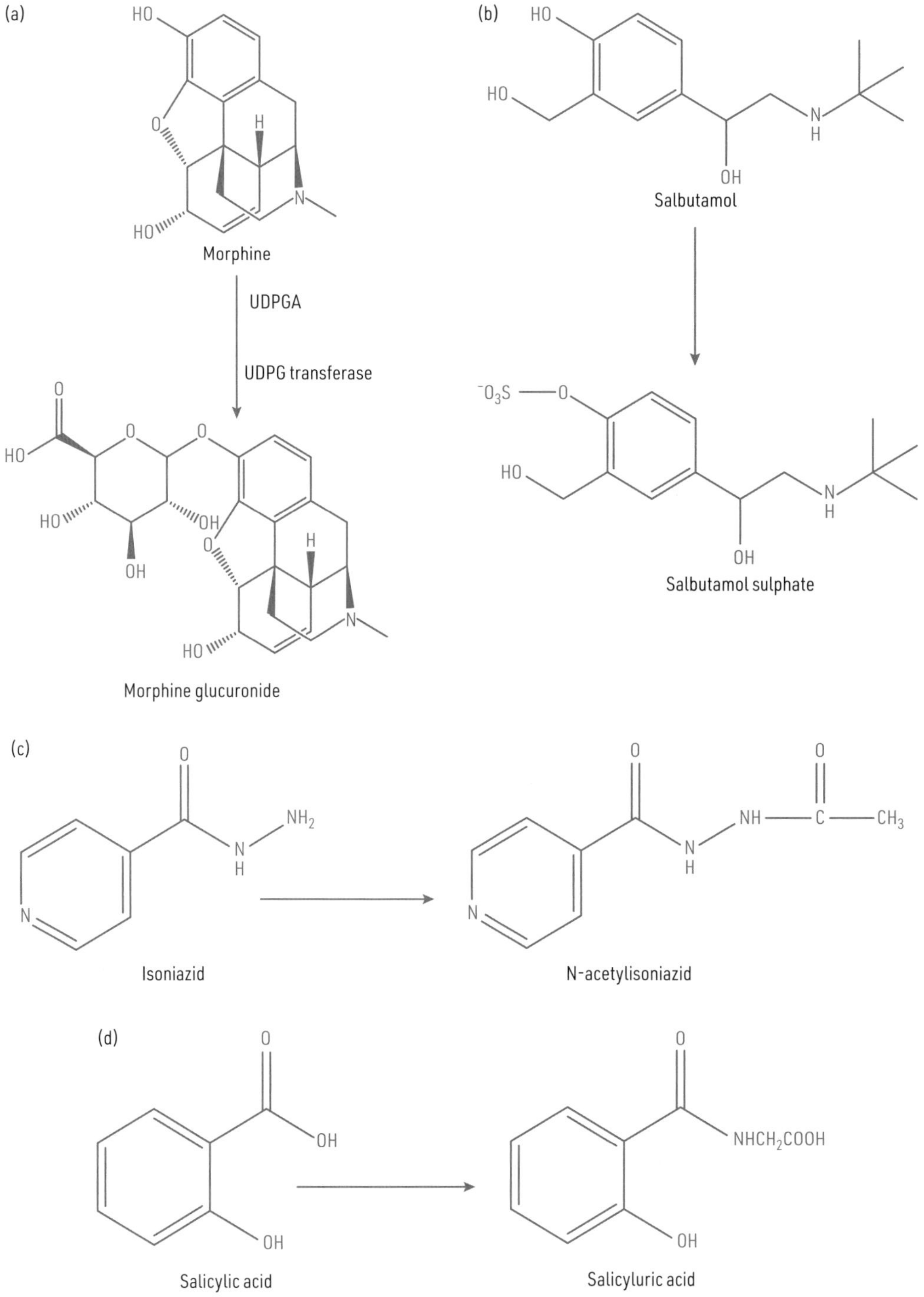

Figure 12.6 (*Continued*)

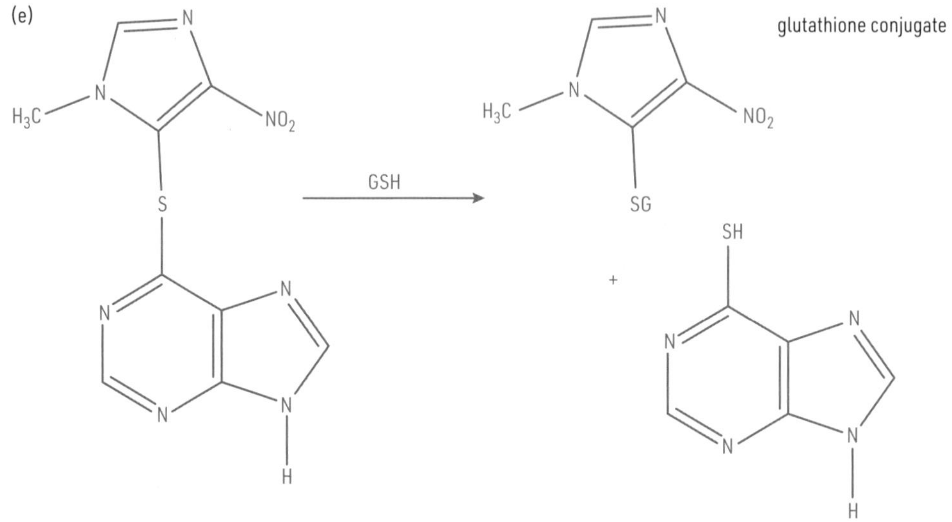

(e)

GSH

glutathione conjugate

Azathioprine

+

6-mercaptopurine

INTEGRATION BOX 12.3   THE SULPHATE POOL

The body's pool of sulphate is quite limited compared to the availability of glucuronic acid. This is because the body's sulphate is used significantly for the metabolism of endogenous molecules such as steroids, catecholamines, heparin and thyroxine, thus reducing the amount available for reaction with xenobiotics.

Acetylation, or rather reaction with activated acetate (acetylCoA), usually involves amines or alcohols. Probably the best-known example is the metabolism of the antitubercular drug isoniazid (see Figure 12.6c and ❯ XR Section 12.5.5).

Conjugation with an amino acid is an important metabolic route for carboxylic acids. The reaction takes place in a series of steps. The carboxylic acid reacts with ATP to form an AMP intermediate. This intermediate is converted to an active CoA intermediate, and this activated intermediate undergoes nucleophilic displacement with the amino acid. The most common amino acid conjugate used by humans is with glycine (see Figure 12.6d), but glutamine conjugates are also formed. Species other than humans use different amino acids—birds use ornithine and rodents use alanine.

Humans also use glutathione (GSH) which is a tripeptide consisting of the amino acids glycine, cysteine and glutamic acid. In this process, however, it is the thiol (SH) group of the cysteine which reacts. This thiol group is very nucleophilic and undergoes conjugation with molecules containing electrophilic centres such as epoxides or haloalkanes. Glutathione conjugates are formed (see Figure 12.6e), and then converted to mercapturic acids which are excreted in the urine (❯ XR Section 12.5.5 and Integration Box 12.4).

 Phase II metabolism involves reaction with an endogenous substance to form a highly water-soluble conjugate. The endogenous compounds are mainly glucuronic acid, sulphate, acetylCoA, amino acids, and glutathione.

| **INTEGRATION BOX 12.4** | **PARACETAMOL TOXICITY** |

The restriction on the quantity of paracetamol tablets that can be sold is related to the serious consequences of paracetamol overdose, even though, at normal doses, paracetamol is a very safe drug. Overdose of paracetamol can cause irreversible liver damage and is potentially fatal. The liver toxicity problem with paracetamol is not due to paracetamol itself but is due to one of its metabolites. A small proportion of paracetamol (~4 per cent) is oxidatively metabolized in the liver to a quinoneimine molecule. This is a very reactive species and could potentially cause damage to liver cells. If the normal doses of paracetamol are taken this is not a problem because this reactive metabolite is deactivated by glutathione (see Figure 12.7). Although only 4 per cent of the reactive metabolite is produced, in an overdose situation this will be a significant amount and may be sufficient to deplete the liver's supply of glutathione. Any remaining reactive metabolite will then cause irreversible damage to the cells of the liver.

Figure 12.7 Paracetamol potential toxicity

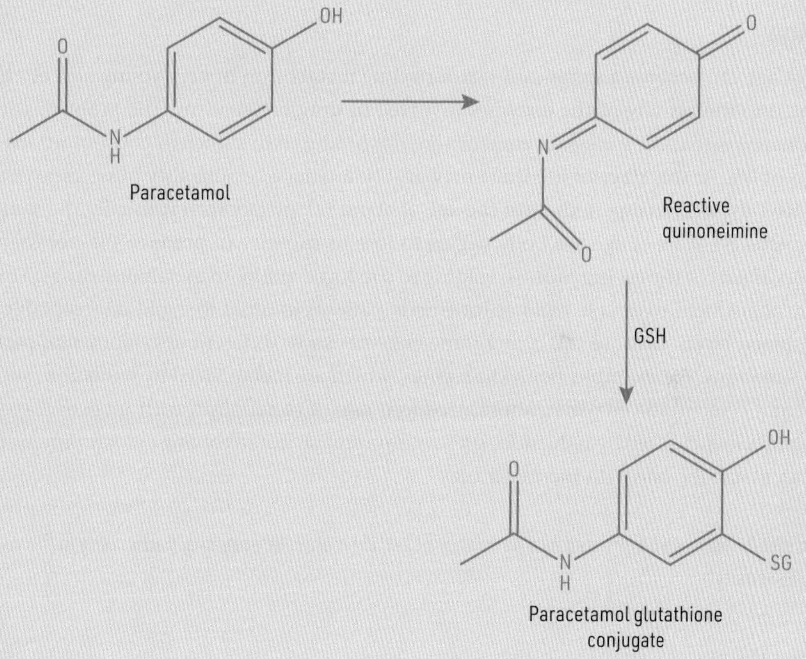

Paracetamol

Reactive quinoneimine

GSH

Paracetamol glutathione conjugate

12.5 **FACTORS AFFECTING METABOLISM**

There are numerous factors which can affect the metabolic fate of a drug. These factors can result in different outcomes—different rates of metabolism, different routes of metabolism—which can have different influences on the pharmacodynamics of a drug. Because drug metabolism is largely dependent on enzymatic reactions, many of these differences result from factors which have direct or indirect influence on these enzymatic reactions. Because of this, these factors need to be controlled in clinical trials of new drugs (❯ **XR Part 5**).

 In the process of drug design it is important to be aware of the factors which can affect drug metabolism.

12.5.1 Disease

Because the majority of drug metabolism takes place in the liver, any condition which affects the liver structure and function will potentially affect drug metabolism. Examples of such diseases are cirrhosis, hepatitis, and liver cancer. Severe cardiac conditions (such as myocardial infarction) which limits blood flow to the liver will affect those drugs whose metabolism is blood flow limited. Additionally, endocrine dysfunction can also have indirect effects on drug metabolism. For example, hyperthyroidism will cause an increase in oxidative metabolism, increasing the metabolism of drugs such as propranolol and theophylline. Chronic illness, leading to general debilitation, can lead to reduced production of metabolic enzymes and their cofactors, resulting in reduced drug metabolism.

 Drug metabolism can be affected by diseases of certain organs, such as the liver and the heart, as well as certain biochemical dysfunctions.

12.5.2 Age

The effect of age can become a significant factor in drug metabolism in very young and old individuals. This is related to the activity of the enzymes involved in drug metabolism. The problem with the very young (neonates) is that the necessary enzymes are not produced in sufficient concentrations in the first few months of life. At this stage of life there may also be a reduced availability of necessary endogenous cofactors. After the neonatal period, until the age of about 60, metabolism is usually the same, irrespective of age. After 60 years of age the body begins to lose its capacity to produce the necessary enzymes and cofactors as part of the ageing process, leading to a reduced ability to metabolize drugs. This situation may require adjustment to dosage regimes for elderly patients in order to avoid unacceptable high, possibly toxic, blood levels. Because the cytochrome enzymes show different developmental patterns there can be age variations. For example, benzodiazepines, which are metabolized by oxidation, such as diazepam, involving cytochrome enzymes, show a reduced rate of metabolism with increased age. However, benzodiazepines metabolized by reduction, such as nitrazepam, not involving cytochrome systems, show no change in metabolic rate with increased age.

 Drug metabolism can be affected by a deficiency of certain metabolic enzymes, particularly in the very young and the elderly.

12.5.3 Gender

In most cases there is no difference in drug metabolism between males and females. However there are a small number of gender differences, usually associated with differing enzyme concentrations. A good example is alcohol dehydrogenase. Women have a lower concentration of this enzyme than men. This means that for equal alcohol intakes, alcohol remains longer in the body in women and hence has the potential to cause more damage. This makes women more susceptible to alcohol-induced liver and heart disease. This is one of the reasons why the recommended weekly intake of units of alcohol is lower for women than for men.

 In most circumstances there are no differences with respect to gender in drug metabolism, although there are a few exceptions.

12.5.4 **Diet**

Diet can affect the metabolism of a drug, either as a result of poor diet or sudden changes in diet. The ultimate in poor diet, i.e. starvation, will lead to reduced drug metabolism as a result of the lack of necessary biochemical energy required for optimal metabolism. Weight reduction diets can also interfere with drug metabolism in some cases. For example, the half-life of theophylline can be doubled by the change from a high to low protein and low to high carbohydrate diet. The metabolism of xanthine alkaloid drugs such as theophylline (an anti-asthmatic drug) can also be affected by high levels of coffee or tea which contain caffeine and theobromine (see Figure 12.8). Both of these substances are structurally related to theophylline and will compete for the same metabolic pathways, thus leading to a decreased capacity to metabolize theophylline. As theophylline has a relatively narrow therapeutic index, this may cause toxicity problems.

A significant intake of cruciferous vegetables (such as broccoli) can cause the induction of intestinal hydroxylase enzymes, leading to metabolism of drugs even before they are absorbed. Although not strictly classified as diet, smoking can affect drug metabolism because the presence of benzo[a]pyrene in cigarette smoke induces cytochrome CYP1A1. Another cytochrome enzyme that is affected by a dietary item is CYP3A4 which is inhibited by compounds present in grapefruit juice. This is the reason why patients on a wide range of drugs (such as amiodarone, diazepam, atorvastatin) are advised to avoid grapefruit juice. This inhibition may be caused by a bioflavonoid, naringenin, formed by gastro-intestinal bacteria from naringin present in grapefruit (see Figure 12.9).

 There are a number of circumstances where dietary items, or a change of diet, can affect drug metabolism.

12.5.5 **Genetics**

The production of the enzymes involved in drug metabolism is controlled by the activity of specific genes within an individual's genetic code. Therefore, a mutation with respect to the gene codifying for an enzyme may lead to an under- or over-production of that particular enzyme. Consequently, individuals may exhibit different rates of metabolism, different routes of metabolism, or even total lack of metabolism of a particular drug. This is best explained by looking at some examples.

Figure 12.8 Xanthine alkaloids

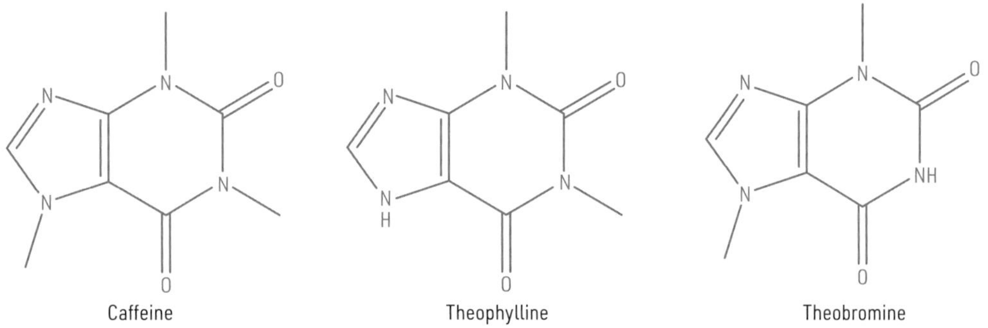

Caffeine   Theophylline   Theobromine

Figure 12.9 Naringenin, a bioflavonoid from grapefruit

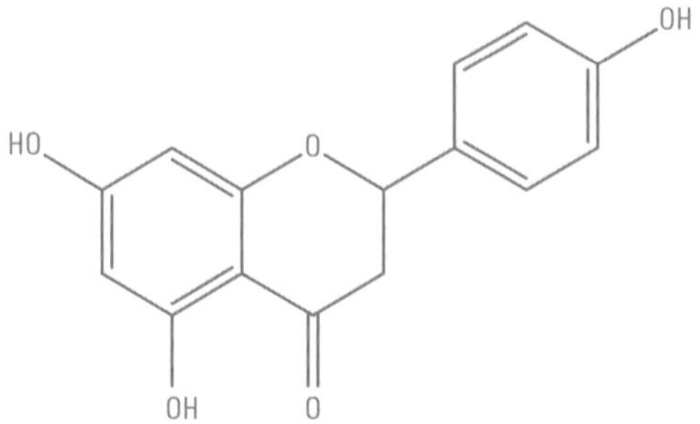

Naringenin

The case with glucose-6-phosphate dehydrogenase deficiency is an interesting one. Over 100 million people are affected worldwide. The proteins of the red blood cell membranes are stabilized by being kept in a reduced and operative state by interaction with reduced glutathione. If drug metabolism leads to the production of reactive metabolites, these metabolites can lead to oxidation of the membrane proteins. In order to remain operative, the oxidized membranes must be reduced by glutathione or haemolysis will occur. As glucose-6-phosphate dehydrogenase is involved in the formation of reduced glutathione, a deficiency of this enzyme can result in haemolysis, in some circumstances. An example of a drug which produces such reactive metabolites is the antimalarial drug primaquine, and it was the use of this drug during World War Two which led, eventually, to the discovery of this particular enzyme deficiency.

The drug suxamethonium (succinylcholine) is a short-acting neuromuscular blocking agent used to prevent voluntary breathing by the patient during periods of artificial ventilation and is administered intravenously in a controlled dosage. When the artificial ventilation is removed the blocking effect of the suxamethonium is required to cease as soon as possible to allow the patient to resume normal respiration. Thus suxamethonium is required to have a very short duration of action and is of the order of a few minutes. This is due to the hydrolysis of the ester groups by the enzyme plasma cholinesterase (see Figure 12.10). However, about 4 per cent of the population have an atypical plasma cholinesterase and this leads to a prolonged action of the suxamethonium and may lead to severe problems with respiration (including death) if the artificial ventilation is not retained for a longer period (❯ XR Section 12.6.1).

Isoniazid, an anti-tubercular drug, is metabolized by the action of a liver acylase enzyme (see ❯ XR Section 12.4.4 and XR Section 12.6 3). In some patients the normal dose of isoniazid is inadequate and in others a normal dose leads to **nephrotoxicity**. This is because the rate of formation of the enzyme responsible, N-acetyltransferase, is genetically controlled. So-called 'fast acetylators' can lead to normal doses being ineffective due to more rapid metabolism and 'slow acetylators' can lead to normal doses being toxic due to very slow metabolism. There are some interesting geographical variations among fast and slow acetylators. Around 50 per cent of Caucasians and African-Americans are slow acetylators, compared with 10–20 per cent of Inuits and Japanese and 80 per cent of Egyptians.

Figure 12.10 Metabolism of suxamethonium

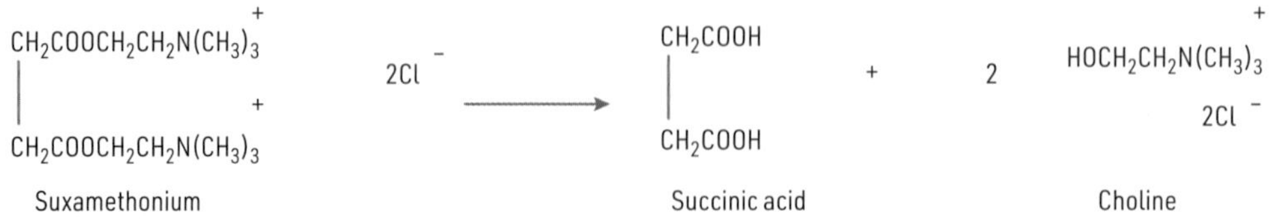

Suxamethonium   Succinic acid   Choline

Because most drug metabolism is enzyme controlled and enzyme production is under genetic control, any genetic variation in this respect can significantly affect drug metabolism.

12.5.6 Enzyme induction and inhibition

There are a number of drugs which are capable of enhancing or reducing the activity of drug-metabolizing enzymes. Because this situation can affect the metabolism of concurrently administered drugs, it is often referred to as drug-drug interaction. The enhancement of enzyme activity is caused by the synthesis of additional enzyme, known as enzyme induction. This will increase the metabolism of the drug and leads to a reduction in the duration of action of that drug and this can be clinically significant. Equally important is the effect that this enzyme induction can have on a co-administered drug. The rate of metabolism of this second drug can also be increased, again with potential clinical consequences.

Alternatively, some drugs can inhibit the activity of metabolizing enzymes, leading to decreased metabolism. Consequently, the drug accumulates, potentially leading to serious side effects (see Integration Box 12.5). Whereas metabolic enzyme enhancement is largely due to new enzyme formation, inhibition can result from a number of situations such as enzyme inactivation, competitive inhibition, or reduction of protein synthesis (❯ XR Section 12.5.5).

 Certain drugs have the potential to increase or decrease the production of metabolic enzymes which can lead to increased or decreased metabolism of these or concurrently administered drugs with potential serious clinical consequences.

12.5.7 Chirality

Xenobiotic-metabolizing enzymes often exhibit enantiomeric differences in the metabolism of enantiomeric drugs. This is because the enzyme active site provides a chiral environment. As enzymes are involved in both Phase I and Phase II pathways, stereochemical effects are often observed, especially when chiral drugs are administered as racemic mixtures. Enantiomers may be metabolized at different rates or by different routes or both. If only one enantiomer is capable of interacting with the enzyme active site, the enantiomers will be metabolized by different routes, i.e. stereospecific routes. If one enantiomer interacts more effectively with the enzyme active site, the enantiomers will be metabolized at different rates, i.e. stereoselective metabolism. Overall, stereospecificity in drug metabolism is unusual as there is usually more than one enzyme involved, and they may exhibit different stereochemical effects, e.g. glucuronidation of propranolol is stereoselective for the S isomer but ring hydroxylation is stereoselective for the R isomer (see Figure 12.11).

The anticoagulant drug warfarin is a good example of different enantiomeric routes of metabolism (see Figure 12.11).

INTEGRATION BOX 12.5 | **WARFARIN AND CIMETIDINE DO NOT MIX**

The anti-ulcer drug cimetidine binds reversibly to the iron atom in a number of CYP450s. It does so by forming a reversible coordinate bond between the iron and the tertiary nitrogen in the imidazole ring of cimetidine. One of the cytochromes it binds to is CYP2C9 which is involved in the metabolism of the anticoagulant drug warfarin. This interaction competitively reduces the metabolism of warfarin and can lead to an accumulation of warfarin in the body, potentially resulting in dangerous internal bleeding.

Figure 12.11 Examples of stereochemical differences in metabolism

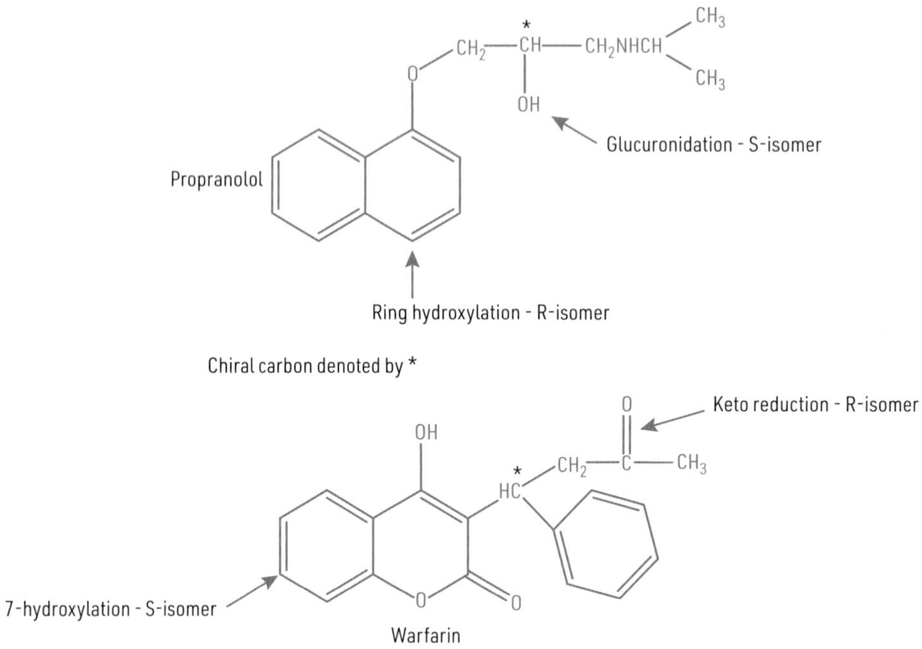

Propranolol

Glucuronidation - S-isomer

Ring hydroxylation - R-isomer

Chiral carbon denoted by *

Keto reduction - R-isomer

7-hydroxylation - S-isomer

Warfarin

Verapamil is a good example of different enantiomeric rates of metabolism, the S-isomer being more rapidly metabolized. As the S-isomer has better therapeutic activity than the R-isomer, a higher oral dose of the drug is required compared with an intravenous dose, due to the excessive first pass metabolism of the S-isomer.

 Enantiomers of chiral drugs can be metabolized by different routes or at different rates.

12.6 METABOLISM AND DRUG DESIGN

From the previous sections of this chapter, it is clear that extensive knowledge of the metabolic profile of a proposed drug substance is of vital importance. The drug licensing authorities, therefore, require a full investigation of the metabolic profile of a new drug. As a result, pharmaceutical companies must fully investigate the metabolism of a new drug and provide the results as part of the submission to the licensing authority. However, knowledge of drug metabolism can often be of great value in the drug design process itself and can be deliberately exploited in the search for new drug candidates. When a pharmacologically active molecule is metabolized by the body, there are a number of potential outcomes. The metabolite(s) may be pharmacologically inactive, they may retain a similar pharmacological activity but with a different potency or they may exhibit a different type of pharmacological activity (and may be potentially toxic as a result). All of these situations can be useful in the drug design process, potentially giving rise to more useful drug candidates.

 Full knowledge of the metabolism of a new drug and its metabolites is required by drug licensing authorities.

12.6.1 Inactive metabolites

The knowledge that a new drug candidate is metabolized to a pharmacologically inactive metabolite is very useful as, providing that metabolite is readily excreted, there is no need to worry about any unforeseen biological activity following metabolism. Indeed, it is sometimes useful to include a metabolically labile functionality in a potential drug candidate if a short duration of action is desirable. A good example of this is the neuromuscular blocking drug succinylcholine. The clinical usage of this drug requires a very short half-life, and this is achieved by the inclusion of the metabolically sensitive ester groups. However, see Section 12.5.5 for potential difficulties (➤ **XR Section 12.5.5**).

 A drug may be metabolized to metabolites that are biologically inactive, a situation which is sometimes exploited by inclusion of a metabolically sensitive group to reduce the duration of action.

12.6.2 Metabolites with similar pharmacological activity but differing in potency

Diazepam has a long duration of action as an anxiolytic. Two of its metabolites (by hydroxylation) are oxazepam and temazepam (N-methyloxazepam) which have shorter half-lives, and this can be clinically useful in some circumstances. The introduction of OH makes the molecule more polar and N-demethylation (in the case of oxazepam) even more polar (see Figure 12.12). Thus, the half-lives of

Figure 12.12 Metabolites of diazepam used as drugs

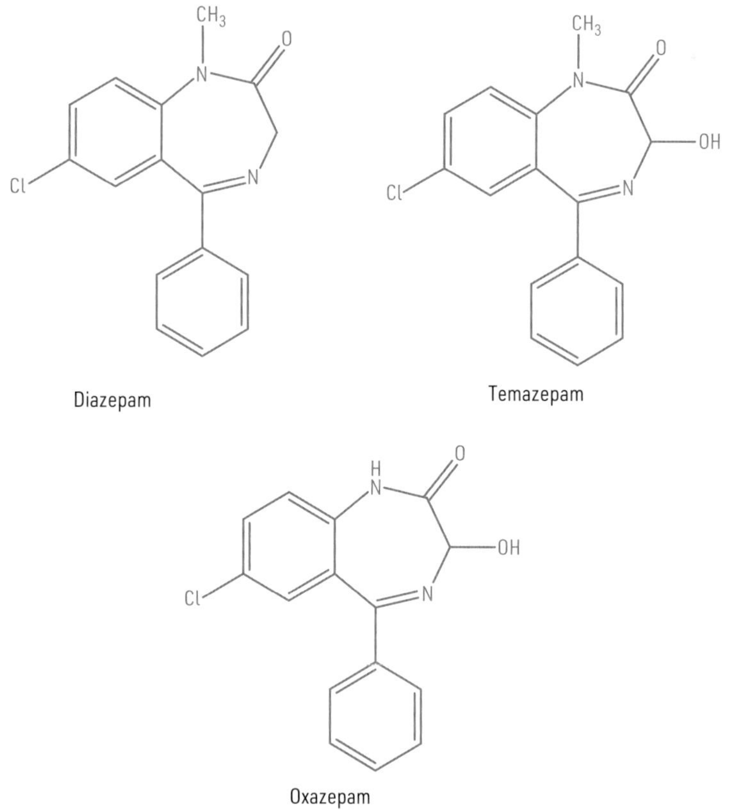

Diazepam

Temazepam

Oxazepam

Figure 12.13 Example of structural changes to retard metabolism

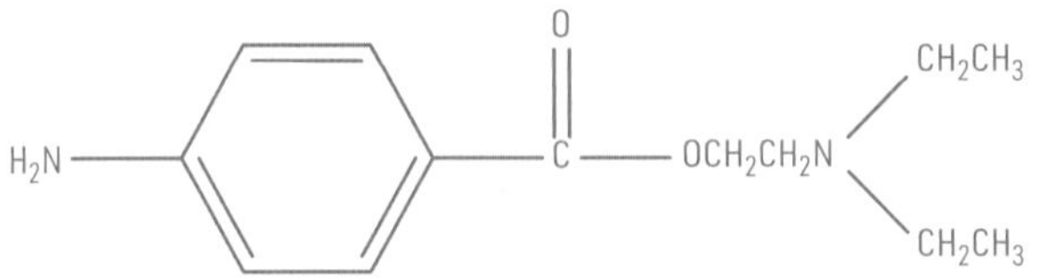

Procaine

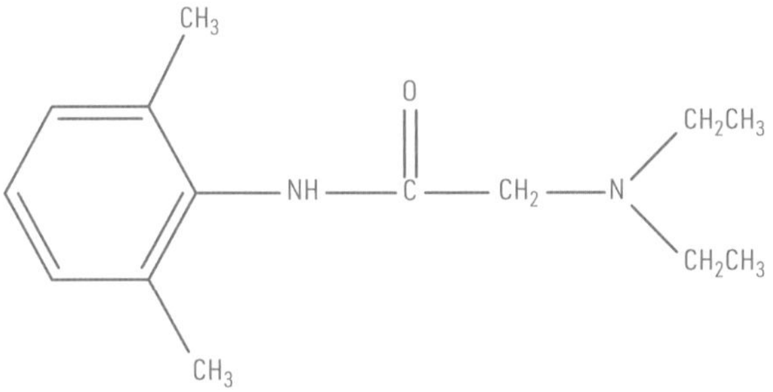

Lidocaine

temazepam and oxazepam are much reduced compared with diazepam itself (diazepam 20–40 hours, temazepam and oxazepam 8–12 hours). This results in a different clinical usage for temazepam and oxazepam, as hypnotics without any residual effects.

Alternatively, the duration of action of a drug can be increased by inclusion of groups which can retard metabolism. The ester group in the local anaesthetic procaine is easily hydrolysed. The duration of action can be increased by replacement of the ester group by an amide group which is more resistant to the action of esterases. The hydrolysis of the amide group can be further retarded by the inclusion of suitably placed bulky groups, leading to the long-acting local anaesthetic lidocaine (see Figure 12.13).

 Useful drugs can be developed by observation and utilization of the drug metabolism process.

12.6.3 **Metabolites with a different pharmacological activity**

From time to time, investigation of the metabolism of a drug candidate can lead to the discovery of a useful drug candidate in a different therapeutic area. Iproniazid, the first monoamine oxidase inhibitor to be used, was developed from structural modification of the anti-tubercular drug isoniazid in attempts to prevent its metabolism by acetylation (see Figure 12.14 and **➤ XR Section 12.4.4**). Sometimes a metabolite with a different pharmacological activity can lead to a situation of increased toxicity (**➤ XR Integration Box 12.4**).

 Useful drugs can be developed from observations that drug metabolites have activity in a different therapeutic area.

12.6.4 **Prodrugs**

Prodrugs are molecules that are pharmacologically inactive themselves but are converted to an active drug in the body, usually by the action of a metabolic enzyme. The prodrug can have a functional group present in

Figure 12.14 Example of a new drug developed from investigation of the metabolism of an existing drug

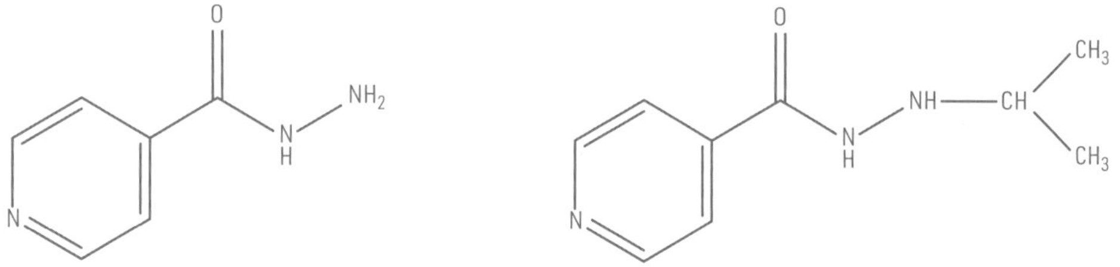

Isoniazid   Iproniazid

the molecule which is metabolically sensitive. Metabolism thus leads to the desired active molecule. Alternatively, the active drug may be combined with a carrier molecule. In this case, it is the link between the drug and the carrier molecule which is metabolically labile. There are a number of reasons why use of a prodrug is desirable, such as improving patient acceptance by masking odour, taste, or certain side effects, altering the drug activity profile (usually producing sustained release) and improving absorption and/or distribution.

 Prodrugs are pharmacologically inactive molecules which are converted to an active form by a metabolic reaction.

12.6.4.1 *Improving patient acceptance*

Drug substances often have a particularly unpleasant taste and prodrugs can be used to mask this taste, making them more acceptable to patients. Erythomycin is widely used to treat infections, particularly those which are resistant to penicillins. The problem with erythromycin, however, is that it tastes absolutely foul. Adults can utilize coated tablets which mask the taste, but children cannot utilize the 250mg tablets that adults can take. Erythromycin can be made tolerable for children by converting it to an ester, usually the ethylsuccinate (see Figure 12.15) and administering it as a suspension. An additional flavouring agent is also included to assist with the masking process. These esters need to be hydrolysed to erythromycin in the body by base-catalysed hydrolysis in the intestine and the bloodstream.

A similar situation arises with chloramphenicol which is converted to the tasteless palmitate ester which is hydrolysed *in vivo* to produce the active drug (see Figure 12.15).

Willow bark extract has been used for centuries to treat mild pain and fever and, in 1828, the active component was shown to be salicin. This is a prodrug, being converted to the active form, salicylic acid, in the body. Attempts to use salicylic acid itself led to serious side effects such as severe irritation of the mouth, throat, and stomach. Acetylation of the phenolic OH group of salicylic acid to form aspirin greatly reduces the side effects (see Figure 12.15).

An injection of the antibiotic clindamycin can be very painful at the site of injection. However, if it is converted to a more water-soluble phosphate ester the irritation due to the low aqueous solubility of clindamycin is reduced (see Figure 12.15).

 Prodrugs are often used to improve patient acceptability.

12.6.4.2 *Improving drug activity profile*

The use of prodrugs in this context involves mainly producing a sustained release profile of the active drug. The immunosuppressant drug azathioprine is very slowly metabolized to the active molecule, 6-mercaptopurine, thus effectively providing a sustained release profile of the drug (see Figure 12.6e).

Figure 12.15 Examples of prodrugs used to improve patient acceptance

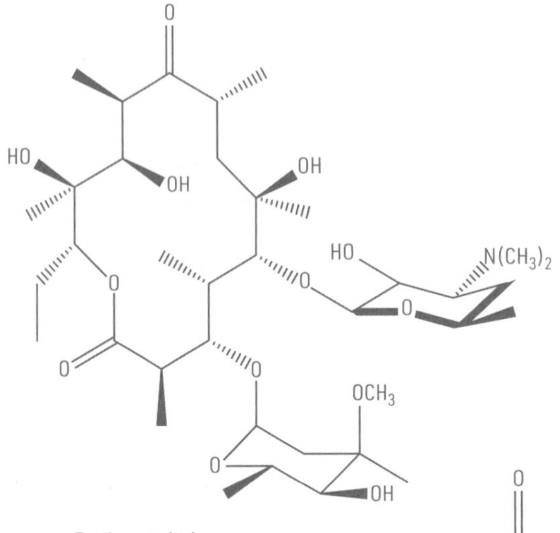

Erythromycin A

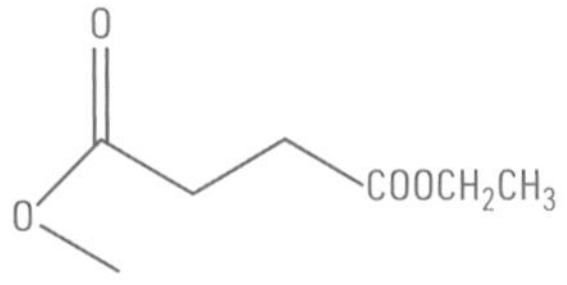

Erythromycin A ethylsuccinate

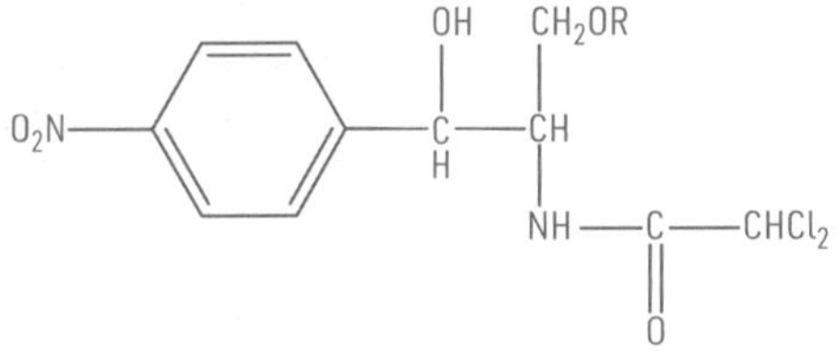

R = H chloramphenicol
R = CO(CH$_2$)$_{14}$CH$_3$
chloramphenicol palmitate

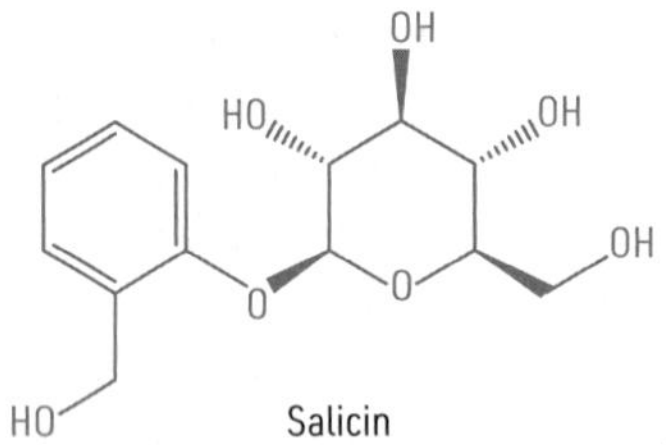

Salicin

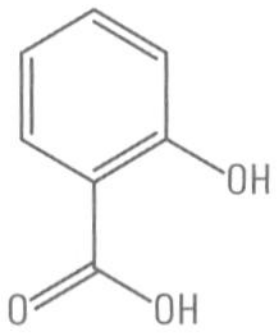

Salicylic acid

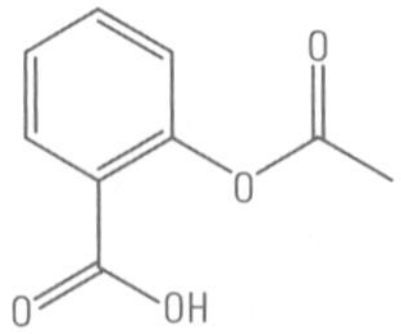

Aspirin

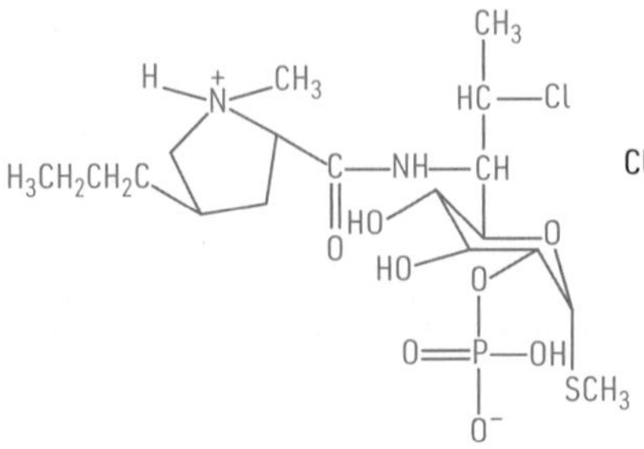

Clindamycin phosphate –
zwitterionic form

The rather slow metabolism is, in this case, due to the metabolic reaction being nucleophilic substitution with glutathione.

Another example of sustained release can be achieved by incorporating esters of steroid drugs into depot preparations. The esters are slowly released from the depot preparations and subsequently hydrolysed to the active steroid by esterases in the body.

 Prodrugs are often used to improve the activity profile of a drug.

12.6.4.3 *Improving absorption and/or distribution*

The parent drug may be too hydrophilic or too lipophilic for appropriate absorption and distribution. For example a drug containing a carboxylic acid group will be ionized at physiological pH, preventing optimum distribution. The angiotensin-converting enzyme (ACE) inhibitor enalaprilic acid is too hydrophilic to be readily absorbed, because of the presence of the carboxylic acid group. Enalapril, the ethyl ester of enalaprilic acid, is readily absorbed orally and then hydrolysed to the pharmacologically active carboxylic acid by esterases (see Figure 12.16).

If the parent drug is too lipid soluble, for example a steroid molecule, this can be dealt with by producing a succinate ester. A good example of this is the conversion of the highly lipophilic methylprednisolone

Figure 12.16 Examples of prodrugs used to improve absorption and distribution

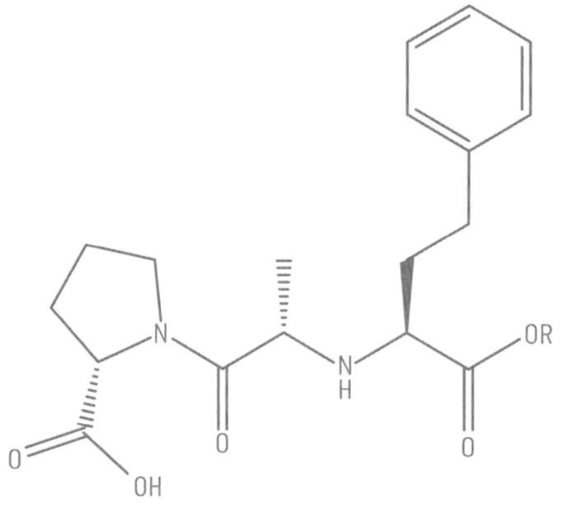

R = CH$_2$CH$_3$ enalapril
R = H enalaprilic acid

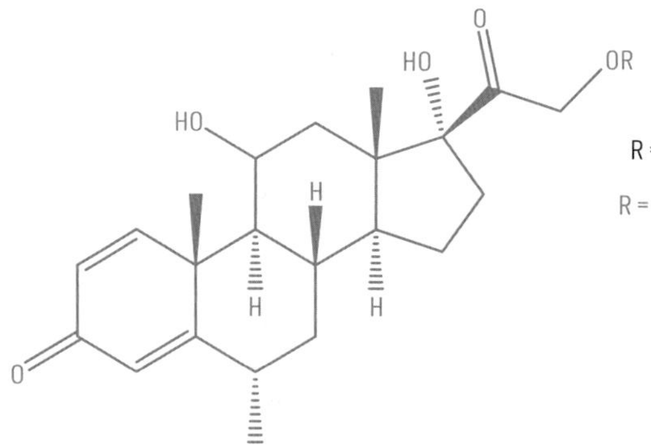

R = H methylprednisolone

R = —— C —— CH$_2$CH$_2$ —— COO⁻Na⁺
           ‖
           O

methylprednisolone
sodium succinate

Figure 12.17 Use of levodopa to deliver dopamine to the brain

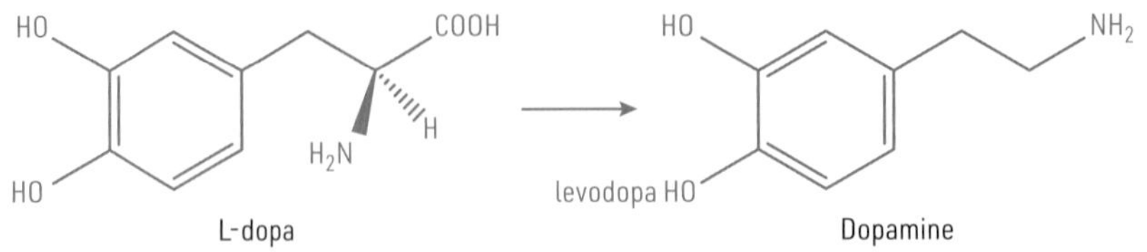

L-dopa → levodopa → Dopamine

into a water-soluble sodium succinate ester (see Figure 12.16). This form can then be formulated in both oral and intravenous dosage forms, whereas methylprednisolone is normally only found in tablet form. Once again, esterases in the body are responsible for producing the active methylprednisolone from the ester prodrug.

An unusual example involves levodopa (L-dopa) as a means of delivering dopamine to the central nervous system. Levodopa is a drug used to treat Parkinsonism which is a disease characterized by degradation of dopaminergic neurones in the brain. Replacement dopamine cannot be administered systemically for delivery to the central nervous system because it is too hydrophilic to cross the blood-brain barrier and is also subject to significant metabolism by oxidative deamination. However, if levodopa is used, delivery across the blood-brain barrier can be achieved. Levodopa is transported across the blood-brain barrier by an active transport system designed to incorporate L-amino acids into the central nervous system. Once across the blood-brain barrier, Levodopa is decarboxylated to produce dopamine (see Figure 12.17).

Prodrugs are often used to improve the absorption and/or distribution of a drug.

? Questions

1. Suggest possible metabolic routes for the following drugs: pethidine, amphetamine, ibuprofen, lidocaine, trimethoprim. Compare your suggestions with the known metabolic routes for these drugs.

2. The metabolism of benzo-[a]-pyrene gives rise to a toxic metabolite containing an epoxide and a diol. What is the structure of this metabolite and why is it toxic?

3. Phenacetin, an analgesic once widely used, was withdrawn from use because of toxicity to the kidney. One suggested reason for this toxicity is related to the metabolism of phenacetin—what is the suggested mechanism for this?

4. Why might it be desirable to design a drug with a very short duration of action?

5. How is UDGPA formed from glucose-1-phosphate?

6. Why is it particularly difficult to find an appropriate animal model to study human drug metabolism?

↻ Chapter summary

- The principal objective of drug metabolism is aiding the removal of the drug from the body by increasing its water solubility.

- Drug design requires a detailed knowledge of drug metabolism.

- The liver is the most important site of drug metabolism, although drug metabolism can take place in other tissues.

- Drug metabolism takes place in two phases—Phase I and Phase II. Both phases are designed to produce metabolites with increased water solubility.
- Phase I metabolism involves the introduction or unmasking of a group with increased water solubility.
- Phase II metabolism involves reaction of a drug and/or its Phase I metabolite with an endogenous molecule to produce a highly water-soluble conjugate.
- The most important Phase I reactions are oxidation reactions, mainly catalysed by cytochrome P450 enzymes. Other Phase I reactions are reduction and hydrolysis.
- The endogenous molecules involved in Phase II reactions are glucuronic acid, sulphate, acetylCoA, amino acids, and glutathione.
- Drug metabolism can be affected by a number of factors including disease, age, gender, diet, and genetics.
- Some drugs are capable of inducing or inhibiting the activity of drug metabolizing enzymes.
- Stereoisomerism can have a significant effect on drug metabolism, resulting in enantiomers being metabolized by different routes or at different rates or both.
- When a pharmacologically active molecule is metabolized, the metabolite(s) may be pharmacologically inactive, may exhibit different potency or may exhibit a different type of pharmacological activity. All these situations can be potentially exploited in drug design.
- Prodrugs are pharmacologically inactive, but are converted to a pharmacologically active molecule by drug metabolism processes.
- Prodrugs may be used for a number of reasons including improving patient acceptance, improving the drug activity profile and improving absorption and distribution properties.

📖 Further reading

Roden, D.M. and George, A.L. (2002) The genetic basis of variability in drug responses, *Nature Reviews Drug Discovery* 1: 37–44.

A review of the genetic influence on drug metabolism.

Jones, S., Preston, C.L., and Sandhu, H. (2014) How fruit juice interacts with common medicines, *Pharmaceutical Journal* 293: 369–72.

An article explaining how fruit juices can affect the metabolism of medicines.

Jenner, P. and Testa, B. (1973) The influence of stereochemical factors on drug disposition, *Drug Metabolism Reviews* 2: 117.

A review in which the impact of stereochemistry on drug metabolism is considered.

Coleman, M. (2010) *Human Drug Metabolism: An Introduction*. 2nd edn, Oxford, UK: Wiley.

An accessible text dealing with all aspects of drug metabolism, including a number of case studies.

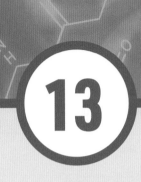

Pharmacogenetics and Pharmacogenomics

The two terms in the title of this chapter are often used interchangeably but there is actually a subtle difference between them. Pharmacogenetics is the study of how variations in a single gene can influence an individual's response to drugs with respect to therapeutic as well as adverse effects. Pharmacogenomics, however, is the study of how all the genes (the genome) can influence responses to drugs. As can be seen in the previous chapter, drug metabolism can be influenced by a number of factors, such as health, age, and diet (➤ XR Section 12.5). Another important influence in this respect is an individual's genetic makeup and the term pharmacogenetics was coined to reflect this relationship between drug response (pharmacology) and genetics. Subsequent sequencing of the human genome has allowed the study of the influence of multiple genes, rather than a single gene, on an individual's response to drugs, hence the term pharmacogenomics. The chapter describes the development of the science of pharmacogenetics (➤ XR Section 13.1), the clinical importance of polymorphisms of certain metabolic enzymes (➤ XR Section 13.2), and the potential and challenges which the relatively new science of pharmacogenomics presents for the process of drug design (➤ XR Section 13.8).

13.1 THE HISTORY OF PHARMACOGENETICS

The development of pharmacogenetics can be traced back to 1932 when Arthur Fox, a chemist working at Du Pont Industries, spilt a quantity of phenylthiocarbamide (PTC) (see Figure 13.1). A colleague complained of a bitter taste in the air, but Fox could taste nothing. What followed was an experiment which would not be allowed under current health and safety legislation—they conducted taste tests on PTC and concluded that there was a significant difference in a 'large sample' of people and that this variation was

Figure 13.1 Phenylthiocarbamide

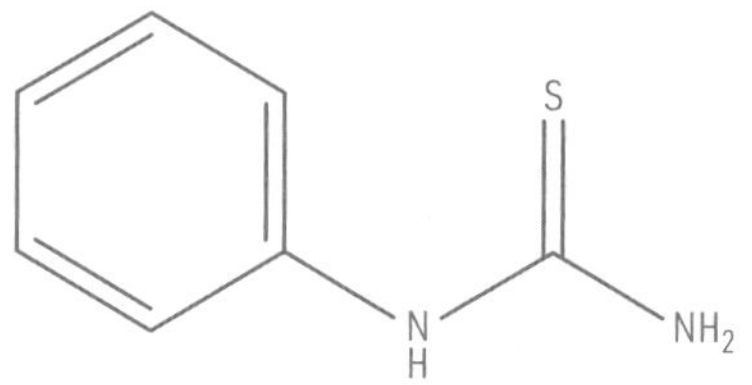

Phenylthiocarbamide

unaffected by factors such as gender, age or ethnicity (see Box 13.1 Toxicity of phenylthiocarbamide). This finding was picked up by geneticists, in particular L.H. Snyder, who subsequently attributed the taste sensitivity to PTC to a single **recessive gene**.

BOX 13.1 TOXICITY OF PHENYLTHIOCARBAMIDE

The testing of sensitivity has been refined from the original taste testing used by Fox in 1932, where tasting of the powdered compound was used. PTC taste sensitivity is tested using small strips of paper impregnated with PTC. This method has been used in schools and colleges as an experiment to demonstrate genetic polymorphism. However, PTC is classed as very toxic and has an LD_{50} of 3mg/kg and has been replaced by the less toxic 6-propylthiouracil (PROP), a drug which has been used to treat hyperthyroidism. PROP, however, does not show as good an association with the PTC taste gene. Compounds with similar structures are to be found in plants of the *Brassica* family, so there is perhaps a good genetic reason if you don't like Brussels sprouts.

Subsequently, in the 1950s, genetic polymorphisms for glucose-6-phosphate dehydrogenase, butyrylcholinesterase and N-acetyltransferase (➤ **XR Section 12.5.5**) were described. However the most significant development took place in the late 1970s and early 1980s with the identification of genetic polymorphisms of cytochrome P450 enzymes. The clinical relevance of these genetic polymorphisms can be both pharmacokinetic and pharmacodynamic. A change in the normal metabolic enzymes can lead to altered drug metabolism. Increased or decreased metabolism will change the concentration of circulating drug in the body and, additionally, may give rise to active, inactive or toxic metabolites. A genetic polymorphism may give rise to an unexpected drug effect outside its normal therapeutic indication (see Integration Box 13.1 Glucose-6-phosphate dehydrogenase deficiency).

INTEGRATION BOX 13.1 GLUCOSE-6-PHOSPHATE DEHYDROGENASE DEFICIENCY

The genetic polymorphism related to glucose-6-phosphate dehydrogenase was discovered during World War Two. American soldiers engaged in conflicts in the Far East were supplied with antimalarial drugs, in particular those based on 8-aminoquinolones such as pamaquine and primaquine. Some soldiers were found to suffer from haemolysis after taking the antimalarial medication. It was observed that only soldiers of black African origin suffered from this side effect. Subsequent testing showed this situation to be caused by a deficiency of glucose-6-phosphate dehydrogenase.

The proteins of the cell membrane of erythrocytes are kept in a reduced and functional state by glutathione. Erythrocyte cell membranes, as oxygen carriers in the blood, are at risk from oxidation, particularly by free radicals unless sufficient glutathione is present. Glucose-6-phosphate dehydrogenase is necessary for maintaining the

→

supply of glutathione. Individuals with glucose-6-phosphate dehydrogenase deficiency are thus at risk of haemolytic anaemia in conditions of oxidative stress. The metabolism of 8-aminoquinolones produces reactive oxidative metabolites which interfere with the malarial parasites but also with the membrane proteins of erythrocytes, causing haemolysis in the case of individuals with glucose-6-phosphate dehydrogenase deficiency. This deficiency is a common genetic trait found in people living in areas where malaria is endemic and provides some resistance against the malarial parasite.

The science of pharmacogenetics has a long history dating back to the 1930s but was initially linked to empirical observations regarding, mainly, drug metabolism.

13.2 CYTOCHROME P450 2D6 (CYP2D6) POLYMORPHISM

CYP2D6 is probably the most widely studied drug metabolic enzyme in humans. CYP2D6 is clinically important as it is responsible for about 25 per cent of the metabolism of known drugs and is involved in the metabolism of drugs used in a wide variety of conditions (see Table 13.1). The genetic polymorphism associated with CYP2D6 was discovered in the 1970s, when individuals were shown to be unable to metabolize the antihypertensive drug debrisoquine (see Figure 13.2). Subsequently it has been shown that individuals can be divided into poor metabolizers (little or no CYP2D6 function), extensive metabolizers (normal CYP2D6 function), and ultra-rapid metabolizers (possess multiple copies of the CYP2D6 gene). Although debrisoquine has been superseded by more useful antihypertensive drugs (because of problems with its metabolism), it has found widespread use for clinical determination of an individual's CYP2D6 phenotype by monitoring the plasma levels of its metabolite, 4-hydroxydebrisoquine (see Figure 13.2) (see Integration Box 13.2 Debrisoquine and sparteine). There are 48 known polymorphisms of CYP2D6. Poor metabolizers are most common in white populations, e.g. approximately 6 per cent of the UK population. Ultra-rapid (also known as enhanced) metabolizers are more common in Middle East and North African populations. A lack of CYP2D6 function is a recessive trait arising from two defective copies of the gene, one from each parent. The next three sub-sections provide examples of the clinical significance of CYP2D6 polymorphism.

Table 13.1 Major substrates and inhibitors of CYP2D6

Substrates	Inhibitors
Tricyclic antidepressants	SSRIs
SSRIs	Amiodarone
Neuroleptics	Methadone
β-blockers	Quinidine
Antiarrythmics	Ritanavir
Chlorpropamide	Trifluperidol
Codeine	

Figure 13.2 a Metabolic hydroxylation of debrisoquine

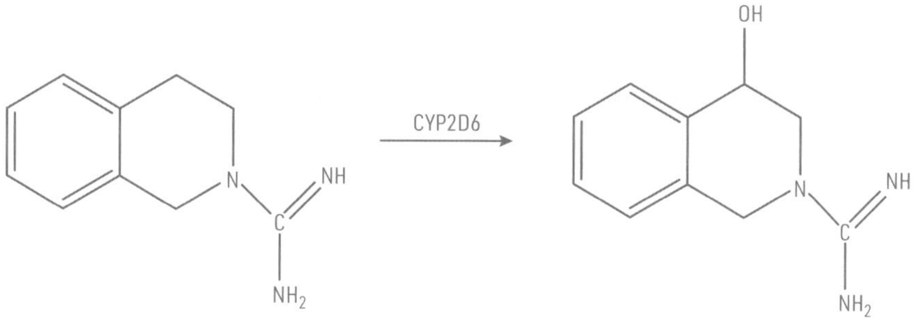

Figure 13.2 b Metabolic oxidation of sparteine

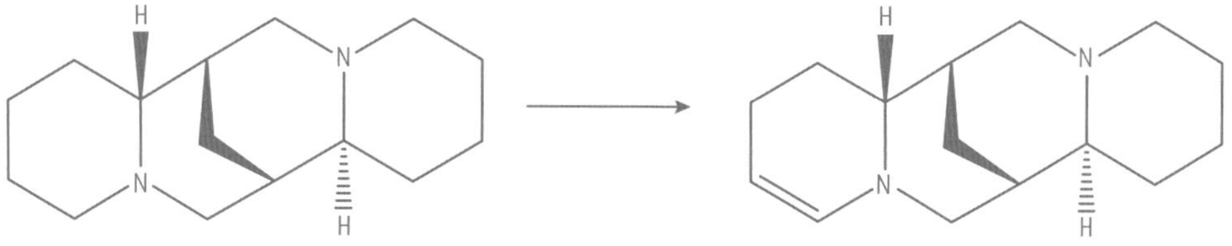

Sparteine   5-dehydrosparteine

INTEGRATION BOX 13.2   **DEBRISOQUINE AND SPARTEINE**

The polymorphism of CYP2D6 was discovered by serendipity in two different situations, almost simultaneously. One commenced with the personal observation of a clinical pharmacologist in London who had taken the antihypertensive drug debrisoquine. He felt dizzy, faint, and experienced serious hypotension. He and co-workers subsequently identified two phenotypes of CYP2D6 by performing a study on the metabolism of debrisoquine on 94 volunteers which was published in 1977. At about the same time a study, in Germany, on the antiarrythmic activity of sparteine produced, in some subjects, severe side effects and it was found that their plasma levels of sparteine were 4–5 times higher than those subjects who did not experience these side effects. Again two phenotypes were identified, and the work was published in 1978. The genetic basis of this polymorphism was finally elucidated about 10 years later. A third study in 1967, on the pharmacokinetics of nortriptyline and desipramine (both CYP2D6 substrates), had shown very significant variations in plasma levels, although at first it was not recognized that these variations were related to genetics.

Genetic polymorphism of cytochrome P450 2D6 is one of the most clinically significant of the drug metabolic enzyme polymorphisms.

13.2.1 Selective serotonin reuptake inhibitors (SSRIs) and CYP2D6

CYP2D6 has a major influence on the metabolism of SSRIs and is involved in the biotransformation of all of the currently used SSRIs (see Figure 13.3). In most cases the main metabolic route is N-demethylation but in the case of paroxetine it is O-demethylation. In polymorphic variants where CYP2D6 is absent, reduced or increased, the risk of adverse drug reactions and decreased efficacy is increased, with a possible influence, in the worst-case scenario, on a patient's suicide risk. There may even be a problem when normal CYP2D6 function is present because SSRIs are known to inhibit CYP2D6.

Figure 13.3 Examples of SSRIs metabolized by CYP2D6

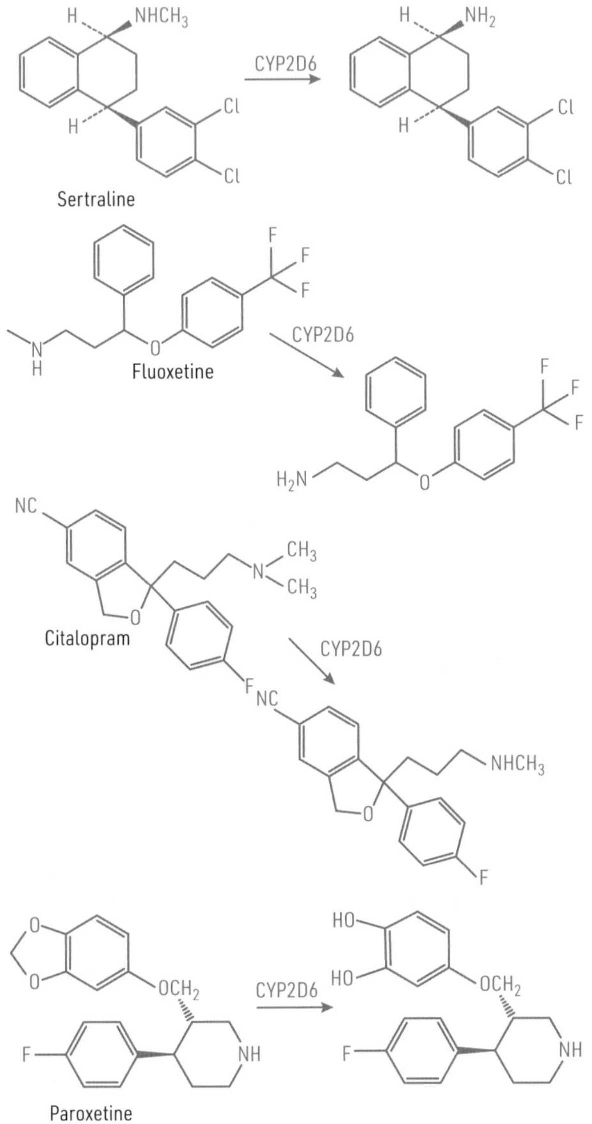

Polymorphisms of CYP2D6 can have a clinically significant effect on the activity of SSRIs.

13.2.2 Tamoxifen and CYP2D6

Tamoxifen, an oestrogen receptor antagonist, is metabolized by CYP2D6 to 4-hydroxydesmethyltamoxifen (endoxifen), its primary active metabolite (see Figure 13.4). Patients identified as poor metabolizers on the basis of a lack of CYP2D6 had lower endoxifen levels than patients with normal CYP2D6 function. Poor metabolizers were shown to have significantly higher relapse rates in breast cancer than extensive metabolizers, although they didn't show significantly reduced survival rates. Clinically, because of the SSRI situation described above, it is suggested that the use of potent CYP2D6-inhibiting SSRIs are avoided with patients taking tamoxifen.

Figure 13.4 Tamoxifen metabolism

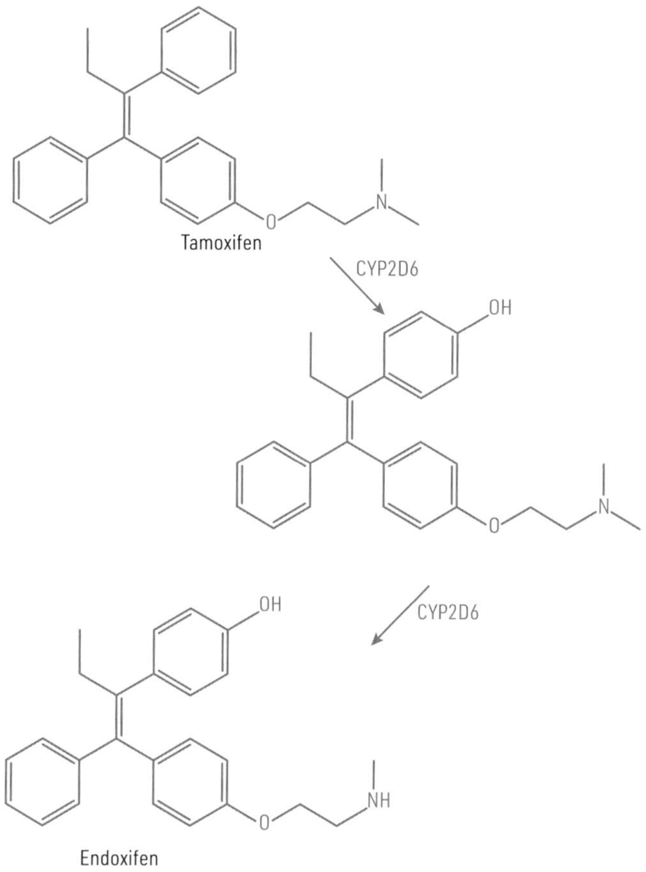

Tamoxifen

CYP2D6

CYP2D6

Endoxifen

 Polymorphisms of CYP2D6 can have clinically significant effects on the activity of tamoxifen.

13.2.3 Codeine and CYP2D6

Codeine is metabolized to morphine and this is catalysed by CYP2D6 (see Figure 13.5). Ultra-rapid (extensive) metabolizers will, therefore, produce higher levels of morphine than usual when taking codeine. Patients taking codeine for serious pain relief (such as post-operative pain) may experience opiate intoxication if they are ultra-rapid metabolizers (see Integration Box 13.3 Mother/baby opiate intoxication).

| INTEGRATION BOX 13.3 | MOTHER/BABY OPIATE INTOXICATION |

A case has been reported where a mother was prescribed codeine for pain relief after giving birth. Unfortunately her baby died 13 days later from morphine intoxication. The mother had been breast-feeding the baby during this time. Subsequent genotyping revealed that the mother had a CYP2D6 polymorphism arising from gene duplication and so was an ultra-rapid metabolizer. Thus, the mother was converting the prescribed codeine very rapidly to morphine which was then excreted in the breast milk. This led to a toxic level of morphine accumulating in the baby who, being a neonate, had not developed the necessary enzymes to metabolize the morphine it was receiving via the breast milk.

Figure 13.5 Metabolism of codeine to morphine

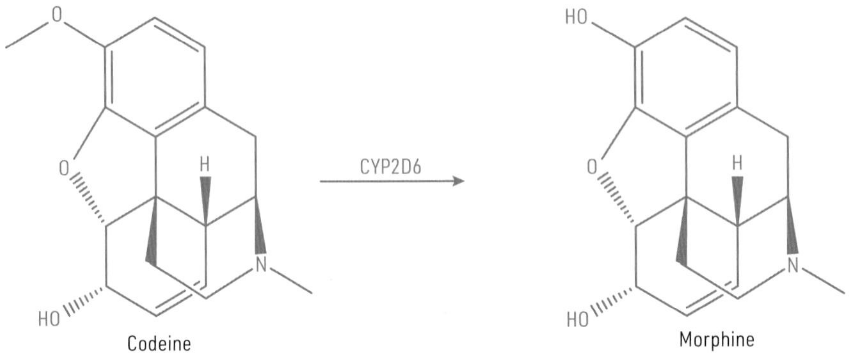

Codeine → CYP2D6 → Morphine

Polymorphisms of CYP2D6 can have significant clinical effects on codeine metabolism.

13.3 CYTOCHROME P450 2C9 (CYP2C9) POLYMORPHISM

CYP2C9 is another important cytochrome P450 enzyme which exhibits polymorphism. Significant drug substrates for this enzyme are warfarin, phenytoin, tolbutamide and NSAIDs such as ibuprofen and diclofenac. Around 40 per cent of Europeans exhibit one or two of the known variants known as CYP2C9*2 and CYP2C9*3. Unlike CYP2D6, these variants were not discovered by drug investigations but were discovered by genetic fingerprinting. The two variants are different in their influence on drugs. CYP2C9*2 is substrate dependent. It has little effect on the metabolism of NSAIDs but causes a reduction in the metabolism of S-warfarin. CYP2C9*3, however, is not substrate dependent but has a much larger effect, reducing hydroxylation of warfarin by about ten-fold (see Figure 13.6).

Figure 13.6 Metabolism of warfarin isomers

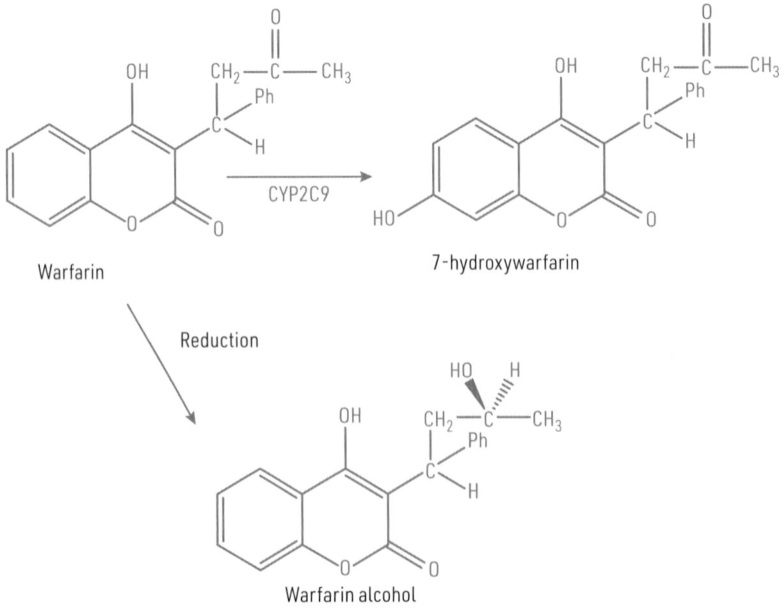

Warfarin → CYP2C9 → 7-hydroxywarfarin

Reduction → Warfarin alcohol

Obviously, this situation is clinically very important from the point of view of getting the correct dose of warfarin for each patient. Too high a dose of the anticoagulant could lead to internal bleeding: too low a dose could result in clot formation. The extent of metabolism, therefore, is vital to this situation. Warfarin is a mixture of R and S isomers; the higher anticoagulant activity being associated with the S isomer. It is this isomer which is metabolized by CYP2C9, whereas the R isomer is metabolized mainly by reduction (see Figure 13.6). In the USA, it is now advised that patients to be prescribed warfarin are phenotyped for CYP2C9 in order to improve the safety and efficacy of their drug usage. It is also important to avoid drug-drug interactions which can arise from the co-administration of drugs which inhibit CYP2C9, such as the H_2-antagonist cimetidine (**> XR Integration Box 12.5**).

 Polymorphism of CYP2C9 can have clinically significant effects, particularly with respect to warfarin therapy.

13.4 METHYLTRANSFERASE POLYMORPHISM

Just as with cytochrome P450 metabolizing enzymes, there is a large number of methyltransferase enzymes, such as O-methyltransferases, N-methyltransferases, and S-methyltransferases. Methyltransferases appear to oppose the general principle of metabolism, i.e. to make xenobiotics more water soluble, the addition of a methyl group generally increasing hydrophobicity. Nevertheless, these enzymes play an important role in metabolism. In particular they play an important role in the activation of physiologically active amines such as noradrenaline, dopamine, serotonin, and histamine.

Catechol-O-methyltransferase (COMT) terminates the activity of noradrenaline and dopamine by O-methylation (see Figure 13.7). COMT will also methylate drugs which contain catechol, phenol, amino, N-heterocyclic, and thiol groups. Examples of such drugs are methyldopa, dopa, isoprotenerol and morphine (see Figure 13.8). Note that all these drugs contain the catechol group except morphine. O-methylation of morphine to produce codeine occurs to a significant extent in morphine-tolerant individuals (up to 10 per cent of the morphine dose).

Whereas N-methylation of endogenous amines occurs to a significant extent, N-methylation of xenobiotics occurs only to a limited extent.

S-methyltransferase methylates 6-mercaptopurine which is used in cancer chemotherapy and as an immunosuppressant (see Figure 13.9). The enzyme involved, thiopurine-S-methyltransferase (TPMT),

Figure 13.7 Metabolism of noradrenaline and dopamine

HO, HO — (Noradrenaline) — NH$_2$, OH → COMT → HO, H$_3$CO — NH$_2$, OH

HO, HO — (Dopamine) — NH$_2$ → COMT → HO, H$_3$CO — NH$_2$

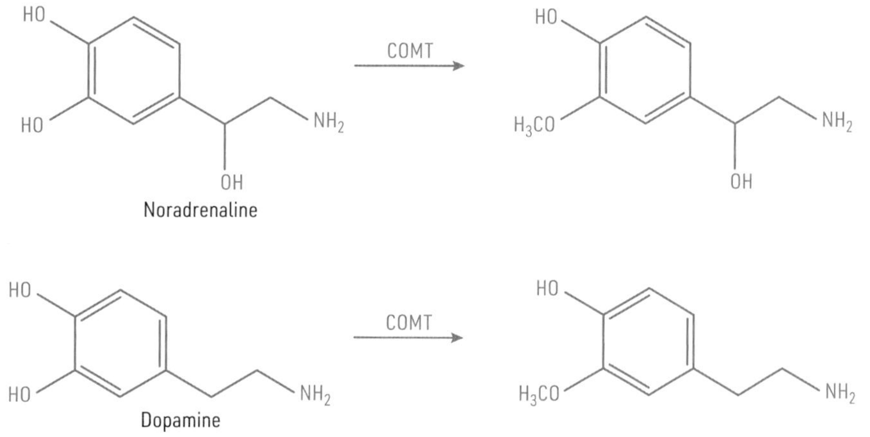

Figure 13.8 Examples of drugs metabolized by COMT

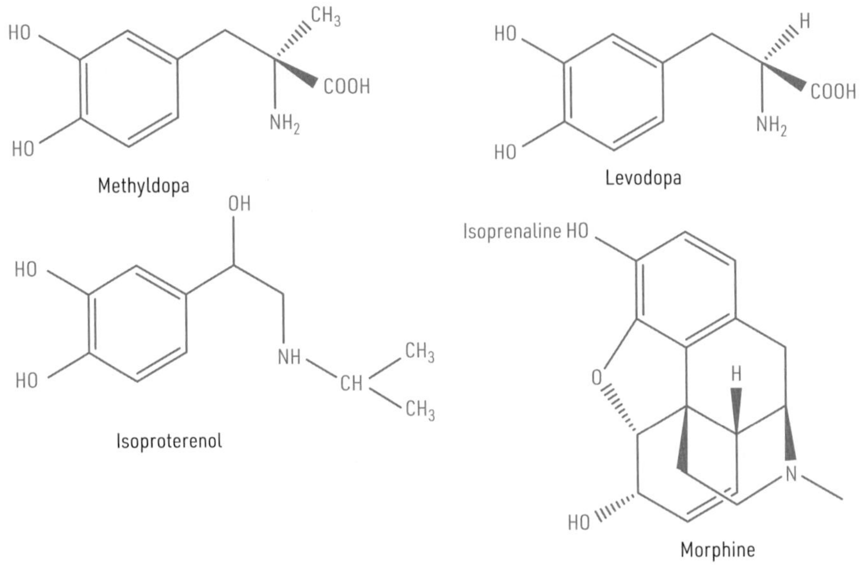

Methyldopa

Levodopa

Isoproterenol

Isoprenaline

Morphine

Figure 13.9 Metabolism of 6-azathioprine and 6-mercaptopurine

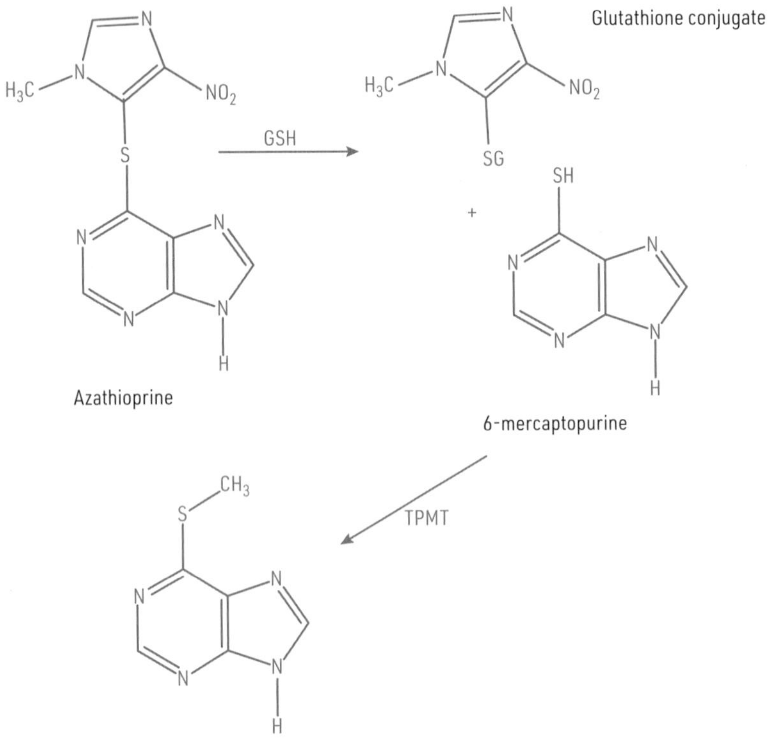

Glutathione conjugate

GSH

Azathioprine

6-mercaptopurine

TPMT

exhibits polymorphism where some individuals lack TPMT activity which puts them at risk of increased toxicity if administered 6-mercaptopurine or azathioprine.

 Polymorphism of thiopurine-S-methyltransferase is the most clinically important within the methyltransferases.

13.5 IDIOSYNCRATIC ADVERSE DRUG REACTIONS

Such reactions are rare but are more difficult to predict than the previously described polymorphism examples, because there appear to be other factors, other than genetic, which have an additional influence, including a possible contribution from the immune system. These are often referred to as genome-wide reactions and are difficult to study because of their rarity. However, pharmacogenetic studies have been used to potentially shed light on these problems.

Flucloxacillin is an antibiotic commonly used to treat staphylococcal infections but can cause liver toxicity which is manifested as jaundice. Normally, this situation is resolved by withdrawal of the drug. However, in a small number of individuals, this resolution does not occur, and this can result in severe liver failure. The individuals in which this has occurred have been shown, by genome-wide association studies, to possess a particular mutated gene known as the human leukocyte antigen-B*5701 gene. A similar situation has been examined with respect to a common side effect of statins—that of myopathy. Again, this is normally resolved by withdrawal of the drug, but in a small number of individuals can persist, potentially leading to death. Again, genome-wide association studies have identified a single defective gene (SLCO1B1 gene) thought to be responsible.

 Some adverse drug reactions are difficult to predict because they involve factors other than genetic polymorphisms.

13.6 PHASE II PHARMACOGENETICS

The enzymes associated with Phase II metabolism exhibit less polymorphism than those associated with Phase I metabolism, although there are a few significant pharmacogenetic variations. The Phase II metabolic reactions associated with polymorphism are those catalysed by sulphotransferases and N-acetyltransferases.

 Phase II metabolic enzymes exhibit less clinically significant polymorphisms than Phase I metabolic enzymes.

13.6.1 Sulphotransferases

There are at least eleven isoforms of human sulphotransferases and several contribute to drug metabolism. The most significant of these is glutathione-S-transferase (GST). There are known to be three polymorphic forms of GST—GSTM1, GSTT1, and GSTP1. Possession of GSTM1 and GSTT1 isoforms results in loss of enzyme activity, whereas possession of GSTP1 results in a slight reduction in catalytic activity.

GSTM1 is involved with the detoxification of the toxic metabolite of benzo-[a]-pyrene (❯ XR Box 12.1) and approximately 50 per cent of Europeans possess this polymorphism (another reason to give up smoking!).

GSTT1 is largely involved in the metabolism of small organic molecules such as simple halogenated hydrocarbons. About 15 per cent of Europeans lack this enzyme but there is no link with the lack of GSTM1 because their synthesis is coded by entirely separate genes. Much less is known about GSTP1, but it is thought to be involved in some xenobiotic metabolism as well as being implicated in a susceptibility to certain cancers such as lung cancer, prostate cancer, and breast cancer.

 Sulphotransferases are mainly involved in the metabolism of toxic organic xenobiotics but may be implicated in the susceptibility to some cancers.

13.6.2 N-acetyltransferases

There are two forms of human N-acetyltransferase (NAT1 and NAT2). These enzymes have different but overlapping substrate specificities. Drugs metabolized by these enzymes include isoniazid (❯ **XR Section 12.5.5**), and sulfanilamides (see Figure 13.10). NAT2 is lacking in about 50 per cent of Europeans and they are referred to as slow acetylators.

Figure 13.10 Examples of drugs metabolized by N-acetyltransferases

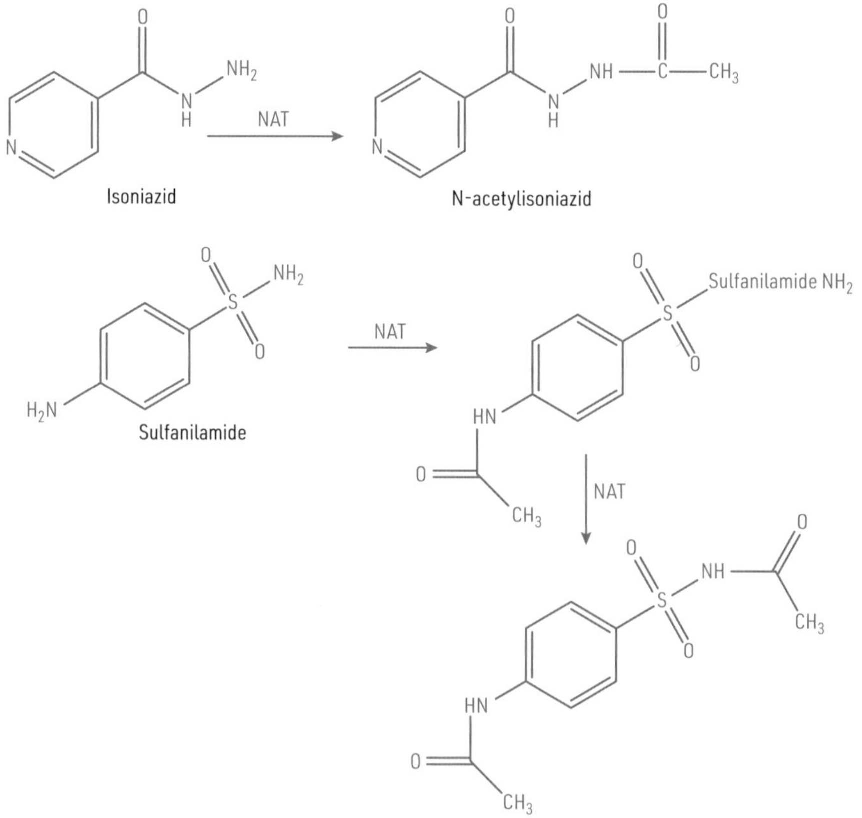

13.7 THE CLINICAL RELEVANCE OF PHARMACOGENETICS

Pharmacogenetic testing is already available and there are a number of areas in which patients can potentially benefit from such testing. Knowledge of an individual's genetic profile could help in deciding the most effective choice from a range of available drugs (it has been suggested that 30–50 per cent of people do not obtain a useful clinical response to drugs). Such genetic knowledge could be used to avoid potentially dangerous side effects. The genetic knowledge could be used to make dose adjustments, such as varying the dose of a drug for particular individuals or changing the dosing interval for different individuals. Genetic information could also be used to diagnose certain disorders, or to develop more effective therapeutic strategies.

There are a number of limitations for genetic-based dose adjustments. Although genetic testing is available (for example for several of the cytochrome P450s), there is still a lack of hard data providing evidence of the usefulness of this approach. Most of the data comes from what are known as association studies. These are studies on groups of patients who are taking a particular drug and an examination is undertaken of individual responses to the drug and related to their genotype. Often these studies have been performed on relatively small sample sizes and, currently, there are very few prospective studies of dose adjustments. However, there are a number of situations where pharmacogenetic-based dose adjustments are already made including oral anticoagulants (CYP2C9), β-blockers (CYP2D6) and 6-mercaptopurine (TPMT).

The areas in which pharmacogenetic testing might make the most impact are those involving long-term drug therapy for drugs with a narrow therapeutic index and those drugs with serious adverse side effects. As ever the cost/benefit relationship has to be investigated with respect to the cost of adverse drug reactions and subsequent hospitalization and the cost of such genetic testing.

 Pharmacogenetic testing could prove useful in making clinically valuable dose adjustments for certain drugs, particularly those with narrow therapeutic indices and with serious side effects.

13.8 PHARMACOGENOMICS

The promise of pharmacogenomics for the future is to be able to move from defining a disease by its symptoms to an understanding of the mechanism of that disease. This will allow the recognition that a disease is not uniform but exhibits heterogeneity between patients. It will also allow the recognition that patients are not uniform and, therefore, that uniform drug treatment is not appropriate, heralding the introduction of individualized therapy. Additionally, if the mechanism of the disease is known there is the potential for preventative cure, as opposed to treatment of an established illness.

The sequencing of the human genome in 2003 has led to the concept of 'druggable' and 'non-druggable' targets. 'Druggable' targets are those which can involve the use of conventional drug interventions. 'Non-druggable' targets are those which are likely to require non-conventional approaches such as anti-sense or gene therapies. In 2006 it was estimated that there were approximately 250 drug targets (300 if you include pathogens as targets) for approved drugs, which is about 1 per cent of the potential targets suggested by the human genome (~25,000 individual genes).

 The science of pharmacogenomics holds much promise for the ways in which diseases are treated in the future.

13.8.1 Phenotyping and genotyping

Within pharmacogenomics there are two techniques which can be used to identify associations between genomic data and drug response patterns—these are known as phenotyping and genotyping. Phenotyping was the first technique to be introduced and is the identification of a gene and its influence on the response to a drug (e.g. polymorphisms of metabolizing enzymes previously discussed). Genotyping involves the identification of a gene (or genes) which relate to a particular function which may be involved in a disease state. The current availability and cost of pharmacogenomic tests means that there is more emphasis on phenotyping than genotyping. With a few exceptions, these types of genetic testing are mainly restricted to patients taking part in academic studies or clinical trials (association studies).

Phenotyping involves the administration of a marker or test drug (e.g. debrisoquine, ❯ XR Section 13.2) and collection and analysis of body fluids, and may have to be repeated at regular intervals. Genotyping is a one in a lifetime test and is unequivocal. Currently the expense of such tests means that they are restricted to individuals considered to be at high risk, such as potential carriers of a potential gene disorder, e.g. cystic fibrosis, breast cancer.

The trend is towards molecular diagnosis of multifactorial diseases such as cardiac disease (there is now a genetic test for inherited cardiovascular disease and sudden death—if you have £2000). Techniques are not yet at the stage where these tests can be offered to all, due to financial restriction, and genetic testing within the NHS is governed by NICE criteria. However, advances in DNA analysis, mutation detection, and the increasing computerization of such tests means that, in the future, genetic testing should become a standard medical tool.

 Phenotyping is already used to provide information about metabolic enzyme polymorphisms and its use will probably expand in the future whereas genotyping is still in its infancy but will also prove very useful in the future.

13.8.2 Pharmacogenomics—the challenges

There are a number of challenges to the increased use of pharmacogenomics with a view to the development of individualized therapy. These challenges can be broadly divided into scientific, ethical, social and legal issues, although most issues do straddle these broad boundaries.

The scientific challenges are probably the easiest to address as these issues will probably be solved as the scientific basis of pharmacogenomics develops. Currently, there is a limited range of situations where genetic testing has been proven to be of clinical value, such as warfarin therapy, 6-mercaptopurine therapy, and the detection of certain single gene disorders such as cystic fibrosis. There still remains much work to be done to improve the evidence that genetic testing can be of greater value in healthcare. There are not yet adequate statistics to support its wider use because most patient studies have been carried out retrospectively on relatively small numbers of individuals. What is required are more prospective studies based on hypotheses about disease states and their links to genetic profiles. This is necessary because with complex disorders like heart disease, diabetes, or cancer, the current level of test validity is only indicative of probability rather than certainty.

One of the most serious challenges to pharmacogenomics is that of privacy of data, i.e. who has the right to the data generated from genetic testing. As things stand, an individual has the right to knowledge of their medical details and this ought to extend to results of genetic testing. The question arises as to who else has a right, or need, to access that data. If the information is to be used in making decisions about therapy, the appropriate healthcare workers need to know. However, is there a case for employers, insurers, and law enforcement agencies to have access to this information, with or without the individual's permission?

Linked to the privacy of genetic data are a number of social issues. We have already seen that there are some significant ethnic and geographical differences in enzyme polymorphisms. A wider availability of such information could lead to patient segmentation, quite possibly on the basis of cost/benefit analysis. This situation could lead, effectively, to the stigmatization of some groups of patients as untreatable. Another social issue relates to the conceptual and philosophical implications of an individual knowing the genetic testing results. Such knowledge may cause changes in the behaviour of individuals in areas such as reproductive issues (to have/not to have children) and lifestyle changes (knowledge of the possession of a gene relating to cancer—what would be the effect on an apparently healthy individual knowing they are likely to develop cancer in the future, see Integration Box 13.4 Angelina Jolie)?

INTEGRATION BOX 13.4 | **ANGELINA JOLIE**

The film star Angelina Jolie had a double mastectomy in 2013 after finding out that she possessed a genetic mutation that greatly increased her risk of developing breast cancer. She had already lost her grandmother, mother, and an aunt to cancer. She was shown to have a mutation of the *BRCA1* gene which gave an estimated 87 per cent risk of developing breast cancer and a 50 per cent risk of ovarian cancer. In 2015 a blood test raised fears that she was in the early stages of ovarian cancer. As her mother had died of ovarian cancer, she chose to have her ovaries removed.

Finally, there are a number of potential legal issues relating to the use of pharmacogenomics. These are mostly related to confidentiality of the genetic data and exactly who has the right to access that data. Currently, scientific studies involving genetic data cannot include patient identifiers but if prospective studies are to be of real value this sort of information needs to be available to groups carrying out such studies.

 There are many challenges regarding pharmacogenomics that still need to be addressed before its use can become widely accepted.

Questions

1. What is a genome-wide association study?
2. What is the difference between a biomarker and a probe drug?
3. Categorize the CYP2D6 polymorphisms (e.g. CYP2D6*1 etc.) into functional, reduced functional and non-functional.
4. Gene therapy is of two types—germline and somatic. What is the difference between them?
5. What information do you think should be given to patients: (a) prior to pharmacogenetic testing and (b) during provision of the results?

Chapter summary

- The original discoveries of pharmacogenetics arose from empirical observations of differences in responses, largely to drugs, between individuals.
- Initially the most clinically significant differences were identified in the cytochrome P450 enzymes.

- The polymorphism of CYP2D6 was the first to be identified and is clinically significant with respect to a number of classes of drugs including antidepressants, SSRIs, tamoxifen and opiates.

- CYP2C9 polymorphism is particularly important with respect to warfarin therapy.

- Methyltransferases, which are important for the metabolism of a number of endogenous molecules, also exhibit polymorphism.

- The polymorphism of S-methyltransferases is particularly important in the use of 6-mercaptopurine and azathioprine therapy.

- Idiosyncratic adverse reactions can be due to genetic influences, but they are often complicated by the involvement of other factors.

- Phase II metabolic enzymes exhibit less clinically significant polymorphisms than phase I metabolic enzymes with sulphotransferases and N-acetyltransferases being the most important.

- Pharmacogenetic testing is already available in several clinical situations.

- Currently pharmacogenetic testing is used mainly in situations where drugs have a narrow therapeutic index or severe adverse effects.

- It is anticipated that the use of pharmacogenomics in the future will lead to a different approach to diseases and their treatment, with the possibility of individualized therapy.

- Phenotyping has been in use for some time in some situations but is likely to become more common, particularly for dose adjustments.

- Genotyping is still restricted to a small number of circumstances but will become more widely available as technology develops.

- There are many challenges associated with the wider use of pharmacogenomics but the majority of these are ethical, social, and legal issues.

📖 Further reading

Yan, Q. (ed.) (2008) Pharmacogenomics in drug design and development, in *Methods in Molecular Biology*, 448. New York: Springer.com.

A book which deals with the potential role of pharmacogenomics in a wide range of disease states.

Ma, Q. and Lu, A.Y.H. (2011) Pharmacogenetics, pharmacogenomics and individualized medicine, *Pharmacological Reviews* 63: 437–59.

A comprehensive review of the role of genetics in the development of individualized therapy.

Scott, S.A. (2012) Personalizing medicine with clinical pharmacogenetics, *Genetic Medicine* 13: 987–95.

A more clinically based review of the development of personalized medicine.

Daly, A.K. and King, B.P. (2003) Pharmacogenetics of oral anticoagulants, *Pharmacogenetics* 13: 247–52.

A paper detailing research work carried out on the pharmacogenetics of oral anticoagulants.

Wallace, S. (2013) *Chemistry World*. podcast, 30 October.

A podcast with some additional information about the role of phenylthiocarbamide in taste genetics.

Toxicity Testing

The testing of the toxicity profile of a potential drug candidate is a vital component of drug development. Toxicological studies are usually carried out at the same time as other aspects of drug development as, if any significant toxicity problems are detected, further development of the drug can be stopped, saving valuable time and expense for the pharmaceutical company. Lead compounds in a drug development process will be subject to *in vitro* toxicity studies. Once potential drug candidates have been identified they will be subjected to preliminary *in vivo* toxicity studies in order to identify potential development candidates (and potential back-up compounds). These toxicity tests will be carried out at the same time as metabolic studies and pre-formulation studies (⊳ XR Part 4).

This chapter will explain why toxicity testing is necessary (⊳ XR Section 14.1) and what is hoped will be achieved during such testing (⊳ XR Section 14.2). The types of tests which may be involved in toxicity testing will be described (⊳ XR Section 14.3) as well as the necessary duration of these tests (⊳ XR Section 14.4). Toxicity tests fall into two categories, namely *in vitro* and *in vivo* tests and rationale for their respective use will be discussed (⊳ XR Section 14.5). The development of more biological and biotechnology derived drug candidates has introduced new challenges with respect to toxicity testing and these will be described (⊳ XR Section 14.6). Not all toxicity tests are required in each circumstance and information about which tests are obligatory and which are elective will be given and so toxicity testing is subject to a variety of regulations and guidelines which will be introduced (⊳ XR Section 14.7).

14.1 THE NEED FOR NON-CLINICAL TOXICITY TESTING

There are a number of reasons for performing non-clinical toxicity testing, or preclinical safety assessment, as it is also known. These reasons include regulatory requirements, the support of clinical trials and to inform future drug development.

As a result of two highly publicized pharmaceutical toxicity issues (see Integration Box 14.1 and Figure 14.1), there has been a regulatory documentation requirement for data from preclinical toxicity

Figure 14.1 Sulphanilamide and thalidomide tragedies

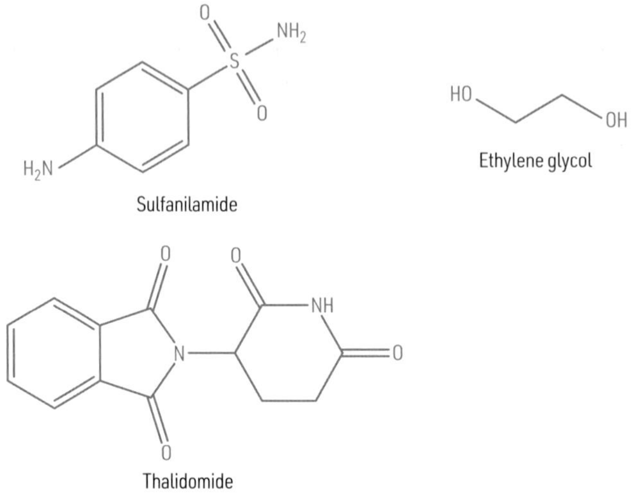

Sulfanilamide

Ethylene glycol

Thalidomide

studies to be included in the process of development and registration of new pharmaceutical products. Preclinical safety assessment can help the prediction of potential human toxicity and can act as a guide for the design, conduct and interpretation of clinical trials (❯ **XR Part 5**) and further toxicological studies. Because toxicity is responsible for about 30 per cent of terminations of new drug development, preclinical toxicity studies and their outcomes can be of great benefit in selecting the best candidates for further drug development.

INTEGRATION BOX 14.1   THE SULFANILAMIDE TRAGEDY

The details of the thalidomide tragedy have been dealt with elsewhere in this volume (❯ **XR Integration Box 6.6**). This tragedy, which occurred in the early 1960s, was pre-dated by the sulfanilamide tragedy which has received much less publicity. Sulfanilamide had been used to treat streptococcal infections for some time and had achieved remarkable success when used in tablet and powder forms. In 1937, a demand, particularly from the southern states of America, for a liquid form of the medication led to the introduction of a sulfanilamide elixir. This new formulation pre-dated the need for toxicity testing (on the principle that selling toxic drugs would be bad for business and, therefore, did not require regulation). Unfortunately, the solvent which was used in the preparation of the elixir was diethylene glycol, which was used for its sweet taste, but is normally used as antifreeze. Diethylene glycol is, however, extremely toxic, and a number of deaths occurred. This toxicity is largely due to its metabolites and the major metabolite is glycolic acid which is cytotoxic via a number of mechanisms. Additionally, glycolic acid is further metabolized to oxalic acid which can cause further damage by the formation of calcium oxalate crystals. Incidentally, the complete loss of confidence in the Austrian wine industry in 1985 was brought about by the adding of diethylene glycol to Austrian wines to improve their sweetness. Fortunately, this adulteration was rapidly discovered, and no deaths occurred, unlike with the sulfanilamide tragedy.

 Non-clinical toxicity is required to satisfy regulatory requirements, to support clinical trials, and to inform drug development.

14.2 **THE OUTCOMES OF TOXICITY TESTING**

The initial outcome to be achieved from toxicity testing is the identification of any biological hazards associated with drug candidates. At a whole body level, this means the identification of any impairment to body organs caused by the drug candidate. There are specific requirements relating to identification of any toxic effects on the cardiovascular and respiratory systems as well as the central nervous system. At a cellular level, the presence of any damage to genetic material (known as genotoxicity) must be identified. This aspect of toxicity testing is also often referred to as mutagenicity testing (❯ XR Secction 14.3.2), although the terms are not strictly interchangeable. All mutagens are genotoxic, whereas not all genotoxic substances are mutagenic. Also often confused with mutagenicity is carcinogenicity (❯ XR Section 14.3.1), the strict meaning of which is causing or contributing to cancer growth. The confusion between the two terms arises because often the cancer growth is caused by damage to the genome. However, cancer growth can also be caused by disruption of cellular metabolic processes. Testing for carcinogenicity is also a regulatory requirement for new pharmaceuticals. The final aspect of hazard identification relates to the testing for any reproductive or developmental toxicity (❯ XR Section 14.3.3).

The outcomes of toxicity testing are to identify biological hazards associated with potential drug candidates, both at the whole body and the cellular level.

Having identified any toxicity hazards, the next step is to attempt to characterize these hazards with respect to any relationships to the dose of the potential drug, and also the probable duration of exposure of any patient to the drug. This is, essentially, a branch of pharmacokinetics and is referred to as toxicokinetics. Investigations must be made in order to establish if there is a dose-dependent relationship with any toxic effects, e.g. does the toxicity occur only at a high dose or does it occur at any dose? It is also important to ascertain whether the toxicity occurs with a short duration of exposure to the drug or whether it occurs only with prolonged exposure. This is significant if the drug is one which is expected to be required to be taken over a long period of time, perhaps requiring a lifetime of therapy.

Once a hazard has been identified and characterized, a risk assessment has to be carried out into the implications of the hazard for patient safety. Initially, this involves a determination of the margin of safety between drug levels required for efficacy and those related to toxic effects. There must also be an investigation into how the toxic effect should be monitored. Additionally, it must be determined if the toxic effect is reversible on withdrawal of the drug treatment. If possible, the mechanism of the toxicity should be established. In particular, it needs to be determined if there is any relationship between the toxicity and the pharmacological mechanism of the therapeutic activity. Because the initial toxicity studies are carried out *in vitro* or in non-human animals, it must be determined if the observed toxicity has any relevance to human usage.

In addition to all the previous aspects, the risk assessment can provide useful guidance for the conduct of clinical trials (❯ XR Chapter 19). It can provide a reasonable estimation of a safe starting dose for any clinical trials as well as guidelines for dose calculations. Knowledge of the monitoring requirements of the toxic effects is useful in establishing guidelines for clinical monitoring.

Any biological hazards which are detected by toxicity testing have to be identified and characterized with respect to the implications for patient safety.

14.3 TYPES OF TOXICITY TESTS

This section will describe the types of tests necessary for investigating toxicity together with the general principles involved in such tests. It is not within the scope of this book to describe the detailed experimental procedures and, if required, these can be found in the Further reading at the end of the chapter.

14.3.1 Carcinogenicity testing

Carcinogenicity is the ability to cause cancer by either changing the genome or disrupting cellular metabolic processes. Because carcinogenesis is such a complex process there is not one single experimental test with the ability to predict the likelihood of carcinogenicity in humans. Currently, the generally minimal acceptable process involves one long-term study in rodents, plus one other study which supplements this long-term study. The additional study is usually a short-term rodent study or a second long-term study in a second rodent species. However, it is likely that, before any biological testing is performed, an analysis of the molecular structure of the potential drug molecule will have been made, comparing its structure to those of chemicals known to interact with DNA. If the structure resembles the structure of a known carcinogen (see Figure 14.2) this is an indication that the molecule may be hazardous and requires further testing. This structural analysis can involve a simple structural comparison or, more likely, a more complex comparison involving determination of certain physicochemical parameters and subsequent computer analysis (❯ XR Section 9.2).

The short-term tests are generally of a few weeks' duration. The tests can be *in vitro* as well as *in vivo* (❯ XR Section 14.4). Both types of test are looking for any chemical interaction with DNA. If there is a positive response in these tests the molecule is deemed to be a potential carcinogen and will, in all likelihood, be abandoned. The long-term study will be carried out in a rodent different from that used in any short-term study, will be of at least 2 years' duration and will be conducted in parallel with further development of the potential drug. The endpoint in these studies is evidence of tumour development.

Figure 14.2 Closely related structures–carcinogens or not?

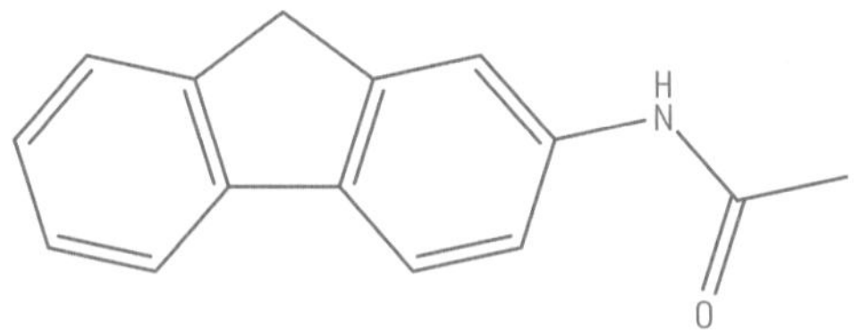

2-acetylaminofluorene

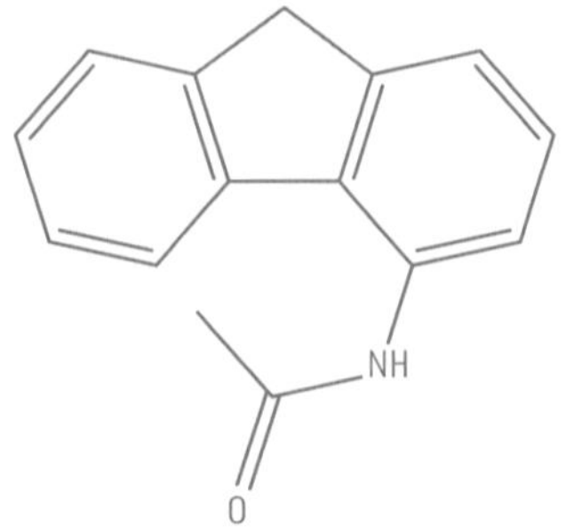

4-acetylaminofluorene

Testing for carcinogenicity usually involves a structural comparison with known carcinogens, a short-term study (of a few weeks' duration), and a long-term *in vivo* animal study (of at least 2 years' duration).

14.3.2 Mutagenicity testing

Mutagenicity is defined as causing a gene mutation leading to structural and/or numerical chromosomal changes. This defined situation can lead to carcinogenicity but, as carcinogenicity can arise by alternative mechanisms, the tests for mutagenicity are separate from those for carcinogenicity. Just as with carcinogenicity testing, prior to commencing testing, a paper or computer-based study should be carried out. As before this will provide useful information with respect to choice of both *in vitro* and *in vivo* studies. The *in vitro* tests usually include two or more of the following: a bacterial test for gene mutation (usually using *Salmonella typhimurium* or *Eschericia coli*) (see Integration Box 14.2 and Figure 14.3), a test for detection of chromosomal mutations, and a mammalian cell mutation assay (e.g. mouse lymphoma assay). Depending on the outcome of these tests, *in vivo* tests may be required. The *in vivo* tests must be carried out in such a way as to avoid any outcome which is uninformative. Therefore aspects such as route of administration and metabolism of the drug candidate must be carefully considered. There are a number of tests available for use, depending on the circumstances. Most commonly a bone marrow micronucleus or a clastogenicity test is performed. Other tests may include mutagenicity studies in transgenic animals or comet assays.

INTEGRATION BOX 14.2 | **THE AMES TEST**

The Ames test is a simple, cheap and widely used mutagenicity test. The test looks for the presence of gene mutations in bacteria, usually in *Salmonella*. Although known not to be 100 per cent accurate, potential drugs that show a positive test are usually rejected for further development. The test employs *Salmonella* strains that have histidine synthesis mutations (known as auxotrophic mutants) which require histidine for growth. The test substance is placed in the centre of an inoculation plate containing minimal histidine. The bacterial strain is inoculated onto the plate which is then incubated overnight at 37°C. A positive result is an increased number of revertants near the test substance. In this simple form the Ames test can give false negative results for compounds that are positive mutagens. The main reason for this is that the test substance may be metabolized in animals and humans and the drug may not cause mutations, but the metabolites might. In order to overcome this situation, fresh liver extracts containing metabolic enzymes are added to the bacterial inoculate. Again a high number of revertants indicate a positive response.

 Mutagenicity testing usually involves a structural analysis, *in vitro* testing (using bacterial cultures), and *in vivo* testing.

14.3.3 Teratogenicity testing

A teratogen is defined as a substance that can induce or increase the incidence of a congenital malformation. Also, included under the general term of teratology is the study of developmental toxicology which includes growth retardation, delayed mental development and other congenital disorders without structural malformations. There are three stages at which a drug can affect foetal development: the fertilization and implantation stage which lasts from conception to 17 days, organogenesis which occurs from 18–55 days during gestation, and growth and development from 56 days onwards. Currently, drugs are

Figure 14.3 The Ames test

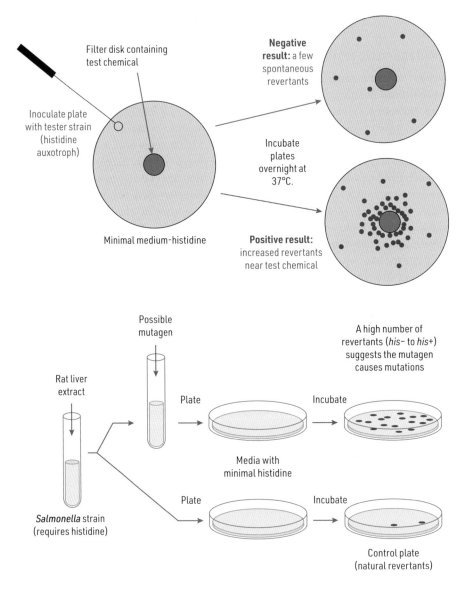

classified with respect to their teratogenicity potential and the classification is based on animal studies. Any such molecule should be avoided during or prior to attempting conception and women should avoid all medication in the first 8 weeks after conception, unless absolutely necessary. Most people will be aware of thalidomide in this respect, but it is, perhaps, surprising just how many currently utilized drugs are included in this category (see Table 14.1).

Teratogenicity studies can only be carried out in mammalian species and generally two species are used (rat and rabbit). The substance under test is given after mating during the period of organogenesis and the foetus is examined for abnormalities. The tests must have been carried out under protocols laid down by the FDA and the ICH. The protocols of the FDA require both single generational studies and multigenerational studies. A single generational study has three stages: an evaluation of fertility and reproductive

Table 14.1 Drugs which are potential teratogens

Class of drug	Example
ACE inhibitors	lisinopril
Acne medication	isotretinoin
Alcohol	
Androgens	
Antibiotics	tetracyclines, doxycycline
Anticoagulants	warfarin
Anticonvulsants	phenytoin, sodium valproate, carbamazepine
Antidepressants	lithium
Anti-cancer agents	methotrexate
Anti-rheumatic chelators	penicillamine
Anti-thyroid agents	propylthiouracil, carbimazole
Oestrogens	diethylstilbestrol
	cocaine
	thalidomide

performance, an assessment of developmental toxicity, and postnatal evaluation. A multigenerational study usually involves a rodent species. The animals are exposed to the test substance shortly after mating and then are mated through three generations and the appropriate parameters (fertility, litter size and neonatal viability) are monitored in each generation. Also required under FDA regulations is an evaluation of fertility and reproductive performance using both male and female rodents. For an assessment of developmental toxicology pregnant female rodents are treated during implantation and organogenesis, the animals are killed one day prior to birth and the subsequent foetuses monitored for viability, body weight and the presence of any malformations. Finally, postnatal monitoring involves observation of parturition, late foetal development, neonatal survival, and growth and the presence of malformations.

The test requirements under ICH are fertility assessment, postnatal evaluation, pregnancy state susceptibility, and an assessment of developmental toxicity. These tests are essentially the same as required by the FDA, although with minor technical differences.

In recent years the strength of feeling about the widespread use of animal testing (even in circumstances such as these) has led to the introduction of alternative tests such as the micromass test, the whole embryo culture test, and the embryonic stem cell test.

 Teratogenicity testing involves only *in vivo* testing, and the requirements are fertility assessment, pregnancy state evaluation, an assessment of developmental toxicity, and postnatal evaluation.

14.3.4 Immunotoxicity testing

Immunotoxicity can manifest itself in any or all of the following responses—immunosuppression, allergic reaction, hypersensitivity, autoimmune disease or an abnormal immune response. Because each of these responses is quite distinct, there is a need for them to be addressed separately. There are a number of tests which can be used in preclinical toxicity testing (see Table 14.2). Usually two or more of these will be

Table 14.2 Immunotoxicity tests

Type of test	Endpoint
Immunosuppression	cytopenias, organ weight decrease, immune organ lymphoid depletion, bacterial sepsis, abcesses, pneumonia
Enhanced immune activation	leucocytosis, neutrophilias, acute phase response, inflammation not associated with organ toxicity
Autoimmunity	haemolysis, thrombocytopenia
Immunostimulation	cytokines
T-cell dependent antibody response	
In vitro cell activity studies	natural killer cells activity

included. However, these tests will only be necessary if there is any evidence of an effect on the immune system during general non-clinical studies. Evidence of immunotoxicity from non-clinical studies may be evidence of **blood dyscrasias**, changes in immune system organs (such as thymus, spleen), decreased serum globulin levels, increased incidence of infections, and/or tumours. It should be recognized, however, that certain drug classes are intended to act on the immune system, e.g. ciclosporin, **HMGCoA** reductase inhibitors (statins), **NSAIDs**.

Once again, the general desire to minimize the use of animal testing has led to the development of a number of new screening tools. These include the use of immune cell lines (T cells, mast cells, monocytes) incorporated into fluorescent cell chips.

 Immunotoxicity testing involves monitoring for immunosuppression, allergic reactions, autoimmune diseases, and abnormal immune responses.

14.3.5 Safety pharmacology testing

Whereas toxicity testing has been an integral part of drug development for many decades, safety pharmacology is a relatively recent addition to the toxicology aspect of drug development, which began to be developed following the problem associated with the drug terfenadine (see Integration Box 14.3 and Figure 14.4). At the time of this problem (1990s) it had started to become apparent that drugs could

Figure 14.4 Structure of terfenadine

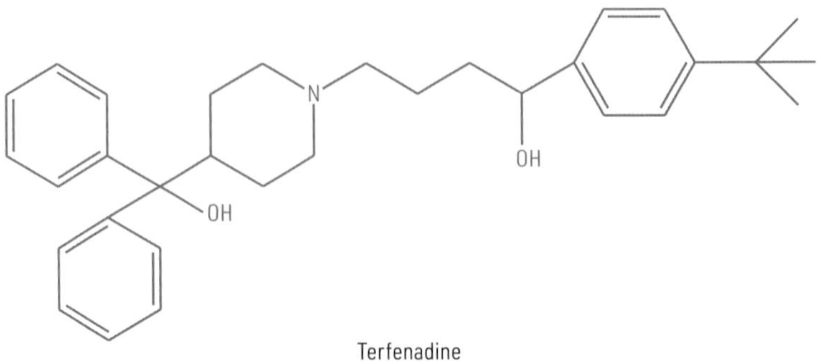

Terfenadine

Table 14.3 Safety pharmacology studies

CNS	Respiratory	Cardiovascular
Motor activity	Respiratory rate	BP and heart rate
Behaviour	Tidal volume	ECG
Coordination	Oxygen saturation	Repolarization
Sensory/motor reflexes		hERG assay
Body temperature		Conduction

reach phase III clinical trials (i.e. involving patients) before potentially dangerous adverse effects became apparent. If an adverse effect is sufficiently rare it may only become apparent during post-marketing surveillance. The terfenadine risk situation could not have been predicted by conventional preclinical toxicity testing. This was because, at that time, adverse effects were determined using chronic high doses of the drug. This would not detect a rare lethal event resulting from therapeutic doses. Safety pharmacology is now used to bridge the gap between preclinical and clinical drug development. The core studies involved in safety pharmacology relate to the central nervous, respiratory and cardiovascular systems (see Table 14.3). The role of safety pharmacology is to determine whether a drug is inherently unsafe or, alternatively, to inform the drug discovery team that the drug is likely to be safe. Of course, the potential therapeutic benefit of a drug may offset the liability of a potentially dangerous adverse effect (risk/benefit analysis).

INTEGRATION BOX 14.3   **TERFENADINE TOXICITY**

The enormous amount of publicity surrounding thalidomide toxicity (**❯ XR Integration Box 6.6**) has led to a wide knowledge of the potential toxicity problems associated with the introduction of a new drug. A situation which is perhaps less well-known is that of the toxicity of terfenadine. Terfenadine, which was marketed in the UK as Tri-ludan®, was the first non-sedating antihistamine when it was introduced in 1980. Previous antihistamines, such as chlorphenamine, had the associated side effects of sedation and psychomotor retardation–serious disadvantages for hay-fever sufferers who relied on such medication. The reason for the lack of CNS side effects was that terfenadine and its active metabolite did not easily cross the blood-brain barrier. Terfenadine was so successful that it soon became established as an over the counter medicine. However, in 1990, reports began to emerge that terfenadine could cause ventricular tachycardia, associated with a prolonged QT interval, particularly in patients taking drugs which had an inhibitory effect on the cytochrome system CYP3A4 by which terfenadine was metabolized. In 1992, the Committee for Safety of Medicines (CSM) issued the first warnings about the cardiovascular problems associated with terfenadine (and related drugs). By 1997 there had been fourteen deaths in the UK linked to terfenadine and the drug was withdrawn. As the cardiotoxicity problems had only been recognized 10 years after the introduction of the drug, safety pharmacology testing (which includes ECG testing) became a standard toxicity study requirement.

 Safety pharmacology testing investigates any adverse effects on the nervous, cardiovascular, and respiratory systems.

14.4 ACUTE AND CHRONIC TOXICITY TESTING

There are very specific requirements for toxicity testing, relating to duration of testing, the species and the number of animals used. These are all laid down as regulations or guidelines by the various regulatory authorities. From a duration point of view, toxicity testing is divided into acute, sub-chronic and chronic testing and there is a progression through these stages with each stage having specific objectives.

14.4.1 Acute toxicity testing

These tests usually consist of a single dose or multiple doses within 24 hours and the objectives are to guide dose selection for subsequent repeat dose studies and to support low dose exploratory clinical trials. This is an area where the regulatory requirements have changed over the years. From 1991 until 2009, acute toxicity studies were performed under ICH guidelines and used two mammalian species and needed to meet GLP requirements. In 1996, the FDA introduced guidelines which required more stringent tests. The tests had to use two species—one rodent and one non-rodent. Two routes of administration were also required—the expected clinical route and the intravenous route. The outcomes of these tests were examined for mortality, any clinical observations and any histopathological changes. However, in 2009 a revision of the ICH guidelines allowed the acceptability of non-GLP dose-ranging studies.

 Acute toxicity testing usually is of 24 hours duration, involves two mammalian species, and two routes of administration.

14.4.2 Sub-chronic testing

The main objectives of these studies are to identify any organs affected by toxicity and to determine any dose dependence, exposure dependence and whether the toxic effects are reversible. These outcomes will inform dose levels for chronic studies and will inform clinical safety levels. Additionally, if toxicity is discovered, this may invoke studies of the mechanism of toxicity and can inform suggestions as to possible endpoints or **biomarkers**. Sub-chronic studies can be of variable duration between 2 weeks and 6 months, but most commonly are between 1 and 3 months. Sub-chronic studies can also be used to support clinical trials of a similar duration.

 Sub-chronic toxicity tests usually last between 1 and 3 months and the objectives are to identify any organs affected, to guide mechanistic studies, and to suggest possible toxicity endpoints or biomarkers.

14.4.3 Chronic testing

The outcomes of chronic toxicity testing are numerous. Primarily they are to determine the long-term safety profile of the drug and to further support the development of biomarkers and clinical endpoints. In addition they may identify new toxicities not previously seen in shorter term studies. Any toxicity that has been previously detected can be observed for further development—either an increase or decrease by comparison with short-term studies. Because chronic studies are designed to support clinical trials of duration of more than 6 months, these studies are of 6 months in rodents and 9 months in non-rodents. The endpoints are more complex than in shorter term studies.

 The primary objective of chronic toxicity testing is to determine the long-term safety profile and is usually of between 6 and 9 months duration.

14.5 *IN VITRO* TOXICITY TESTING

The use of animals in assessing the toxicity of drugs under development has been subject to much criticism for a number of years. This criticism was based not only on ethical grounds but also on the scientific basis that the difference between humans and test animals was significant. These differences can be structural, physiological and biochemical. Because of these issues a number of *in vitro* cell culture toxicity tests have been developed.

The proposed benefits of *in vitro* tests are numerous. *In vitro* testing is considerably less expensive than animal testing because the overall number of animals needed for toxicity testing can be substantially reduced but not completely eliminated (❯ XR Section 14.5.2). *In vitro* testing, because of its relative simplicity, can help to predict the toxicity of a drug candidate at a much earlier stage in the drug development process. Additionally, in many cases, they can also predict the likely effectiveness of the drug *in vivo*.

14.5.1 Cell culture toxicity tests

In vitro cell culture cytotoxicity tests have been proven to be reliable indicators of *in vivo* toxicity and have now become widely used as acceptable alternatives to (but not replacements for) animal testing. These cell culture assays use eukaryotic cells unlike the prokaryotic cells used in the Ames test (❯ XR Integration Box 14.2). These cells will have been derived from specific animal or human tissues. They can be cells derived from the drug target tissue or from the target disease. A cell line needs to fulfil certain criteria. They must be morphologically similar to the cells from which they were derived. The cells must function in a similar manner to the tissues from which they were derived. Finally, the cells should retain the structural and functional similarities through repeated cycles of growth. Examples of *in vitro* cell culture assays can be seen in Table 14.4. The principle, for most cell culture toxicity assays, is that cytotoxic molecules cause cell damage and cell death and thus, these molecules will interfere with the continuous growth and division of the culture cells.

 Cell culture toxicity tests, introduced initially to reduce animal toxicity testing, are widely used and have proved useful indicators of *in vivo* toxicity.

14.5.2 Why animal toxicity testing is still necessary

Although there is much useful information that can be obtained from *in vitro* testing, the use of cell cultures does not replicate the complex multi-organ events that occur *in vivo*. Additionally, because metabolic capacity is much reduced or absent in cell culture, assessment of any metabolite toxicity is extremely difficult. Animal assays are able to test the toxicity of a drug and its metabolites (often responsible for

Table 14.4 *In vitro* cell culture-based toxicity assays

Test	Outcome measured	Basis
MTT assay	Cell viability	Colorimetric determination of cell metabolic activity
Alamar Blue assay	Cell viability	Colorimetric determination of cell metabolic activity
NRU assay	Cell viability	Colorimetric determination of cell metabolic activity
ATP assay	Cell viability	Luminescence determination of cellular ATP content
ELISA assay	Antibody detection	Enzyme immunoassay

the toxic effects). In addition to toxicological information, animal testing can provide information on absorption and distribution of the drug candidate, the extent and site of metabolism, and the clearance of the drug candidate from the body.

 Because cell culture toxicity testing cannot provide information about whole organ toxicity and metabolite toxicity, animal toxicity testing is still necessary.

14.5.3 *In silico* toxicity prediction

The utilization of predictive QSAR studies has been applied to the prediction of toxicity of potential drug candidates. There are a number of these computer programs available, e.g. Derek Nexus, available from the software development company Lhasa. Programs such as this enable the prediction of a variety of toxicological endpoints, such as mutagenicity and skin sensitization, and enable prediction of which compounds are likely to have more favourable toxicity profiles. This enables actual toxicity tests to be carried out on those compounds which are likely to have the most favourable outcomes. Additionally compounds thought likely to be toxic can be identified earlier in the drug design process, thus saving time and resources.

14.6 TOXICITY TESTING OF BIOPHARMACEUTICALS

Conventional pharmaceuticals are generally small molecules (usually a maximum of ~ 500 Da) and are usually in a relatively high state of purity. Biopharmaceuticals are large molecules, increasingly of high purity (although high purity biologicals are difficult to produce). Biopharmaceuticals also include what can be classed as hybrid entities between proteins and chemicals, such as synthetic peptides, oligonucleotides, synthetic RNA and **immunoconjugates**.

The goals of toxicity testing for biopharmaceuticals are the same as for small organic molecules. The desired outcomes are to identify target organs for toxicity, whether the toxicity is reversible, to identify safety parameters for clinical monitoring, and to determine safe doses for clinical trials. However, the methods by which the safety evaluations are achieved are different because biopharmaceuticals are highly selective and specific for humans, often being less active or inactive in animals. Toxicity studies on biopharmaceuticals are usually carried out on a single animal species and that species must be one which is deemed to be pharmacologically relevant to humans. Rodents are often not relevant and non-human primates are most often used, with reproductive studies being carried out simultaneously. Interferons and monoclonal antibodies are active only in primates but other biologicals have cross-reactivity such as insulin and **filgrastim** which are active in rats and dogs as well as non-human primates.

One area of toxicity that requires specific attention with biopharmaceuticals is immunogenicity. An immune response to a biopharmaceutical in an animal is to be expected because the product has been designed to be specific for humans (however see Integration Box 14.4 TGN1412). The formation of anti-drug antibodies (ADA) must be carefully monitored. The consequences of any ADA formation may alter pharmacokinetics and may mask or exacerbate other toxicities. It should be recognized, however, that the evidence of immunogenicity in animals is not necessarily reflective of a human response.

INTEGRATION BOX 14.4	TGN1412

TGN1412 (theralizumab) was an immunomodulatory drug which binds to the CD28 receptor of the immune system's T cells. It is, as the name suggests, a humanized monoclonal antibody. The original intention was to use it to treat chronic lymphocytic leukaemia and rheumatoid arthritis. When first trialled in humans in 2006, the drug caused catastrophic organ dysfunction in the subjects (six healthy volunteers), even though it was administered at a sub-clinical dose. TGN1412 had not been previously given to humans, although this clinical trial had been preceded by testing in non-human primates without any similar outcomes. After much investigation, it was concluded that the likely cause of the reaction was an unpredicted biological action in humans. Subsequently, it was shown that the non-human primate species used lacked expression of the CD28 receptor and so the T cells would not be stimulated by the drug, unlike in humans.

Although the objectives of toxicity testing are the same for both small organic molecules and biopharmaceuticals, the methods used are different and more complex.

14.7 **REGULATIONS OR GUIDELINES**

The conduct of toxicity testing of proposed new drugs is governed by a mixture of regulations and guidelines (as are many other aspects of drug development). Regulations provide information regarding what is legally required. Guidelines provide information as to what are considered reasonable courses of action and are not legally binding. In the United States the regulations are set out in the Code of Federal Regulations (CFR). Similar regulations exist in the EU and Japan. In terms of toxicity testing, these regulations describe what is required for non-clinical studies in order to support clinical trials and registration of a new drug.

For many years the guidelines provided by different countries varied considerably and, as the pharmaceutical industry became more globalized, it became obvious that some form of worldwide guidelines would be helpful in the drug development and registration process. This led to the International Conference on Harmonisation (ICH) project which involved the regulators and pharmaceutical industry bodies from the United States, the EU and Japan. The project started in 1990 and has the WHO and the EFTA as overseeing bodies. The objectives of the project were to improve the efficiency of new drug development and registration processes, to promote public health, to prevent duplication of clinical trials, and to minimize the use of animal testing without compromising safety and effectiveness. These objectives were achieved by the development and implementation of harmonized guidelines and standards. Additionally, the FDA has a Center for Drug Evaluation and Research (CDER) which provides guidelines on a wide range of drug-related topics, including toxicity testing. These guidelines are generally produced by a committee of scientists and/or other experts. The ICH guidance documents, which are revised on a regular basis, cover four areas—quality, safety, efficacy and multidisciplinary topics. Toxicity testing falls within the safety area and relates to both *in vitro* and *in vivo* preclinical studies.

From all the preceding material it should be apparent that there is not a 'one size fits all' process and it is important to keep up to date with ICH and regional guidelines because they are changing continually.

Regulations indicate what is legally required with respect to toxicity testing, whilst guidelines indicate what are regarded as reasonable although not legally required.

? Questions

1. What is the mechanism of toxicity of glycolic acid?

2. Explain the specific differences between carcinogenicity, genotoxicity and mutagenicity.

3. The two structures in Figure 14.2 are very similar. However one of the molecules is much more carcinogenic than the other. What is the key structural difference which is responsible for this difference in carcinogenicity?

4. What is the structure of the active metabolite of terfenadine?

5. What are the chemical reactions which form the basis of the cell culture toxicity assays in Table 14.4?

⟳ Chapter summary

- Non-clinical toxicity testing is a necessary aspect of drug development and registration.

- Non-clinical toxicity testing is of great value in guiding the design, conduct, and evaluation of clinical trials.

- One of the objectives of toxicity testing is to identify any hazards associated with body organs, particularly those associated with the central nervous, cardiovascular, and respiratory systems.

- Another objective of toxicity testing is to identify any damage to genetic material.

- A final objective of toxicity testing is to identify any reproductive or developmental toxicity.

- Any hazards identified must be characterized, particularly with respect to patient safety.

- Toxicity tests which are required are those for carcinogenicity, mutagenicity, teratogenicity, and immunotoxicity.

- Safety pharmacology testing on the central nervous, cardiovascular, and respiratory systems is also required.

- Toxicity testing involving different timescales (acute, sub-chronic, and chronic) are required, each of which have different objectives.

- *In vitro* cell culture toxicity tests have been developed to reduce the extent of animal testing.

- Cell culture toxicity testing is much less expensive than animal testing, can be carried out at a much earlier stage in the drug development process, and has been shown to be a reliable predictor of *in vivo* toxicity.

- Animal testing is still required, however, as cell culture assays cannot predict whole body toxic events or metabolite toxicity.

- The toxicity testing of biopharmaceuticals, whilst it has the same objectives as the testing for small organic molecules, has more complex requirements and most often involves non-human primates.

- The regulations associated with toxicity testing in the United States are laid down by the Code of Federal Regulations and similar regulations apply in the EU and Japan.

- Guidelines regarding toxicity testing are provided by the International Conference on Harmonisation and the Center for Drug Evaluation and Research.

📖 Further reading

Eastwood, D.A. et al. (2009) Mutagenicity testing for chemical risk assessment: Update of WHO/IPCS harmonised scheme, *Mutagenesis* 24: 341–9.

A comprehensive account of the current state of mutagenicity testing.

Collins, A R. (2004) The Comet assay for DNA damage and repair: principles, applications and limitations, *Molecular Biotechnology* 26: 249–61.

An account of one of the more recent assays for mutagenicity.

Anbach, A. (2014) Fundamental approaches to immunotoxicity assessment in preclinical safety studies, www.actox.org/meetcourses/webinar_immunotox_assess.

An excellent webinar presentation about immunotoxicity testing.

Pugsley, M.K., Authien, S., and Curtis, M.J. (2008) Principles of safety pharmacology, *British Journal of Pharmacology* 154: 1382–99.

A comprehensive account of safety pharmacology testing.

Graziuw, M.J. and Jacobsen-Kram, D (eds) (2015) *Genotoxicity and Carcinogenicity of Pharmaceuticals*. Switzerland: Springer International Publishing.

A comprehensive textbook dealing with these topics from a pharmaceutical manufacturing viewpoint.

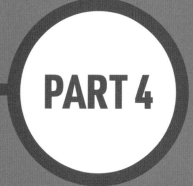

PART 4

Preformulation Studies

At some stage in the drug development process a lead compound (or its derivatives) will show sufficient promise in the appropriate pharmacological screening systems to warrant investigation in humans. At this stage, it becomes necessary to produce a formulation of the potential new drug in order for it to be administered. Preformulation is that component of drug development which is necessary to allow the development of suitable formulations of the drug for use in clinical trials and, ultimately, in the final marketable product. Preformulation studies involve the investigation of the properties of a new drug molecule which could influence the efficacy of that drug and the development of a suitable formulation. There are three aspects to preformulation studies: the determination of physicochemical properties, particularly relating to drug solubility (▶ XR Chapter 15), the solid state properties of the drug, often referred to as micromeritics (▶ XR Chapter 16), and the physical and chemical stability of the drug and its compatibility with commonly used excipients (▶ XR Chapter 17).

Solubility and Drug Development

In order to be absorbed from the gastro-intestinal tract, an orally administered drug has to be soluble in the gastro-intestinal fluid. The drug, in solution, can be absorbed through the gastro-intestinal membrane into the general circulation. Thus the solubility of a potential drug molecule is a critical physicochemical property, and the solubility characteristics of a new drug is one of the most important, and usually the first, preformulation parameters to be investigated (❯ XR Section 15.2). In order to assist in the design of a suitable formulation, use can be made of solubility classification systems which employ specific criteria (❯ XR Section 15.1). There are numerous factors which affect the solubility (❯ XR Section 15.3), such as temperature (❯ XR Section 15.3 1), the nature of the solute and solvent (❯ XR Section 15.3.2), pH and the dissociation constants if the drug is ionizable (❯ XR Section 15.3.3), and salt formation (❯ XR Section 15.3.4). All these previous aspects relate largely to aqueous solubility, but equally important is the lipid solubility of a drug as represented by partition coefficient and log P (❯ XR Section 15.4). Whereas the processes of solubility and dissociation are equilibrium situations, the process of dissolution is a kinetic situation, i.e. it occurs at a particular rate and measurement of dissolution rate is another important preformulation parameter (❯ XR 15.5), as are the factors affecting dissolution rate (❯ XR Section 15.5.1). More recently discovered drug molecules are demonstrating increased lipophilicity and decreased aqueous solubility. In the past, this situation has led to the rejection of drug candidates on the grounds of poor solubility but, increasingly, techniques are being employed to overcome these solubility challenges (❯ XR Section 15.6).

15.1 SOLUBILITY CHARACTERISTICS

For drugs which are the subject of pharmacopoeial monographs solubility is defined in descriptive terms each of which is related to a particular concentration range (Table 15.1). This description of solubility is in terms of quantity of solvent by volume to one part by weight of solute and this can utilized for water and

Table 15.1 Descriptive solubility terms and their meaning

Solubility at 20°C	Volume of solvent per g of solute (ml)	Solubility range (mg ml^{-1})
Practically insoluble	>10000	< 0.1
Very slightly soluble	1000–10000	0.1–1
Slightly soluble	100–1000	1–10
Sparingly soluble	30–100	10–33
Soluble	10–30	33–100
Freely soluble	1–10	100–1000
Very soluble	<1	>1000

other solvents. This classification is essentially the same in the British Pharmacopoeia (BP), the United States Pharmacopoeia (USP), and the European Pharmacopeia (PhEur).

A more useful classification method, from the point of view of assessing the potential development of a new drug substance, is the biopharmaceutical classification system (BCS). This system looks at both solubility and intestinal permeability, which is defined as the ratio of drug absorbed from the gastro-intestinal tract after oral administration to intravenous delivery of the drug. On this basis drug substances can be placed into one of four categories (Table 15.2). High solubility is defined as when the highest dose strength of a drug substance will dissolve in less than 250ml of water over a pH range of 1–7.5. High permeability is when the absorption of the orally administered drug is greater than 90 per cent when compared with the same intravenous dose. Low solubility is defined as requiring more than 250ml of water to dissolve the highest drug dose. Low permeability is when the absorption rate after oral administration is less than 90 per cent of the intravenous dose. Although these categories may appear somewhat empirical, they do provide useful guidelines as to what is required for successful formulation of a drug (Table 15.3). These values are essentially a measure of a drug's bioavailability, i.e. the fraction of a dose that enters the general circulation. Thus a drug that is administered intravenously has a bioavailability of 100 per cent. When a drug is given orally, generally the bioavailability is reduced as a result of low solubility, the extent of gastro-intestinal permeability and first pass metabolism (❯ XR Section 12.3).

While more related to permeability than solubility, Lipinski's rule of five can also be used to give some indication of the likelihood of a potential drug being orally active. Lipinski and co-workers looked at data for ~2500 drug-like molecules and, based on their observations, produced the rule of five which states that poor permeability is more likely when the molecular weight is greater than 500, the log P is greater than 5, there are more than 5 hydrogen bond donor groups and more than 10 hydrogen bond acceptor groups in the molecule. There are an increasing number of exceptions to the rule but, nevertheless, it still provides useful guidelines relatively early in the drug development process.

Table 15.2 Biopharmaceutical classification system (BCS)

BCS class	Solubility	Intestinal permeability
1	High	High
2	Low	High
3	High	Low
4	Low	Low

Table 15.3 Distribution of BCS classes among marketed drugs and drugs in development

BCS class	% marketed drugs	% drugs in development
1	35	5
2	30	70
3	25	5
4	10	20

 Pharmacopoeias utilize descriptive terms to define solubility, but a more relevant classification method of describing solubility is the biopharmaceutical classification system (BCS).

15.2 DETERMINATION OF SOLUBILITY CHARACTERISTICS

An orally administered drug has to be in solution in the gastro-intestinal fluid in order to be absorbed. Once in solution it can permeate the gastro-intestinal membrane to reach the systemic circulation. Solubility, therefore, is one of the most important properties investigated during preformulation studies and is usually the first parameter to be investigated. The definition of solubility of an unionized substance is the concentration of a substance in a solution that is in equilibrium with an excess of the undissolved substance. In other words, the term solubility usually refers to equilibrium solubility, also known as intrinsic solubility. It should be realized, however, that, *in vivo,* the solubility situation is unlikely to be an equilibrium situation. The drug within a dosage form may exist as an unstable polymorph (❯ **XR Section 16.2.2**) and the solubility may change as the polymorphic form reverts to a more stable form. Additionally, the drug in solution will be being removed from the site of dissolution by permeation, removal by the systemic circulation, binding to protein or deposition in lipid storage sites. Thus solubility *in vivo* should be regarded as kinetic rather than equilibrium solubility. Nevertheless, as it is difficult to accurately replicate kinetic solubility, determination of equilibrium solubility usually gives a reasonable indication of the solubility properties of a potential drug substance.

 Intrinsic solubility, determined *in vitro*, refers to an equilibrium situation but solubility *in vivo* is likely to be a kinetic property.

The solubility profile of a potential drug substance will be determined using a variety of solvents. Various aqueous-based solvents will be used, ranging from pure water to simulated biological fluids (Table 15.4) (see Integration Box 15.1). Composition of simulated biological fluids). Additionally, solubility in a range of non-aqueous solvents will be investigated, as well as solubility in a range of surfactant solvents, the latter providing useful information for formulation of poorly soluble drugs.

The actual method for determining equilibrium solubility used will be a variation of the method represented diagrammatically in Figure 15.1. Essentially the method involves preparing a saturated solution of the drug substance under carefully controlled conditions, in which equilibrium is established between dissolved and undissolved solute over a prolonged period of time (generally 72 hours). The most significant differences in methodology will relate to the method used for the determination of the concentration of the drug substances in solution. The analytical method chosen will depend on the chemical nature of the substance being examined and will require only minimal amounts of sample (only small amounts of the potential drug substance will be available at this stage of the development process). The method will also need to be rapid and suitable for automation. The most widely used methods are ultraviolet and fluorescence spectrophotometry usually linked to high performance liquid chromatography (HPLC).

Table 15.4 Solvents commonly used in drug solubility profiling

Solvent
Water
Polyethylene glycol
Propylene glycol
Glycerol
Sorbitol
Ethanol
Methanol
Benzyl alcohol
Isopropanol
Tweens
Polysorbates
Castor oil
Peanut oil
Sesame oil
Buffers of various pHs

INTEGRATION BOX 15.1 **COMPOSITION OF SIMULATED BIOLOGICAL FLUIDS**

For examination of the solubility of an orally delivered drug, the typical simulated biological fluids used would be simulated gastric fluid, fed state simulated gastric fluid, fasted state simulated intestinal fluid, and fed state simulated intestinal fluid.

Simulated gastric fluid is a dissolution medium that is described in the USP and the European Pharmacopoeia and is intended to simulate gastric acid. It is prepared by dissolving 2g sodium chloride and 3.2g purified pepsin (porcine-derived with an activity of 800–2500 units per mg of protein) in 7ml HCl and adding water to 1000ml. The pKa of the solution should be ~1.2. A more relevant gastric medium can be formed by adding small amounts of natural surfactants such as sodium taurocholate and lecithin (to account for back flow into the stomach from the intestine). The equivalent fed state fluid is quite different, with a composition of 17.12 mM glacial acetic acid, 29.75mM sodium acetate, 237.02mM sodium chloride, and water to 1000ml. This solution is then mixed 50:50 with milk.

Simulated intestinal fluid is essentially a phosphate buffer solution containing 0.2M sodium hydroxide with pancreatin added, adjusted to pH 6.5 and diluted to 1000ml. The fasted state fluid also contains sodium taurocholate and lecithin. The fed state fluid is an acetate buffer with added sodium chloride, sodium taurocholate, lecithin and pancreatin and adjusted to pH 5.0.

15.3 FACTORS AFFECTING SOLUBILITY

There are a number of factors which can influence the aqueous solubility of a drug, such as temperature, the chemical nature of the solute and solvent, the physical state of the solute, and the pH and dissociation constant of the drug. All of these factors can influence the availability of a drug from a formulation and, therefore, must be investigated during preformulation.

Figure 15.1 Representation of shake flask method of solubility determination

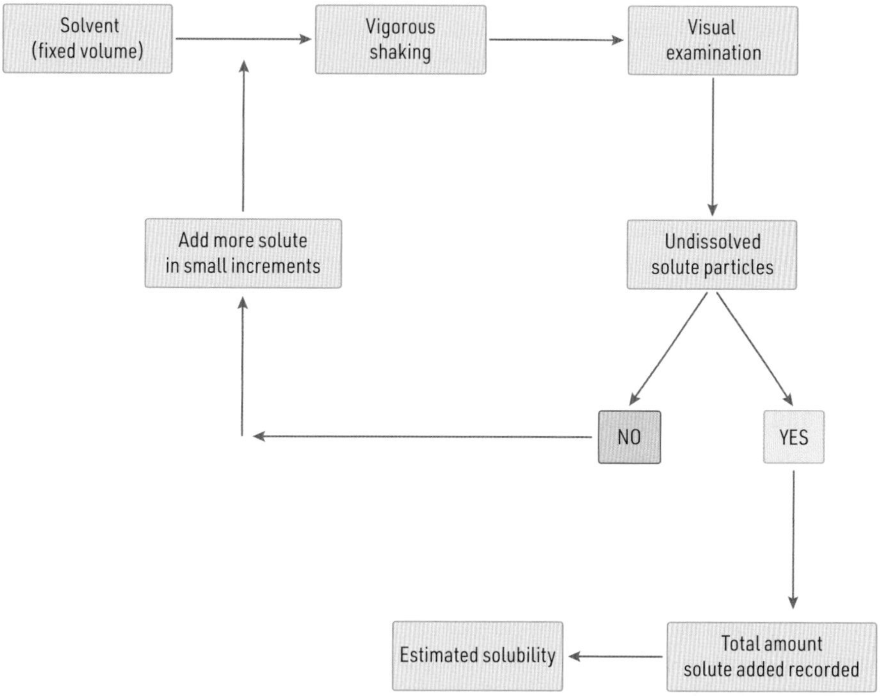

```
Solvent          ──→   Vigorous        ──→   Visual
(fixed volume)          shaking                examination
    ↑
Add more solute                              Undissolved
in small increments                          solute particles
    ↑                                         ↙        ↘
    └──────────────────────  NO              YES
                                              ↓
Estimated solubility ←──  Total amount
                          solute added recorded
```

 During preformulation studies, solubility will be determined in a variety of solvents, including simulated gastro-intestinal fluids.

15.3.1 **Temperature**

Generally speaking, if the potential drug substance is a solid, solubility will increase with an increased temperature, although there are a few exceptions (see Integration Box 15.2 Decreased solubility with increased temperature). Normally solubility studies will be carried out at three temperatures: 4°C where the density of water is at its greatest (which presents the worst-case scenario for solubility) which may relate to storage conditions for the drug, 25°C (standard room temperature) and 37°C (normal body temperature) which will provide an indication of solubility *in vivo*.

INTEGRATION BOX 15.2 **DECREASED SOLUBILITY WITH INCREASED TEMPERATURE**

During dissolution energy is absorbed in order to break bonds between the solute molecules and energy is released by the formation of new bonds between the solute and solvent molecules. If the heat energy absorbed is greater than the heat energy given off, the process of dissolution will be endothermic. For an endothermic reaction an increase in temperature (adding heat energy) drives the forward reaction towards the products (a solution) and hence the solubility of the solute will increase. If the heat energy given off is greater than the heat energy absorbed, then the reaction is exothermic. In an exothermic reaction an increase in temperature drives the reverse reaction towards the reactants (solvent and undissolved solute), hence decreasing the solubility of the solute.

15.3.2 Nature of solute and solvent

The polarity of a drug substance can have a significant influence on the nature of the solvent used in solubility studies. The adage of 'like dissolves like' means that, if the potential drug molecule is polar in nature, then solubility in water (a polar solvent) will be utilized. If the drug molecule is non-polar it is likely to have poor aqueous solubility, but this is not necessarily an insurmountable problem, especially if the required dose of the drug is very small. In addition to aqueous solubility, the solubility of a potential drug molecule will be assessed in a variety of other solvents, including water and other co-solvents mixture such as methanol-water, ethanol-water and tetrahydrofuran-water. This investigation of mixtures of solvents can facilitate drug extraction and separation in assay development, can improve on simple aqueous solubility, and assist in formulation development, particularly for preclinical evaluation of the potential drug. Occasionally, a suitable aqueous-based solvent cannot be used (very poor solubility or hydrolytic instability) leading to the use of more hydrophobic solvents such as oils (❯ XR Section 15.4).

15.3.3 pH and dissociation constants

The intrinsic solubility of a potential new drug substance which is measured in preformulation studies represents the unionized form of the drug. For non-ionizable molecules this relates directly to the actual solubility of the molecule in aqueous media. However, a significant number of existing drugs, and potential new drugs, are ionizable molecules (~90 per cent of existing drugs are either acidic or basic). The intrinsic solubility of an ionizable potential drug (i.e. the solubility of the unionized form) will be determined in an acidic medium for acidic molecules and in an alkaline medium for basic drugs. In addition to the solubility determination, it is important to determine the dissociation constant (pKa) of a potential new drug. The pKa of a molecule is the pH at which unionized and ionized forms of the molecule exist in equal amounts. Knowledge of the pKa of a potential new drug is important because, although the ionized species will be more soluble in aqueous media, it is the unionized species which will be absorbed across the gastro-intestinal membrane. The gastro-intestinal tract will expose the drug to a range of pH values (stomach pH 2, small intestine pH 8), which will influence the site of absorption of the drug. Having determined the pKa, the concentration of the ionized and unionized species can be determined at a particular pH by use of the Henderson–Hasselbalch equation:

$$pH = pK_a + \log_{10}\frac{[A^-]}{[HA]}$$

This information can assist in the choice of the appropriate pH to ensure sufficient drug solubility and the possibility of solubility improvement by use of salt formation (❯ XR Section 15.3.4).

The methods that are used for pKa determination are based on conductance measurement such as **potentiometric titration** (Figure 15.2) or change of a physicochemical property, such as ultraviolet absorbance or fluorescence intensity, with varying pH. It must be recognized, however, that methods which rely on pH measurement can only be considered accurate to ± 0.02 pH units.

There are an increasing number of new drugs which are biologically-based substances (such as **monoclonal antibodies**). Drugs such as these usually have a high aqueous solubility but have no measurable pKa. As such, drugs like these provide a different formulation challenge. Although aqueous solubility is high, they are protein in nature and, consequently, maintaining their **tertiary structure** (and thus activity) is important during formulation despite their good solubility characteristics.

15.3.4 Salt formation

If a potential new drug substance possesses one (or more) ionizable group(s), the aqueous solubility of that molecule can often be increased by the preparation of a salt. Salt formation may also be useful in assisting purification at the isolation stage of drug production or may increase stability. In addition to

Figure 15.2 Potentiometric titration curve

(Credit: From Harvey, D. (2019). 9.2: Acid–Base Titrations. [online] Chemistry LibreTexts. Available at: https://chem.libretexts.org/Bookshelves/
Analytical_Chemistry/Book%3A_Analytical_Chemistry_2.0_(Harvey)/09_Titrimetric_Methods/9.2%3A_Acid%E2%80%93Base_Titrations
[Accessed 22 Aug. 2019]. (CC BY-NC-SA 4.0))

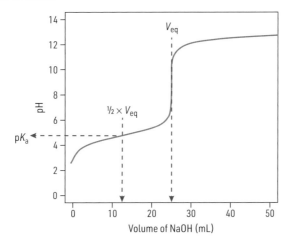

There are a variety of factors which can affect solubility, such as temperature, the nature of the solute and solvent, and pH.

changing the solubility of a drug, salt formation can also change a number of other important preformulation parameters (Table 15.5). Many of these changes are advantageous but, equally, there may be disadvantages associated with salt formation. A balanced decision, therefore, about salt formation needs to be taken relatively early in the drug development process and certainly before any toxicity testing is carried out, as a subsequent change of salt would require further toxicity testing on the new salt. However, the marketing of so many drugs as salts would indicate that, to a large extent, the advantages outweigh the disadvantages.

Salt formation is a relatively simple process whereby an acid reacts with a base, forming a salt where the two counter-ions are held together by ionic bonds. In theory, any weak acid or base can react to form a salt but, in reality, a stable salt will only be formed when there is a difference of at least three pKa units between the free base/acid and its salt co-former. It is also suggested that a basic drug with a pKa value below 5 (rule of five again) will probably be unstable at physiological pH.

Initially, a process known as salt screening will take place, whereby potential salt formers are reacted with the potential drug substance to check that salt formation does take place. This process can be carried out using a 96-well plate, making it possible to examine the salt formation of a number of counter-ions and a number of solvents simultaneously. The decision as to which potential salt formers to include in salt screening can be informed by the classification of salt formers in three categories as specified by Stahl

Table 15.5 Effect of salt formation of a drug

Potential positive effects	Potential negative effects
Increased solubility	Increased hygroscopicity
Increased dissolution rate	Decreased chemical stability
Higher melting point	Increased number of polymorphs
Lower hygroscopicity	Reduced dissolution in gastric media
Higher bioavailability	Increased toxicity

and Wermuth in the Handbook of Pharmaceutical Salts (see further reading at end of chapter). First-class salt formers are produced from ions that are physiologically present or occur as metabolites in biochemical pathways (such as hydrochloride or sodium salts). Because of their physiological existence there is no restriction on their use. Second-class salt formers are not naturally occurring but are already commonly used and have not demonstrated any significant toxicological issues. Third-class salt formers are only resorted to in order to solve a particular problem, are not naturally occurring and are not in common usage. This process can, potentially, give rise to a significant number of candidate salts and a logical process of examination needs to take place to identify candidates for further development. In such circumstances use will be made of a decision tree process based on measurable physicochemical characteristics (Figure 15.3). Once the candidates with the most appropriate physicochemical properties have been identified by use of the decision tree (usually about two or three candidates), they must be tested for bioavailability in animals against a suspension of the unionized form of the drug at the projected clinical dose. This is necessary because an increase in aqueous solubility does not guarantee increased bioavailability. For example, if a hydrochloride salt is formed there may be reduced solubility *in vivo* due to the common ion effect (see Integration Box 15.3 The common ion effect).

Care must be exercised when utilizing salts of **zwitterionic** molecules like ciprofloxacin. This is a fluoroquinolone antibiotic which has an amino group with a pKa of 8.8 and a carboxylic acid group with a pKa of 6.0. The **isoelectric point** of the zwitterionic form is pH(I) 7.4. Therefore, at a pH of ~7.4, ciprofloxacin will have minimal water solubility. Ciprofloxacin is used as the water-soluble lactate which has a positively charged ammonium salt. If ciprofloxacin is to be infused intravenously, then it must be ensured that the pH of the infusion fluid is well above pH 7.4 by use of a suitable excess of sodium bicarbonate. This ensures the conversion of ciprofloxacin lactate to its water-soluble sodium carboxylate salt instead of the water insoluble zwitterionic form.

Figure 15.3 Decision tree for salt selection in preformulation studies

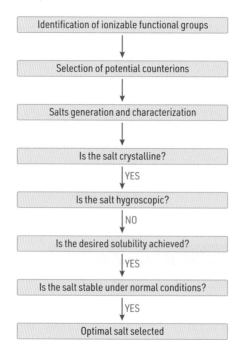

The solubility of an acidic or basic drug can often be increased by formation of a soluble salt. The nature of the salt to be used is selected by a process known as salt screening.

INTEGRATION BOX 15.3   THE COMMON ION EFFECT

When a shift in an ionic equilibrium takes place because of the addition of an ion already in the equilibrium, this is known as the common ion effect. One of the most important examples of this in drug development can occur when the hydrochloride salt of a poorly water-soluble drug is used. Because of the presence of a high concentration of chloride ions in the gastric fluid, the total concentration of chloride ions may cause the solubility product to be exceeded (see equation)—the equilibrium will shift to the left hand side and the solubility of the hydrochloride salt will be reduced,.

$$K_{sp} = [BH^+][Cl^-] \text{ where } K_{sp} \text{ is the solubility product}$$

$$BH^+Cl^-_{(s)} \rightleftharpoons BH^+_{(aq)} + Cl^-_{(aq)}$$

15.4 PARTITIONING AND LOG *P*

The majority of the preceding material in this chapter has been concerned with aqueous solubility of potential drug molecules and the factors which affect this solubility. However, also of significance is the lipid solubility of such molecules. The hydrophobic character of a potential drug molecule is very important with respect to absorption across biological membranes, which are lipid in nature. Therefore, the measurement of the partition coefficient is one of the physicochemical parameters determined during preformulation. The partition coefficient (P) represents the relative affinity of the potential drug substance for aqueous and organic phases.

$$P = C_o/C_w$$

where P is the partition coefficient, C_o is the concentration of the substance in the organic phase and C_w is the concentration of the substance in the aqueous phase.

The partition coefficient is usually represented as log *P* (❯ **XR Section 9.2.2.1**), as use of this logarithmic scale is better able to represent the large range of partition coefficients. Hydrophobic molecules will possess a positive log *P* value and hydrophilic molecules will possess a negative log *P* value (see Table 15.6).

The partition coefficient represents the relative distribution of a single species of the potential drug substance between two immiscible phases. This representation is acceptable when the molecule in question is non-ionizable, as only a single species will exist in solution. Because, in these circumstances, the partition coefficient measures only the unionized species in solution the value will be unaffected by pH.

Table 15.6 Examples of log *P* values

Positive values	Negative values
Benzocaine 1.9	Theophylline −0.02
Methadone 3.9	Vildagliptin −0.16
Hydrocortisone 4.7	Levodopa −2.7

However, many potential drug molecules will be acids or bases (or both) and will exist in solution as both ionized and unionized species. In this circumstance the partition coefficient is replaced by the distribution coefficient (D) which is defined as the ratio of the total analytical concentration of a species in one phase (regardless of its chemical form) to the total analytical concentration in the other phase.

$$D_{o,w} = \frac{C_o}{C_{w,ionized} + C_{w,unionized}}$$

D is also usually represented on the log scale. When both ionized and unionized species are present in solution the value of the distribution coefficient will vary with pH (see Figure 15.4). As a result, when values for the distribution coefficient are used, the pH of the aqueous phase used in the determination must be quoted. If the pKa of a molecule is known, then log P can be calculated from the measured log D using the equations for acidic and basic drugs.

$$logP = logD - log\left(\frac{1}{1+10^{pH-pKa}}\right) \text{ for acidic drugs}$$

$$logP = logD - log\left(\frac{1}{1+10^{pKa-pH}}\right) \text{ for basic drugs}$$

The standard method for determining log P or log D is known as the shake flask method. In this technique, the potential drug substance is introduced into either the aqueous or the organic phase (whichever is more appropriate for the molecule under investigation). The aqueous and organic phases are mixed and shaken together until equilibrium is obtained. Once equilibrium is reached (normally no more than 72 hours), the concentration of the molecule in each phase is determined and the appropriate coefficient calculated. Although the method is relatively simple from a practical viewpoint, there are a number of factors which have led to the introduction of other methods. At the formulation stage of drug development, there may only be a small amount of the potential drug available leading to analytical difficulties. The method is also relatively time-consuming in ensuring equilibrium has been reached. For these reasons, chromatographic methods have been developed, in particular the use of reverse-phase HPLC. Indeed, *in silico* methods are often used to generate calculated values, e.g. Clog P (▶ **XR Integration Box 9.3**).

 During preformulation studies the hydrophobic character of a drug is investigated by determination of the partition coefficient or distribution coefficient, as appropriate.

Figure 15.4 Variation of D with pH for **(a)** a weakly acidic drug and **(b)** a weakly basic drug

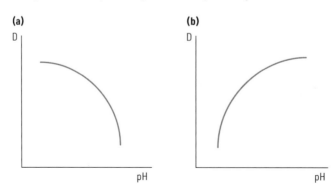

15.5 **DISSOLUTION RATE**

As can be seen from Figure 15.5, the process of dissolution is extremely important with respect to the absorption of a drug from the gastro-intestinal tract. Whereas the previous physicochemical parameters in this chapter (solubility, dissociation, partition and distribution) are all equilibrium-based parameters, dissolution is a kinetic parameter (Integration Box 15.4 Dissolution-limited vs solubility-limited absorption).

Often, a fast dissolution rate equates to good bioavailability and so is a desirable feature to be achieved during preformulation. When a solid particle composed of a soluble potential drug is placed in a liquid medium (e.g. the gastro-intestinal fluid), a diffusion layer forms around the particle (see Figure 15.6). This layer contains dissolved drug which has not yet entered the bulk of the dissolution medium. The concentration of the drug in this layer will be high and probably equal to the maximum solubility of the drug in that medium. Between the diffusion layer and the bulk liquid is a boundary layer of intermediate drug concentration. The dissolution rate is represented as the mass (m) of solid entering the liquid phase per unit time (t) and is calculated by the Noyes–Whitney equation (Integration Box 15.5).

Dissolution testing has been a pharmacopoeial requirement for many years and the type of apparatus to be used is specified in the relevant pharmacopoeia. When dissolution testing was first introduced it was primarily aimed at monitoring batch to batch variations in the production process of solid dosage forms. In preformulation studies the use of dissolution testing is used to provide information about any potential problems with poor absorption from the gastro-intestinal tract (usually only a problem if the

---

INTEGRATION BOX 15.4   **DISSOLUTION-LIMITED VS SOLUBILITY-LIMITED ABSORPTION**

An oral solid dosage form first has to disintegrate into particles from which dissolution takes place, followed by absorption. It is possible for there to be different rate-limiting steps controlling the rate of absorption of the drug. If the rate-limiting step is dissolution, the amount of absorbed drug can be increased by increasing the dose of the drug. In this situation the dissolution time will be greater than 3 hours. If the absorption of the drug is solubility-limited, the dissolution time will be less than 1 hour and the amount of drug absorbed will not increase by increasing the dose. An example of a drug which has dissolution-limited absorption is digoxin and an example of a drug which has solubility-limited absorption is griseofulvin.

Figure 15.5 Absorption of drug from a solid dosage form

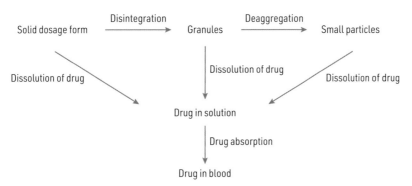

Figure 15.6 Diffusion layer surrounding a solid particle

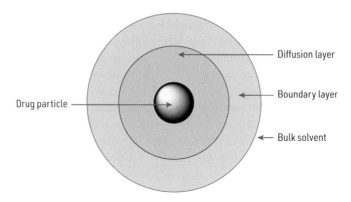

Diffusion layer

Boundary layer

Drug particle

Bulk solvent

INTEGRATION BOX 15.5   **THE NOYES-WHITNEY EQUATION**

The Noyes-Whitney equation was first derived in 1897, following work on two model compounds—benzoic acid and lead chloride. The equation gave rise to a general law whereby the rate of dissolution is proportional to the difference of solution concentration (C), relative to the solubility (S_t):

$$dC/dt = K(S_t - C)$$

Further work investigated the factors which contributed to the proportionality constant (K) which produced the Noyes-Whitney equation used today.

$$dm/dt = DA/h(S_t - C)$$ where dm/dt is the rate dissolution of the solid

D is the diffusion coefficient

A is the solid/liquid interface area

h is the thickness of the diffusion layer

S_t is the concentration of the solid in the diffusion layer

C is the concentration of the solid in the bulk solvent

The workers who first carried out these investigations (Brunner and Nernst) produced their own version of the equation known as the Noyes-Whitney-Nernst-Brunner (NWNB) equation:

$$dm/dt = DA/Vh(S_t - C)$$ where dm/dt is the rate dissolution of the solid

D is the diffusion coefficient

A is the solid/liquid interface area

h is the thickness of the diffusion layer

S_t is the concentration of the solid in the diffusion layer

C is the concentration of the solid in the bulk solvent

V is the volume of the bulk solvent

This is the equation most often used today.

drug solubility is below 1mg/ml at pH 7). Dissolution testing is also used to assist in investigating the effect on solubility and bioavailability of the drug of particle size, available surface area and the presence of excipients (Integration Box 15.6 Dissolution testing apparatus).

An assumption in the use of the Noyes–Whitney equation is that the parameters D, A, and h are constant. This is a reasonable assumption for D and h, but A will change as the solid being tested dissolves, and this will affect the dissolution rate. In order for A to be constant throughout the test the material must be able to dissolve from only one face of a **compact**. This is usually achieved by placing the compact in a specially designed holder. Under these conditions, and if **sink conditions** are maintained (i.e. the concentration of the dissolving solid is never greater than 10 per cent of the equilibrium solubility), then the measured dissolution rate is known as the intrinsic dissolution rate (IDR).

INTEGRATION BOX 15.6 | **DISSOLUTION TESTING APPARATUS**

There is quite a variety of forms of dissolution testing apparatus which are specified in the various pharmacopoeias (see Table 15.7). The two which are most often used for tablet formulations are the basket and the paddle (see Figure 15.7 and photos). The paddle apparatus operates at 50rpm and the basket at 50-100rpm.

Table 15.7 Examples of dissolution apparatus

Apparatus	Volume	Examples of application
Basket	900–1000ml	Tablets, capsules
Paddle	900–1000ml	Tablets, capsules
Reciprocating cylinder	200–50ml	Tablets, controlled release products
Flow-through cell	Unlimited volume	Implants, suppositories
Paddle/disc	900ml	Transdermal patches
Rotating cylinder	900ml	Transdermal patches

Figure 15.7 Dissolution apparatus, Paddle apparatus, Basket apparatus, Photograph of dissolution apparatus

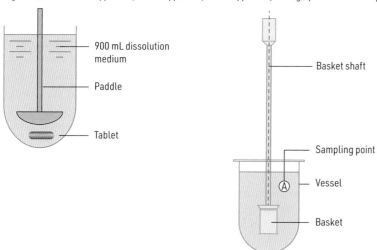

Figure 15.7 (*Continued*)

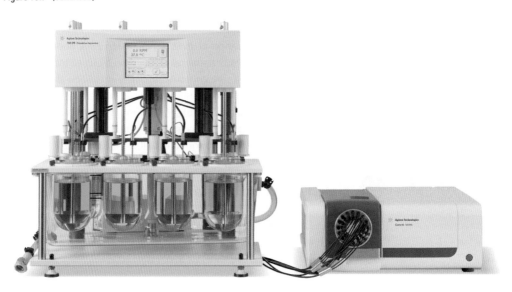

 The dissolution rate of a drug is important with respect to its bioavailability and the determination of dissolution rate is a key parameter in preformulation studies.

15.5.1 **Factors affecting dissolution rate**

In order for the measured dissolution rate of a potential new drug to give a realistic indication of *in vivo* dissolution rate, it is important that dissolution testing utilizes appropriate conditions. When a dosage form is taken orally it will encounter a variety of conditions during the passage through the gastro-intestinal tract, all of which can influence the dissolution rate. This is particularly important if the drug is to be formulated as a **modified** or **sustained release** product. The usual volume for a standard pharmacopoeial dissolution test is 900 or 1000ml, whereas the average volume of the human stomach in the fed state is ~650-700ml and can be as little as 50ml in the fasted state. The volumes in the intestines continue to reduce lower down the gastro-intestinal tract, with the small intestine being around 100ml and the large intestine around 30ml. In addition to difference in volume, the composition of gastro-intestinal fluids is much more complex than standard dissolution media (0.1M HCl, phosphate buffer). Simulated gastro-intestinal fluid can be used but this almost always complicates the analytical process involved. If the drug is an acid or a base the high concentration of drug in the diffusion layer will result in a different pH to that in the surrounding liquid and may lead to unexpected results. The presence of chloride ions is high in some of the gastro-intestinal fluids (e.g. gastric fluid) and this may lead to a reduction in dissolution of hydrochloride salts as a result of the common ion effect (❯ **XR Integration Box 15.3**).

 In order for the measured dissolution rate to give a realistic indication of what will happen *in vivo*, it is vital to use appropriate volumes of simulated gastro-intestinal fluids.

15.6 **DEALING WITH POORLY SOLUBLE MOLECULES**

In the past, many potential new drugs have been relatively simple organic molecules with few solubility problems. In recent years, however, there has been an increase in the number of poorly soluble molecules coming into drug development. These molecules typically belong to classes 2 and 4 of the BCS classification. Class 4 compounds, with both low solubility and low permeability, are particularly poor drug candidates, unless the dose is expected to be particularly low. The performance of class 2 compounds, however, can often be improved by utilizing appropriate formulation strategies to achieve consistent bioavailability. It is estimated that approximately 40 per cent of new drug molecules fall into this category, with an even higher percentage in some therapeutic areas. It is vital, therefore, that pharmaceutical companies can improve the oral absorption and bioavailability of poorly soluble drugs.

A pharmaceutical industry survey in 2013 identified the major types of problems faced in formulating poorly soluble potential new drugs (see Table 15.8). Although there are a number of potential solutions to the formulation of poorly soluble drugs, these solutions present a number of challenges, with the physicochemical properties and safety of the potential drug product being of greatest significance. These potential solutions utilize a wide range of approaches (see Table 15.9), with the most common being particle engineering, solid dispersions, nanoparticles, lipid-based delivery systems (including micelles), and salt formation and screening.

Table 15.8 Problems encountered with poorly soluble drugs

Problems encountered in formulation
Poor drug release profile
Poor stability in processing
Poor stability in gastro-intestinal fluids
Poor permeability and absorption
Polymorph formation
Drug precipitation
Food effects

Table 15.9 Potential formulation approaches to formulation of poorly soluble drugs

Potential formulation approaches
Particle engineering
Solid dispersions
Lipid-based systems
Micellular systems
Salt screening and selection
Cosolvent systems
Complex formation (e.g. with cyclodextrins)

? Questions

1. To which BCS classes do the following drugs belong: propranolol, felodipine, captopril, furosemide, carbamazepine, hydrochlorthiazide, verapamil, ranitidine?

2. What is the rationale for the inclusion of sodium taurocholate, lecithin, and pancreatin in simulated fed state intestinal fluid?

3. Give examples of second-class and third-class salt formers.

4. Why would a drug with a log P of greater than 5 be poorly absorbed?

5. What percentage of aspirin (pKa 3.5) would be ionized in the stomach, given that the pH of the stomach is 2?

6. For the amino acid alanine the pKa of the COOH group is 2.35 and the NH_2 group is 9.69. What is the isoelectric point for alanine?

↻ Chapter summary

- Investigation of the solubility characteristics of a potential new drug is a key aspect of preformulation studies.

- Solubility can be represented in descriptive terms which are based on ranges of numerical values.

- The biopharmaceutical classification system (BCS) is useful because it includes permeability as well as solubility when determining the class to which a drug belongs.

- Intrinsic solubility or equilibrium solubility is determined experimentally *in vitro* because *in vivo* or kinetic solubility is extremely difficult to replicate.

- Intrinsic solubility is determined in a range of solvents, including simulated gastro-intestinal fluids.

- The effect of temperature on intrinsic solubility is determined at three temperatures: 4^0C, 25^0C, and 37^0C.

- The polarity of the potential new drug may determine the nature of the solvent used in solubility studies.

- If a potential new drug is ionizable it is important to determine the solubility at a range of pHs which reflect the pHs within the gastro-intestinal tract.

- If a potential new drug is ionizable, its solubility can often be improved by the formation of a salt using a process known as salt screening.

- The lipophilicity of a potential new drug molecule can be represented by a log P value, or log D if the molecule is ionizable.

- The dissolution rate of a potential new drug molecule is another key property determined during preformulation studies.

- Appropriate volumes and pHs of the solvents used in dissolution testing are important in order to better reflect the *in vivo* conditions.

📖 Further reading

Gaisford, S. and Saunders, M. (2013) *Essentials of Pharmaceutical Preformulation*. Chichester, UK: Wiley-Blackwell, ISBN 978-0-470-97636-4.

A comprehensive account of preformulation studies including all aspects of solubility studies.

Amidon, G.L., Lennemäs, H., Shah, V.P., and Crison, J.R. (1995) A theoretical basis for a biopharmaceutic drug classification: The correlation of *in vitro* product dissolution and *in vivo* bioavailability, *Pharmaceutical Research*. 12: 413–20.

The original publication on which the Biopharmaceutical Classification System is based.

Stahl, P.H. and Wermuth, C.G. (eds) (2011) *Handbook of Pharmaceutical Salts: Properties, Selection and Use*. 2nd edn, Chichester, UK: Wiley, ISBN 978-3-90639-051-2.

A book containing all the necessary information regarding the use of salts in drug formulation.

Lipinski, C.A., Lombardo, F., Dominy, B.W., and Feeney, P.J. (2001) Experimental and computational approaches to estimate solubility and permeability in drug discovery and development settings, *Advanced Drug Delivery Reviews* 46: 3–26.

The origin of Lipinski's rule of five.

Dokoumetzidis, A. and Macheras, P. (2006) A century of dissolution research: From Noyes-Whitney to the biopharmaceutical classification system, *International Journal of Pharmaceutics*. 321: 1–11.

A comprehensive review of the development of dissolution testing.

Solid State Characteristics

The previous chapter describes the important physicochemical parameters of potential drugs, their determination and their significance within preformulation studies. This chapter describes another important aspect of preformulation studies, namely the investigation of the solid-state properties of a potential new drug. These solid-state properties are important with respect to the development of a suitable dosage form. The physical form of the potential drug substance will affect the dissolution rate, bioavailability and production processes. The drug molecule may exist in several solid states and each of these is considered individually–crystalline state (▶ **XR Section 16.1**), polymorphic states (▶ **XR Section 16.2**), pseudopolymorphs (▶ **XR Section 16.3**), or amorphous state (▶ **XR Section 16.4**). Each of these states exhibits different characteristics which can have a significant effect on solubility, bioavailability and production processing. The investigation of the characteristics of the solid state of the potential drug (also known as micromeritics) is also important, as the size, shape and surface area of the particles (▶ **XR Section 16.5**) can influence the dissolution rate and physical stability of a formulation (▶ **XR Chapter 17**). Of less importance in choosing a suitable drug candidate, but very important from the point of view of developing a suitable product, are the powder flow properties (▶ **XR Section 16.6**), including powder density and compressibility.

16.1 CRYSTAL STATES

Crystals are formed when molecules form into a defined order and this order is repeated throughout the entire physical structure. In order for this to happen the sample of the material must first be molten or in a supersaturated solution. The three-dimensional order is composed of a number of repeating structures known as the unit cell, of which there are seven types (see Figure 16.1).

The unit cell is repeated in three dimensions to yield the macroscopic crystal, the exterior of which is known as the crystal habit, of which there are six basis types (see Figure 16.2).

Figure 16.1 Crystal lattice unit cells

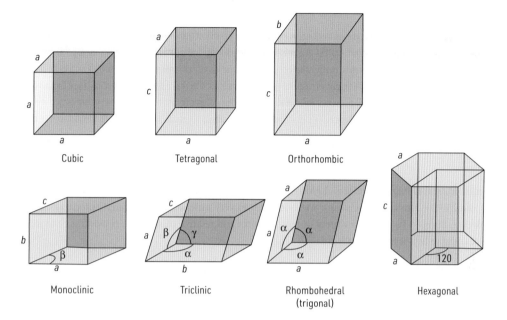

Figure 16.2 Crystal habits

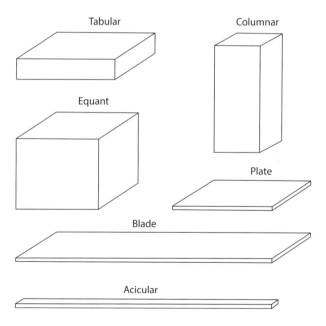

It should be noted that the crystal habit significantly influences particle (❯ **XR Section 16.5**) and bulk powder (❯ **XR Section 16.6**) properties. Crystal growth occurs in two stages—nucleation and crystal growth. The first of these stages is nucleation in which a small mass (nucleus) is formed to which further molecules can condense, which is known as crystal growth. The nature of the crystal structure is usually

---

INTEGRATION BOX 16.1   XRD AND XRPD

X-ray diffraction (XRD) is a broad term describing all types of diffraction measurements such as single crystal diffraction and thin film diffraction. XRPD is a method of measuring the scattering of X-rays by a polycrystalline sample. An XRPD sample consists of many small crystal units randomly oriented and is regarded as a bulk characterization technique. The diffraction pattern so obtained is considered to represent a 'fingerprint' (see Figures 16.4 and 16.9) for a given material. It provides information about the polymorphic form and the crystallinity (or otherwise) of the material under examination. The instrumentation is similar for both XRD and XRPD, the difference being the form of the sample—a single crystal in the case of XRD and a fine powder for XRPD.

---

determined, at this stage in preformulation, by X-ray powder diffraction (XRPD) (see Integration Box 16.1 XRD and XRPD). This relatively simple method requires very little sample, no sample preparation beyond powdering, and can be used at a variety of temperatures and relative humidities, providing good information of the stability of the crystal form.

 Crystal structure is composed of repeating unit cells which form a three-dimensional structure known as the crystal habit. The crystal habit determines particle bulk powder properties.

16.2 POLYMORPHISM

It is possible for the same substance to crystallize into different unit cells and these different crystalline forms are known as polymorphs (see Integration Box 16.2 Formation of different polymorphs).

Chemically, the unit cells are identical, but they have different packing structures. If only one polymorphic form is stable under changing temperature and pressure (temperature is particularly important in preformulation studies) this is known as monotropic polymorphism. If one form can change to another with changing conditions this is known as enantiotropic polymorphism. For monotropic polymorphism only one form is stable under all conditions (and has the highest melting temperature) and all other forms are referred to as metastable polymorphs (see Box 16.1 Diamond and graphite).

Over time metastable forms will convert to the most stable form. Different polymorphic forms have different properties such as melting temperature and solubility which can lead to differences in bioavailability. For example the antibiotic oxytetracycline exists as two polymorphs which exhibit differences in *in vitro* dissolution tests and also result in different blood levels. It is vital that during preformulation as much information about the polymorphism of a potential new drug is obtained, to inform the decision as to which polymorphic form is to be used (usually but not always the most stable (❯ XR Integration Box 16.3)).

INTEGRATION BOX 16.2   FORMATION OF DIFFERENT POLYMORPHS

The formation of different polymorphs is related to the rate of cooling of the liquid form. If the rate of cooling of the liquid is particularly slow, the molecules will have time to organize themselves in the most energy efficient way. This will produce a stable polymorph. At a more rapid rate of cooling, the molecules will not have time to arrange themselves into the most energy efficient crystal structure, but they still have time to organize themselves into a crystal structure. However, this will not be the most energy efficient structure, thus leading to the formation of a metastable polymorph.

BOX 16.1   DIAMOND AND GRAPHITE

Diamond and graphite are known as allotropes of carbon. Allotropy is where an element can exist in two or more physical forms, whereas polymorphism applies to any crystalline material, including compounds. The atoms of carbon are arranged differently in space in diamond and graphite. In diamond, the carbon atoms are arranged tetrahedrally. This results in a rigid, strong three-dimensional structure which is the reason for the strength, hardness, and durability of diamond. The carbon atoms in graphite are in a layer arrangement. These planar layers are held together by relatively weak forces. The layers slide easily over each other and thus graphite is soft and slippery and can be used as a lubricant. There is a third arrangement of carbon atoms which is a football-shaped arrangement of sixty carbon atoms known as buckminsterfullerene (or 'buckyball') but that is another story!

There are a number of additional important properties that may differ between polymorphic forms such as dissolution rate, **hygroscopicity**, degradation and compressibility. Additionally, each polymorphic form is patentable, so it is vital that all polymorphic forms are identified and included in the patent for the new drug product. At least sixty different polymorphs/hydrates of atorvastatin calcium have been patented and so different drug companies have generic drug formulations based of different polymorphs.

 Molecules can crystallize in different ways to produce different crystal forms known as polymorphs which may be stable, metastable, or unstable.

16.2.1 Polymorphic screening and characterization

The process of polymorphic screening entails the crystallization of the potential drug from a range of solvents and solvent mixtures. The process is carried out using a 96-well plate using about 0.5mg of the substance under investigation to which is added a small volume of solvent or solvent mixture. Each well is examined microscopically, after a suitable period of time, for the presence of crystals. If there has been no crystal formation the 96-well plate is stored at a lower temperature and/or the plate heated to remove some of the solvent and then cooled. The crystals formed can be examined by X-ray powder diffraction (XRPD) or hot stage microscopy. Differential scanning calorimetry (DSC) can also be used but has the disadvantage of being a potentially destructive method of analysis. However it does provide information about any phase changes associated with metastable polymorphs (see Figure 16.3). In DSC the amount of heat required to increase the temperature of a sample and reference material is measured over a range of temperatures. This allows the determination of the location of important transition temperatures such as melting points.

It should be noted that XRPD and DSC, as the most commonly used characterization techniques for polymorphs, provide different information. XRPD provides structural information and is the most useful technique for identifying and differentiating polymorphic forms (see Figure 16.4). Actually carbamazepine has four polymorphic forms (I, II, III, and IV). The dissolution rate was in the order of III>I but the total amount reaching the general circulation was I>III. This was probably due to the conversion of III to a dihydrate in gastro-intestinal fluids.

Each polymorph exhibits a unique set of intensity peaks in the diffractogram, providing a 'fingerprint' for each polymorph formed and, if appropriate experimental conditions are used, can provide a quantitative measurement of each form. DSC, on the other hand, provides thermodynamic information but no

Figure 16.3 DSC trace of polymorphs of ethambutol

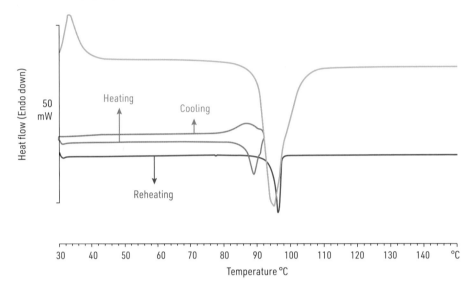

Figure 16.4 XRPD trace of two polymorphic forms of carbamazepine

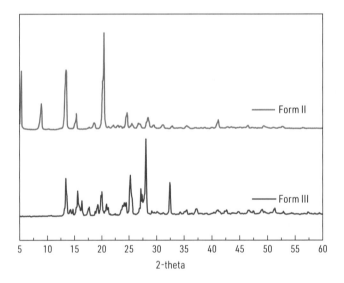

structural information. It does allow the identification of the stable and metastable polymorphs (which XRPD does not) and identification of polymorphs as monotropic or enantiotropic. A stable polymorph will show a single **melting endotherm** (see Figure 16.5a). A metastable polymorph will exhibit a number of transitions, characteristically a melting endotherm of the metastable form, a crystallization exotherm as the stable polymorph solidifies and a second endotherm as the stable form melts (see Figure 16.5b). This pattern of transitions is obtained for monotropic polymorphs. For enantiotropic polymorphs the DSC trace will exhibit two separate endothermic events as one stable form is converted into the other one and then melts (see Figure 16.5c).

Figure 16.5 DSC scans of various polymorphs: (a) Stable polymorph, (b) Metastable monotropic polymorph, (c) Metastable enantio-tropic polymorph

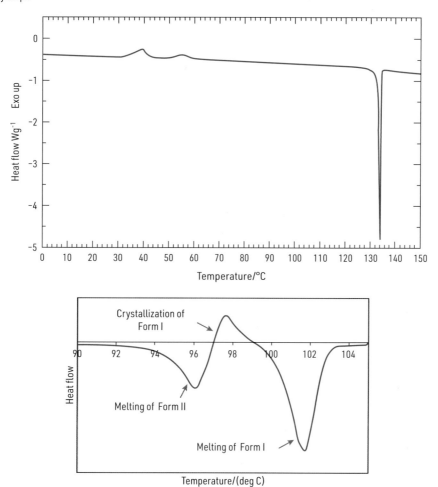

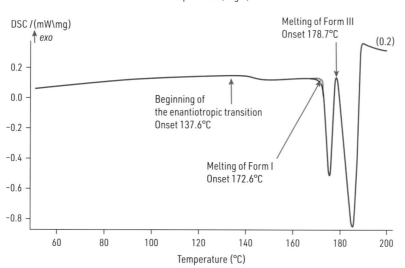

Detailed polymorphic screening is vital when attempting to bring a new drug product to market. Several batches of ritonavir, the antiretroviral drug used to treat HIV/AIDS, failed dissolution specifications. These failures were found to be due to the presence of a different polymorphic form which had 50 per cent lower intrinsic solubility than the reference form. This situation led to a recall and a reformulation of the product.

 Both XRPD and DSC can be used to characterize polymorphic forms but they provide different information. XRPD provides structural information and DSC provides thermodynamic information.

16.2.2 Use of metastable polymorphs

If the most stable polymorph has acceptable properties, in terms of solubility, dissolution rate and bioavailability, then this will be the form most likely to be taken further for product development. However, if the stable form has poor solubility or processing properties, then a metastable polymorph may be used (see Figure 16.6).

The figure shows that the metastable form (B) dissolves more rapidly (initially) leading to a faster dissolution rate, although the maximum equilibrium solubility is that of the stable polymorph (A) to which the metastable form is converted. When a metastable polymorph is used to improve bioavailability or ease of processing, care must be taken to ensure the metastable form doesn't undergo conversion during manipulation and storage—a balance has to be achieved between the benefit of improved bioavailability and potential physical instability (see Integration Box 16.3 Chloramphenicol palmitate).

INTEGRATION BOX 16.3   **CHLORAMPHENICOL PALMITATE**

Chloramphenicol palmitate, an antibiotic, is a good example of the use of a metastable polymorph in order to increase bioavailability. Chloramphenicol palmitate exists in three polymorphic forms—a stable polymorph, a metastable polymorph and a very unstable polymorph. The stable polymorph is only poorly soluble and provides very poor blood levels. The metastable polymorph provides much higher blood levels because of its rapid dissolution rate. This is the polymorphic form used in the dosage form—indeed there are pharmacopoeial limits for the presence of the stable polymorph. The very unstable polymorph is too unstable to be used and cannot be present in the dosage form.

Figure 16.6 Faster dissolution rate of metastable polymorph

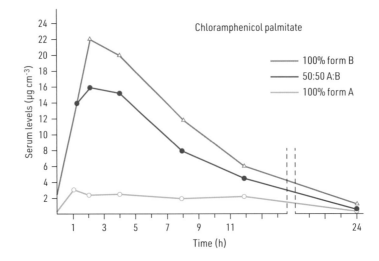

Metastable polymorphs usually have a faster dissolution rate and can be used to improve the bioavailability of a poorly soluble drug substance.

16.3 **PSEUDOPOLYMORPHISM**

Unit cells, as previously described, were considered to contain only one species. It is possible, however, under certain conditions, that crystal lattices can be formed in which there are more than one species present. The second species is the solvent from which crystallization has taken place—the crystal form is known as a solvate. If the second species is water, the crystal is known as a hydrate. Collectively solvates and hydrates are referred to as pseudopolymorphs. It is unlikely that a solvate will become a drug candidate due to potential toxicity problems associated with the solvent. Although hydrates do not pose a toxicity problem, nevertheless they will have different properties from other crystal forms. In particular they will be susceptible to dehydration/rehydration under changing conditions of temperature and relative humidity which is undesirable from a production/storage point of view. In addition, the presence of water in a crystal lattice tends to form hydrogen bonds between the components of the lattice, thus requiring more energy to disrupt the lattice. This will result in reduced solubility. For all these reasons it is important that pseudopolymorphs are identified during polymorphic screening as their presence is likely to lead to a number of difficulties in the drug development process. The presence of a hydrate can be detected in a DSC trace by the appearance of a broad endotherm around 100°C (although it can occur at higher temperatures if the water is tightly bound), which is due to the loss of water from the hydrate (see Figure 16.7). Heating cycle 1 shows a broad endotherm due to loss of water which is absent in the second heating cycle (cycle 3). Cycle 2 is a cooling cycle. The same result would be seen with a solvate, although the endotherm would appear at a lower temperature owing to solvents having lower boiling temperatures.

Figure 16.7 DSC trace of carbamazepine hydrate

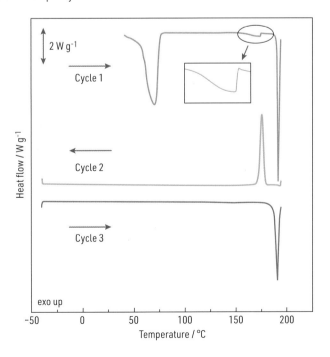

Crystals which include water or a solvent in the crystal lattice are called hydrates or solvates and are collectively referred to as pseudopolymorphs.

16.4 AMORPHOUS MATERIAL

Whereas a crystalline material possesses an ordered arrangement of molecules within the lattice, in a non-crystalline (or amorphous) material the molecules are randomly arranged (see Figure 16.8).

Because less energy is required to disrupt this arrangement than a crystalline one, amorphous materials are more soluble and have a faster dissolution rate. This feature can be used to improve the bioavailability of drugs, particularly poorly soluble ones. However, it must be recognized that amorphous materials can gradually restructure, ultimately achieving the crystalline state. There is, therefore, the challenge of keeping the drug in the amorphous state during processing and storage and this risk must be weighed against the possible benefits of using the amorphous form.

 The molecules within an amorphous material are randomly arranged, unlike the ordered arrangement in crystalline material.

16.4.1 Formation of amorphous material

Under normal circumstances, when materials form a solid phase, they will do so by arranging the molecules in a defined order (crystal formation). However, there can be a number of circumstances in which it is difficult for the molecules to array themselves in this defined order to any significant extent. If the solid phase is formed rapidly (precipitation or **quench-cooling**) the molecules will not have sufficient time to align themselves in an ordered fashion. In certain processes during drug manufacture (e.g. particle size reduction) the existing crystalline structure can be disrupted to form, at least partially, amorphous material. Of increasing significance is the failure to crystallize if the potential drug compound has a very high molecular weight (such as biological materials like proteins).

If the rate of cooling of a solution is very rapid the molecules do not have time to form a crystal and become a **supercooled liquid**. If the cooling process continues this supercooled liquid becomes 'frozen' and is referred to as a glass. The temperature at which this occurs is known as the glass transition temperature (T_g). Below the glass transition temperature, materials are described as glassy or brittle and above the glass transition temperature, they are described as rubbery. These terms originated in polymer science and do not describe the actual physical appearance of the material (see Box 16.2 Glassy and rubbery materials).

Figure 16.8 Difference between crystalline and amorphous material

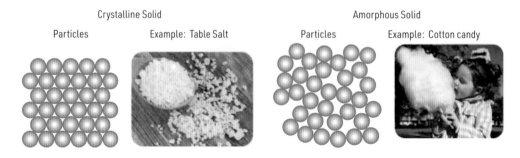

BOX 16.2   GLASSY AND RUBBERY MATERIALS

The terms glassy and rubbery are derived from polymer science and do not strictly describe the macroscopic character of a powder. Glassy materials have a microscopically disordered structure like a liquid and are the state in which an amorphous solid exists below the glass transition temperature. In its glassy state an amorphous solid is hard and brittle. Above the glass transition temperature an amorphous solid becomes soft and flexible and is described as rubbery. An example of a glassy polymer is poly(methyl methacrylate) and an example of a rubbery polymer is polyethylene.

 Amorphous materials are formed when the rate of cooling to form a solid phase is too rapid to allow an ordered arrangement to form.

16.4.2 Ageing and relaxation

In amorphous material all three types of molecular movement (vibration, rotation, and translation) are able to occur. Only vibration is possible in crystalline material because of the strong intermolecular attractions in the crystal lattice. Because of the freedom of movement in amorphous materials they will gradually change structure with time—a process known as relaxation. This will, in time, result in crystallization. This change in structure with time is often referred to as ageing (a process with which we are all familiar!). As a result of these structural changes the physicochemical properties will change and the understanding of how to control these changes is vital if a drug is to be used in its amorphous form for its increased bioavailability.

 Amorphous materials can change structure over time and the process is known as relaxation or ageing.

16.4.3 Characterization of amorphous material

Both XRPD and DSC can be used to identify the presence of amorphous material. In XRPD, because there is no ordered structure to amorphous material, no characteristic peaks will be seen. Instead a broad diffraction pattern, known as a halo, will be obtained (see Figure 16.9). DSC can be used to identify the glass transition temperature (see Figure 16.10) whence the rate of relaxation can be determined and so DSC can be used to study the ageing process of amorphous material. This, however, is a rather complex process and further details can be found in the Further reading at the end of the chapter.

 DSC provides more useful information about amorphous material than does XRPD.

16.4.4 Formation of amorphous material during processing

Although the processing of a drug substance into a drug product may start with a crystalline material, there are a number of pharmaceutical processes which can lead to the formation of amorphous material. Essentially, any process which exerts a force on a crystalline material has the potential to lead to the

Figure 16.9 XRPD of amorphous material

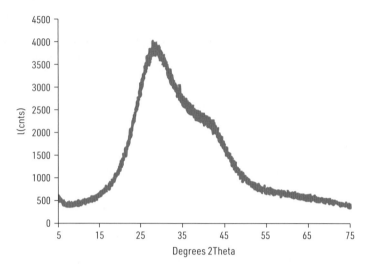

Figure 16.10 DSC of amorphous material

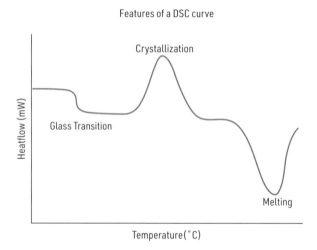

formation of amorphous material. These processes can be divided into those which are likely to produce entirely amorphous material (**spray-drying, freeze-drying,** quench-cooling) and those likely to form partially amorphous material (**milling, compaction**). The former processes are ones in which solvent removal is very rapid, inevitably leading to the production of entirely amorphous material. The latter processes are ones in which the normal crystalline structure can be disrupted to form a relatively small amount (up to 5 per cent) of amorphous material.

 Certain pharmaceutical manufacturing processes can produce amorphous material from crystalline material, either intentionally or unintentionally.

16.5 **PARTICLE SIZE AND SHAPE**

The previous sections of this chapter have been concerned with the polymorphic characteristics and their significance with respect to solubility, dissolution, and bioavailability. This section considers the macroscopic (i.e. bulk) properties and their importance with respect to bioavailability and drug processing. These macroscopic properties include particle size, shape and surface area. As we have already seen, the unit cell of a crystal will expand in three dimensions to produce a macroscopic particle known as the crystal habit (❯ **XR Section 16.1**). It is important to know the crystal habit because, as they will possess different geometrical shapes, the dissolution rate will differ because of different surface area to size ratio. The most common particle shapes are shown in Figure 16.11.

Once the particle shape has been identified, the next step is determination of particle size which is relatively easy for regular shapes and spherical particles but is considerably more difficult for irregular shaped particles.

 The bulk properties of powders can influence both drug processing and bioavailability.

16.5.1 **Particle size determination and distribution**

There are a number of methods for determination of particle size, but they all have their specific drawbacks. The methods include sieve analysis, the use of a Coulter counter, and photon correlation spectroscopy. From a preformulation point of view all these methods utilize significant amounts of sample, usually not available at this stage. The best option at this stage in drug development is visual inspection by use of some form of microscopy, such as light microscopy or scanning electron microscopy. The specific problem with visual inspection is ensuring that the sample observed is truly representative of the entire material.

It is also important to be aware of the distribution of different particle sizes within the sample and this can be represented as a histogram (see Figure 16.12a). From this a cumulative distribution plot can be produced (see Figure 16.12b), yielding a median particle size. However, this does not reflect the amount of scatter in the data, and it is important to have a relatively narrow distribution range. This range should tend towards the smaller particle size (faster dissolution rate), rather than the larger particle size (reduction in overall surface area of the sample).

Figure 16.11 Common particle shapes

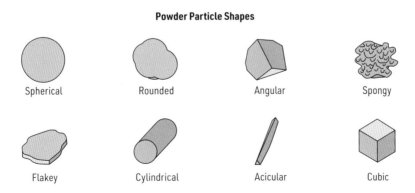

Powder Particle Shapes

Spherical · Rounded · Angular · Spongy

Flakey · Cylindrical · Acicular · Cubic

Figure 16.12 (a) Particle size distribution histogram and (b) cumulative distribution plot

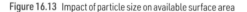

16.5.2 Effects of particle size and shape

As previously mentioned, the particle size and shape can have a significant influence on dissolution rate and hence bioavailability. Smaller particles have an overall greater surface area (see Figure 16.13) and this leads to an increased dissolution rate. However, fine particles are more susceptible to instability, having a greater surface area with which humidity and air can interact.

 The size and shape of particles can significantly affect dissolution rate and hence bioavailability.

Production processes can also be affected by particle size and shape. Powder flow and mixing efficiency can be affected (❯ **XR Section 16.6**) and fine powders are difficult to handle due to the creation of dust because of the ease of suspendability in air (see Integration Box 16.4 The influence of particle size and distribution on dosage forms).

Figure 16.13 Impact of particle size on available surface area

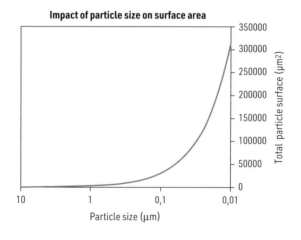

INTEGRATION BOX 16.4	THE INFLUENCE OF PARTICLE SIZE AND DISTRIBUTION ON DOSAGE FORMS

Particle size is an important property of pharmaceutical ingredients (both active drug and excipients) and having an appropriate particle size distribution is an important factor in pharmaceutical manufacturing. Particle size distribution will influence key factors such as dissolution, bioavailability and stability. Additionally, manufacturing aspects such as flowability, uniformity of content and compactability will also be affected. Particle size distribution will influence many steps of the manufacture of a solid dosage form such as powder mixing, wet or dry granulation, blending, tableting, encapsulation, and coating. The determination of an appropriate particle size distribution thus forms a key element of preformulation.

 Pharmaceutical production processes are affected significantly by particle size and shape.

16.6 POWDER FLOW PROPERTIES

Powder flow properties would not normally form part of preformulation studies, but they are included here, briefly, because they will influence the drug production process. Powder flow is dependent on a number of factors, some of which are related to the properties of the powder such as particle shape, particle-particle interactions, and water content. Also influential are environmental factors such as temperature and relative humidity. Because of the influence of these multiple factors powder flow properties cannot be predicted and so must be measured empirically. Because only relatively small amounts of material are available during preformulation studies, some indication of powder flow properties can be gained by measurement of bulk density and angle of repose, both of which are non-destructive methods requiring only small amounts of sample.

16.6.1 Bulk density

The measurement of the bulk density of a powder will give an indication of its compressibility, i.e. how it will behave under the influence of an applied force. Density is defined as mass per unit volume. Because powders consist of particles with air between the particles, the density of the powder will be lower than the true density of the particles and is known as the bulk density. When a powder is poured into a container, its bulk density will be at its lowest value and this is known as the poured or 'fluff' density. The air between the particles can be released by tapping the container, allowing the particles to consolidate, at which point the bulk density is highest and this is known as the final or 'tapped' density. Use of the equation

$$\text{Compressibility}\,(\%) = \frac{\text{Tapped density} - \text{Fluff density}}{\text{Tapped density}} \times 100$$

will give an indication of the compressibility of a powder. A value of less than ten for the compressibility index would indicate excellent flow properties, whereas a compressibility index of greater than forty indicates poor flow properties.

16.6.2 Angle of repose

The angle of repose is the angle (θ) a cone of powder makes when a mass of that powder is poured onto a horizontal surface (see Figure 16.14). The angle will be small if the powder is free-flowing and large when the powder has poor flow properties.

Figure 16.14 Angle of repose

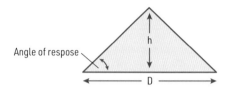

Table 16.1 Flow properties related to bulk powder properties

Flow properties	Compressibility index %	Angle of repose θ
Very poor	32–39	>56
Poor	26–31	46–55
Passable	21–25	41–45
Fair	16–20	36–40
Good	11–15	31–35
Excellent	< 10	< 30

Again, as for bulk density, a reasonable prediction of powder flow characteristics can be obtained by this method, utilizing a small amount of sample in a non-destructive way (see Table 16.1). Usually, compressibility index and angle of repose are considered in conjunction with each other when predicting the flow properties of a powder (see Table 16.1) and the extent to which excipients may be needed.

 Measurement of bulk density and angle of repose can give an indication of powder flow properties.

? Questions

1. Which analytical techniques can be used to differentiate between polymorphs?
2. Why would the DSC scan for a metastable polymorph and a hydrate be similar?
3. What analytical technique could be used to distinguish between a metastable polymorph and a hydrate?
4. How does the process of making candy floss make it an amorphous material?
5. Would you expect a spherical particle or an acyclical particle to have the faster dissolution rate?
6. What type of excipient is added to improve the flow of a powder?

↻ Chapter summary

- Crystals are formed when molecules become arranged in a defined order know as unit cells.
- The unit cells form a three-dimensional arrangement known as the crystal habit.
- Molecules can form different unit cells resulting in different crystalline structures known as polymorphs.
- The different polymorphs of a substance can be stable, metastable, and unstable.
- XRPD and DSC are techniques used to characterize polymorphs.

- Metastable polymorphs have a higher dissolution rate than stable polymorphs and are sometimes used to increase the bioavailability of a poorly soluble drug.

- Amorphous material is formed when the rate of formation of the solid phase occurs too rapidly to allow the formation of an ordered crystal structure.

- Bulk properties of powders such as particle size and shape can affect dissolution rate and bioavailability.

- It is important to measure the particle sizes and the particle size distribution of a pharmaceutical powder because they can affect a number of pharmaceutical processes.

- The two powder flow properties usually determined during preformulation are bulk density and angle of repose.

📖 Further reading

Florence, A.T. and Attwood, D. (2015) *Physicochemical Principles of Pharmacy*. 6th edn, London: Pharmaceutical Press, ISBN 978-0-85711-174-6.

The first chapter in this book deals with crystal structures, crystal habits and their relevance to drug development.

Omar, M., Makary, P., and Wlodanski, M. (2015) A review of polymorphism and the amorphous state in the formulation strategy of medicines and marketed drugs, *UK Journal of Pharmaceutics and Biosciences* 3: 60–6.

This recent review includes a number of pharmaceutically relevant examples.

Gaisford, S. and Saunders, M. (2013) *Essentials of Pharmaceutical Preformulation*. Chichester, UK: Wiley-Blackwell, ISBN 978-0-470-97636-4.

Chapter 8 of this book deals with the measurement of ageing of amorphous materials.

Sun, Z., Ya, N., Adams, R.C., and Fang, F.S. (2010) Particle size specifications for solid oral dosage forms: A regulatory perspective, *American Pharmaceutical Reviews* 13: 4.

An article emphasizing the regulatory importance of investigating particle size properties.

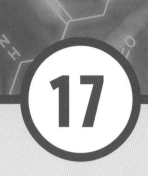

17

Drug Stability

A vital aspect of drug development is the investigation of the stability, or otherwise, of the drug and, subsequently, its formulation. The types of stability that will need to be examined are physical stability (**> XR Section 17.1**), and chemical stability (**> XR Section 17.2**) In particular it is important, at an early stage, to determine the mechanism of any instability, the reaction kinetics involved in any instability (**> XR Section 17.3**) and the factors which can influence such reactions (**> XR Section 17.4**). The submission of a new drug product is required to present the results of any stability studies undertaken and the range of these is specified by International Conference on Harmonisation (ICH) regulations. During preformulation studies the most important stability studies to be carried out are stress testing (**> XR Section 17.5**) in order to identify degradation pathways and mechanisms. The results from the stress testing can then be used to inform the design of longer-term and accelerated stability testing (**> XR Section 17.6**) and determination of shelf life which is necessary for regulatory submission.

17.1 PHYSICAL STABILITY

There are a number of possible physical instability situations which may occur, although most of these relate to dosage forms rather than the drug substance alone. If the drug substance can exist in different polymorphic forms, it is possible that the desired polymorphic form may change, over time, to a polymorph that has less desirable solubility properties. This is particularly likely if a metastable polymorph has been chosen for its enhanced solubility characteristics (**> XR Integration Box 16.3** Chloramphenicol palmitate). Over time the metastable polymorph will revert to the more stable polymorph. This process will occur more rapidly if storage conditions are less than appropriate, such as with increased temperature or relative humidity. Elevated temperatures may lead to the loss of water from a crystal hydrate or, if the relative humidity is high, a hydrate may be formed.

Physical instability of drug substances largely relates to the stability of polymorphic forms.

17.2 **CHEMICAL STABILITY**

There are three main types of reactions which can be the cause of chemical instability—hydrolysis (or solvolysis), oxidation, and photo-degradation. There are also two more unusual causes of chemical instability, namely polymerization and isomerization. All these reactions can occur with the pure drug substance or within a variety of formulations. Preformulation studies should investigate the potential for each of these reactions to take place, the mechanisms of such reactions, the kinetics of the reactions, and the factors affecting them.

 Drug degradation usually occurs by hydrolysis, oxidation, or photo-degradation.

17.2.1 **Hydrolysis and solvolysis**

Hydrolysis is the reaction of a molecule with water, usually resulting in the molecule splitting into two species. Certain functional groups often found in drug molecules are susceptible to hydrolysis, such as esters, amides and β-lactams (see Figure 17.1). Hydrolysis may be catalysed by the presence of acid and/ or base. Construction of a pH-stability profile is often useful in identifying the precise mechanism of the hydrolysis reaction. Solvolysis is the same type of reaction, except that the attacking species is an organic solvent rather than water.

 Hydrolysis is the degradation of a drug substance by reaction with water.

17.2.2 **Oxidation**

Strictly speaking, oxidation refers to a reaction whereby a species loses one or more electrons. However, from a drug stability perspective, oxidation which takes place with atmospheric or dissolved oxygen is of most significance. In this circumstance, oxidation usually occurs via a free radical reaction and is known as autoxidation. Drugs with certain functional groups present, such as phenols, tertiary amines, primary alcohols, and enols are particularly susceptible to this process. Examples of drugs which tend to oxidize in this way are adrenaline, morphine, hydrocortisone, and certain vitamins such as vitamin C (see Figure 17.2). Although free radical oxidation tends to occur spontaneously, it can be speeded up by exposure to heat, light, or the presence of trace metals.

 Oxidative degradation of a drug substance usually involves reaction with oxygen via a free radical reaction.

17.2.3 **Photo-degradation**

If degradation reactions are initiated by exposure to visible or ultraviolet light, the material is said to be photosensitive. The degradation reactions initiated are essentially similar to free radical oxidation. They proceed via an initiation reaction in which the light is responsible for the production of a free radical which

Figure 17.1 Examples of hydrolysis degradation reactions

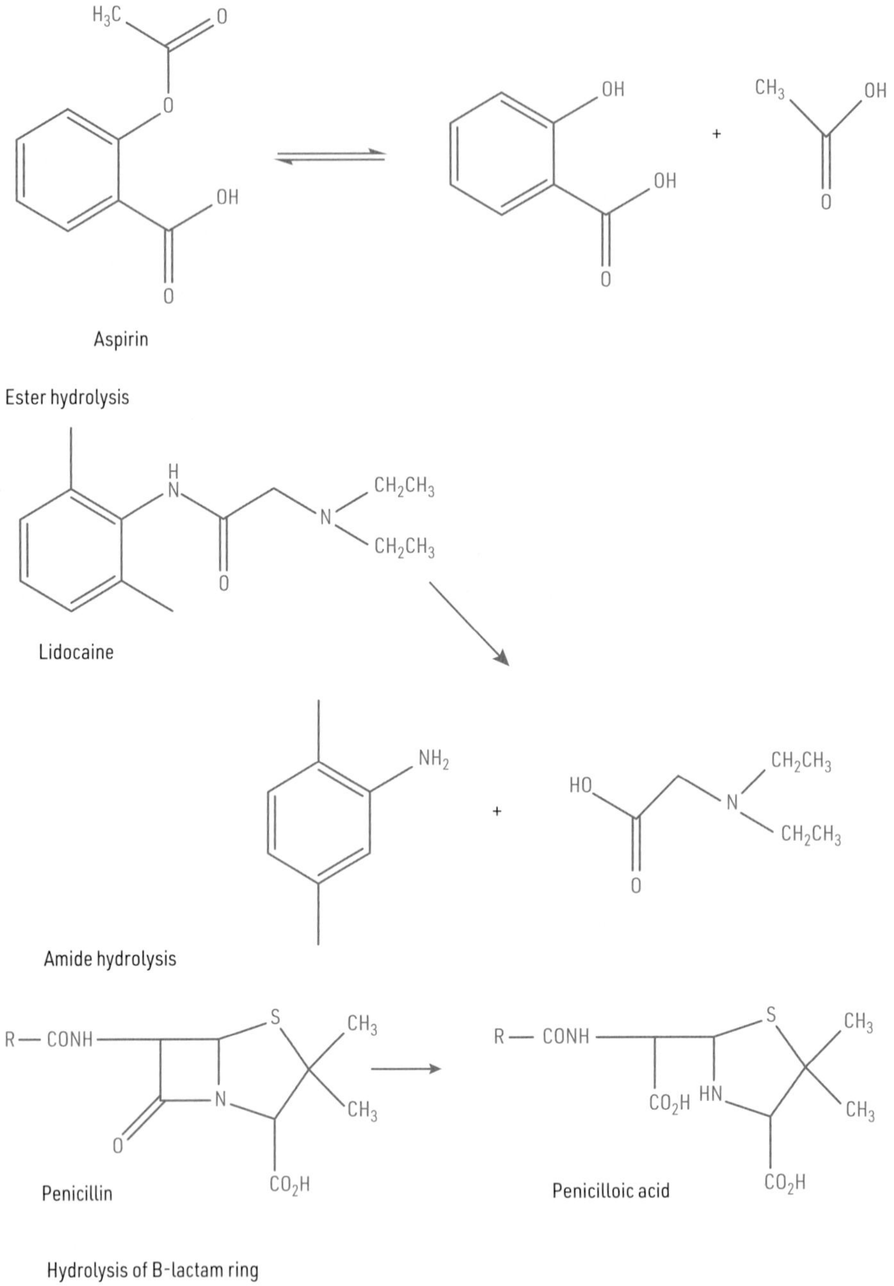

Aspirin

Ester hydrolysis

Lidocaine

Amide hydrolysis

Penicillin

Penicilloic acid

Hydrolysis of B-lactam ring

Figure 17.2 Examples of drugs susceptible to oxidation

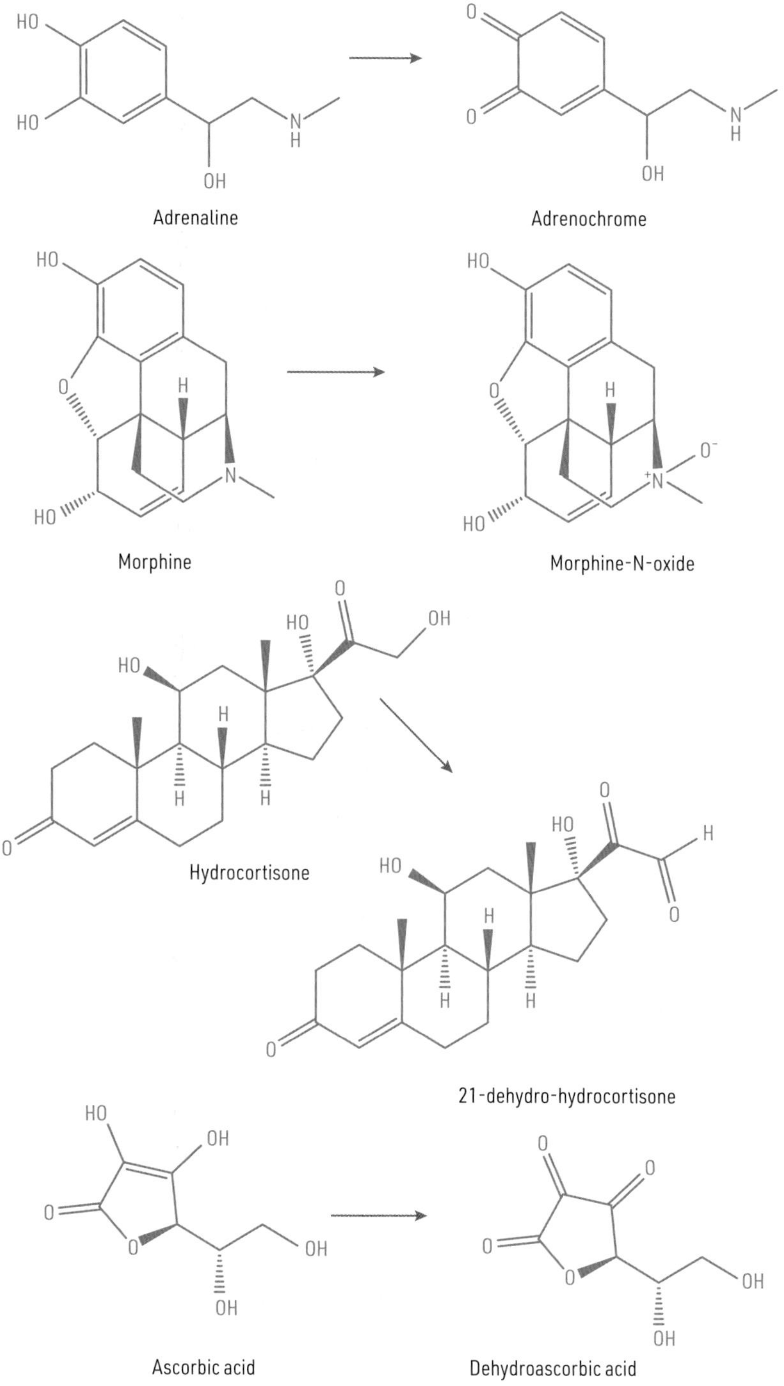

Adrenaline → Adrenochrome

Morphine → Morphine-N-oxide

Hydrocortisone → 21-dehydro-hydrocortisone

Ascorbic acid → Dehydroascorbic acid

Figure 17.3 Free radical reaction

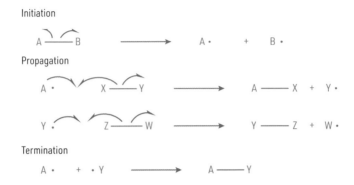

then propagates a chain of degradation reactions (see Figure 17.3). Examples of drug substances which are known to be photosensitive are folic acid, nifedipine, and citalopram (see Figure 17.4). Protection against photo-degradation can be relatively simple, such as storage in amber glass bottles which protect against wavelengths below 470nm, and so protect against ultraviolet and a large proportion of visible light.

 Photo-degradation of a drug substance is usually via a free radical reaction initiated by visible or ultraviolet light.

17.2.4 Polymerization

Occasionally, the new drug substance can be seen to form dimers when stored in solution over an extended period of time. Ampicillin is an example where this can occur (see Figure 17.5), as well as other β-lactam antibiotics. It is thought that the formation of these dimers may possibly be responsible for the allergic reaction to penicillins in humans.

17.2.5 Isomerization

If a potential drug substance can exist as geometrical or optical isomers, there is a possibility that the active isomer, in solution, may be converted to a less active or more toxic isomer, resulting in a reduction in therapeutic activity or an increase in toxicity. Examples of drugs where this is known to occur are adrenaline and tetracycline (see Figure 17.6). R-adrenaline is converted to a 50:50 racemic mixture of R- and S-adrenaline. Note that only one of the chiral centres in tetracycline is affected, and this is known as epimerization. In both these cases, the isomerization is pH-dependent and can be controlled by the use of appropriate buffers.

 Isomerization sometimes takes place at a chiral centre within a drug substance.

Figure 17.4 Examples of photosensitive drugs

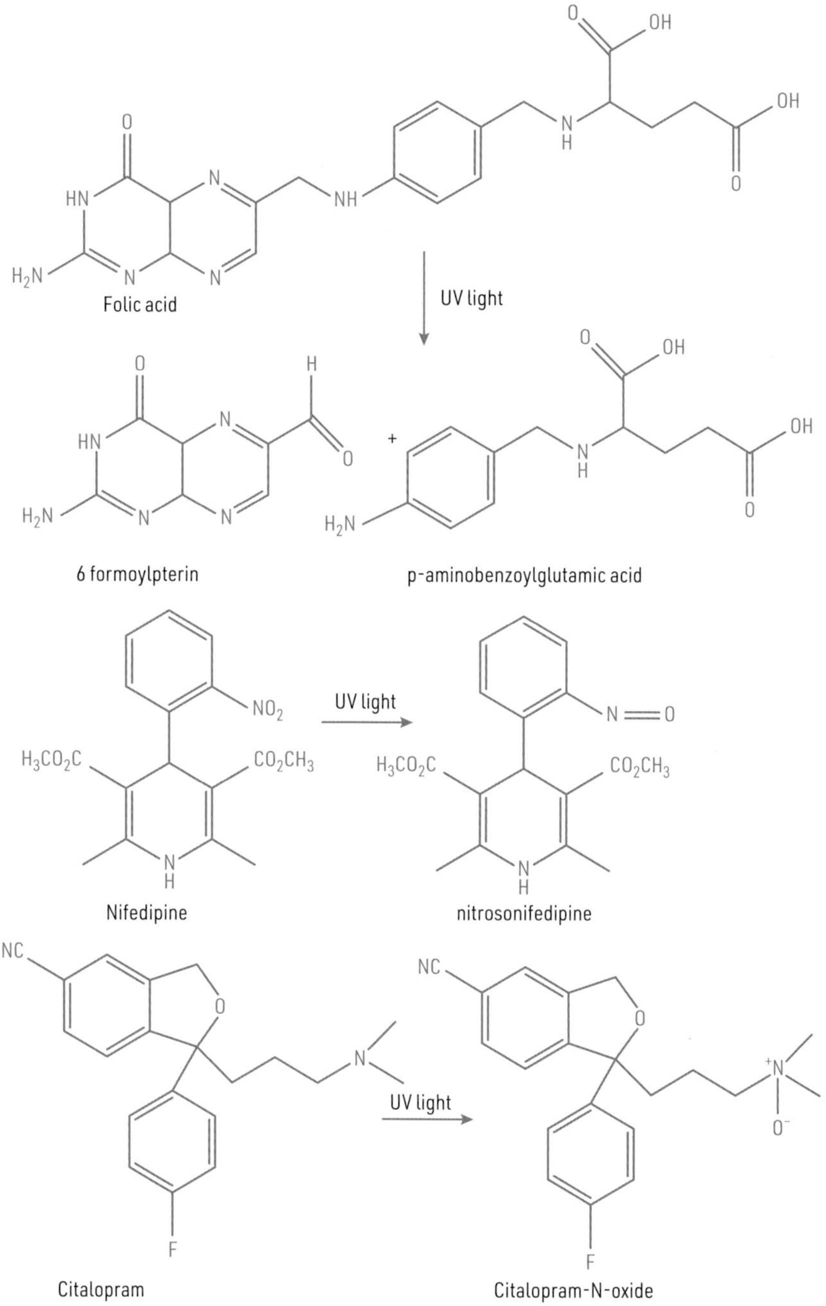

Figure 17.5 Dimerization of ampicillin

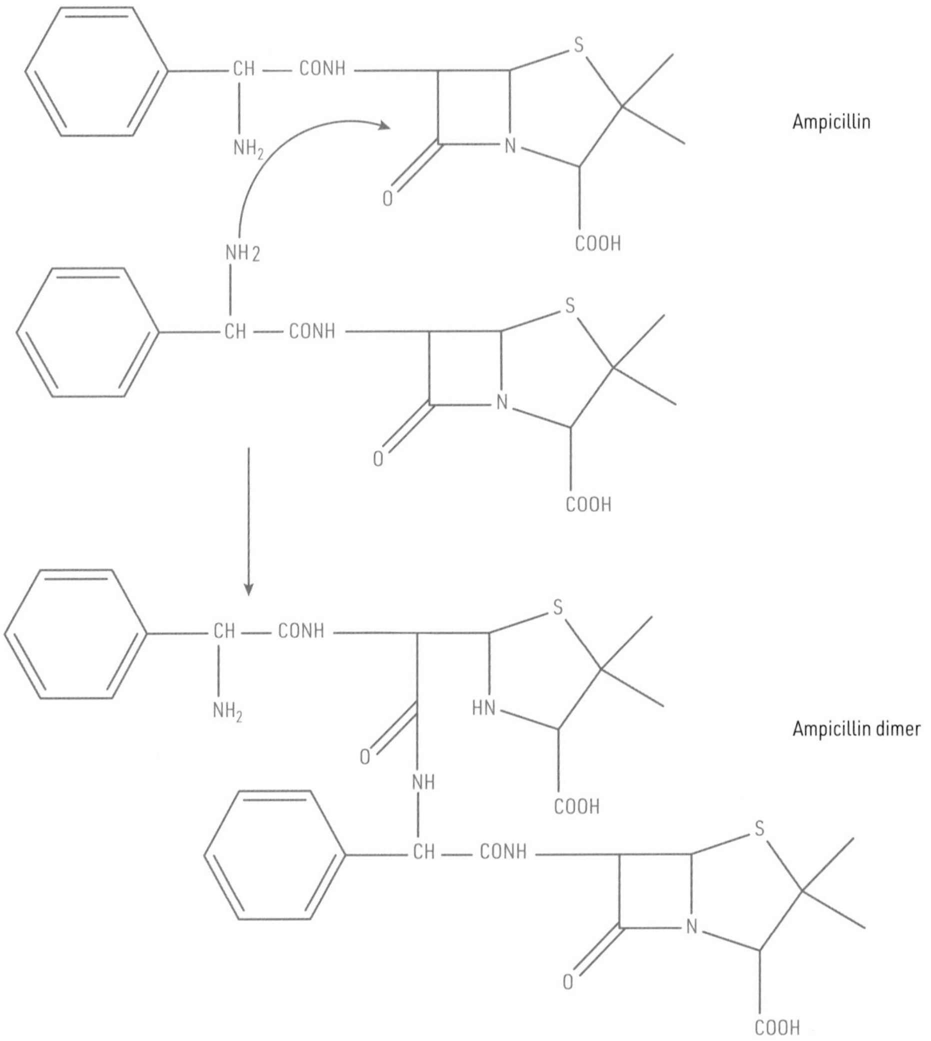

Ampicillin

Ampicillin dimer

17.3 **REACTION KINETICS**

Kinetic studies can provide information on the mechanism by which a reaction proceeds. In terms of drug development, this is important for studying drug dissolution, for developing a formulation that is suitably stable and determining the shelf life of a drug.

An investigation of the reaction kinetics of any identified degradation reaction can prove useful in establishing the mechanism of that reaction, thus assisting the prevention of such a reaction. Reaction kinetics relates to the rate at which a reaction takes place. The rate of a reaction is determined by monitoring the change in concentration of a reactant or product. The reaction can be represented by:

$$v = -\frac{d|\text{reactant}|}{dt} = \frac{d|\text{product}|}{dt}$$

Figure 17.6 Examples of drug isomerization

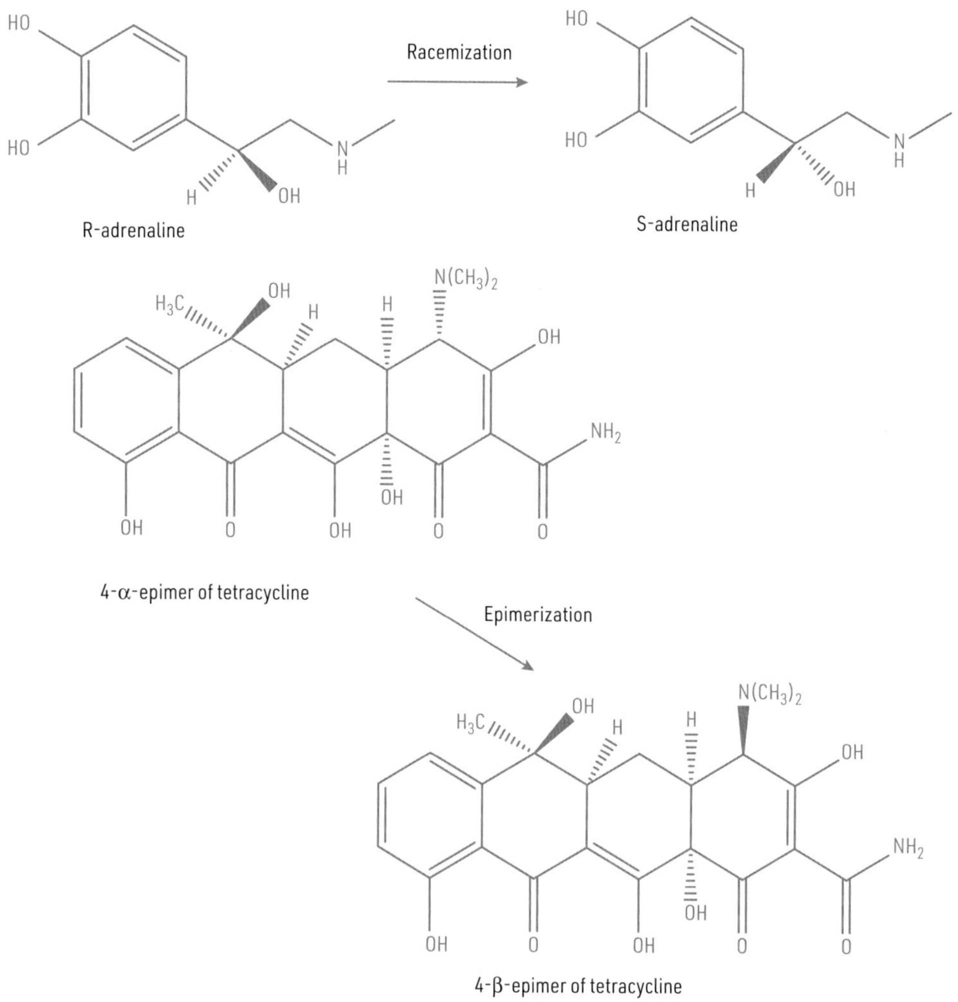

R-adrenaline

Racemization

S-adrenaline

4-α-epimer of tetracycline

Epimerization

4-β-epimer of tetracycline

Often, a reaction occurs in a number of individual steps, and these are what are referred to as the reaction mechanism. The number of species involved in any particular step is termed the **molecularity** of that step. The slowest reaction step is referred to as the rate-limiting step and will, therefore, be responsible for the overall rate of reaction. According to the number of species taking part in the rate-limiting step, a reaction may be unimolecular or bimolecular (e.g. S_N1 or S_N2). Molecularity assumes that the reactions are taking place in solution, and this will probably be the case in preformulation studies. However, solid state reactions cannot be described in terms of molecularity, but rather in terms of the fraction of the reaction that has taken place expressed as a function of time ($f(\alpha)$). Diffusion is often the rate-limiting step in solid-state reactions.

$$\text{Rate} = d[A]/dt = kf(\alpha)$$

where [A] is the concentration of reactant A remaining at time t and k is the rate constant.

Solution phase reaction kinetics assumes that the reactants can exhibit free movement and thus the reaction rate is related to the number of collisions between the reactants. Thus, for a reaction where A reacts with B to form products C and D,

$$A + B \rightarrow C + D$$

the reaction rate is defined by the reacting species (A and B),

$$Rate = k[A]^a[B]^b$$

where the exponents a and b represent the order of reaction for each of the reactants and k is the rate constant for the reaction. The sum of the exponents (a + b) represents the overall reaction order. Many reactions associated with pharmaceutical solutions are zero-, first- or second-order. Order of reaction is usually an integer. If orders are determined which are non-integer values, this is an indication that the degradation is taking place by more than one pathway (see Integration Box 17.1 Complex reactions).

 Investigation of the reaction kinetics of any degradation reaction of a drug substance is important in understanding and preventing such a reaction.

17.3.1 Zero-order reactions

When a reaction takes place at a rate that is constant and not dependent on the concentration of any of the reactants, this is known as a zero-order reaction and the reaction rate is expressed as:

$$-d[A]/dt = k$$

where [A] is the concentration of reactant A remaining at time t and k is the rate constant. After integration between time t and time zero t_0, this becomes:

$$[A]_t = -kt + [A]_0$$

INTEGRATION BOX 17.1   COMPLEX REACTIONS

Reactions which do not follow zero-, first- or second-order reaction kinetics are referred to as complex reactions and the most common examples are reversible reactions, parallel reactions and consecutive, or serial, reactions. In reversible reactions the overall reaction rate will be dependent on both the forward and reverse reaction rates.

$$A + B \rightleftharpoons C + D$$

In parallel reactions, a reactant may react in different ways simultaneously and produce different products.

$$A \underset{F}{\overset{E}{\rightleftharpoons}}$$

Both reaction rates will contribute to the overall reaction rate. In consecutive reactions the overall reaction proceeds through a sequence of reactions.

$$A \rightarrow G \rightarrow H \rightarrow I$$

Usually one reaction will proceed at a slower rate than all the others and hence this rate-limiting step will determine the overall reaction rate.

Figure 17.7 Graph of zero-order reaction kinetics

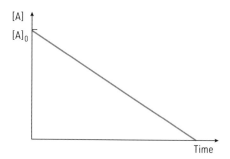

where $[A]_t$ is the concentration of reactant A at time t and $[A]_0$ is the initial concentration. The graphical form of this equation is linear (see Figure 17.7) and the gradient is equal to $-k$ (the rate constant) which has units of concentration time^{-1}.

Most pharmaceutical examples of zero-order reactions are actually pseudo zero-order because one of the reactants is in huge excess, such as degradation of a drug in suspension (see Integration Box 17.2 Degradation of a drug in suspension).

An important concept in stability studies is that of half-life—the time taken for half of the initial concentration of the drug to react ($t_{0.5}$). Insertion of $t_{0.5}$ into the zero-order rate equation yields:

$$[A]_0 / 2 = -kt_{0.5} + [A]_0 \text{ which gives } t_{0.5} = [A]_0 / 2k$$

The rate of a zero-order reaction is independent of the concentration of the reactants.

17.3.2 First-order reactions

The majority of degradation reactions in pharmaceutical systems are first-order reactions where the reaction rate is dependent on the concentration of one reactant only. The rate equation is:

$$-d[A]/dt = k[A]$$

and integration and taking logarithms produces:

$$\ln[A] = -kt + \ln[A]_0$$

where ln is the natural logarithm. In this instance a plot of concentration vs time will show an exponential decay which means that the slope cannot be used to calculate the rate constant. However, a plot of ln [A] against time will produce a straight line with a gradient of $-k$ (see Figure 17.8).

INTEGRATION BOX 17.2   **DEGRADATION OF A DRUG IN SUSPENSION**

If a drug is present in a suspension, it exists as a solid suspended in a liquid (usually aqueous in nature). Some of the drug will be dissolved in the liquid (although only a small amount), forming a saturated solution, and the remainder of the drug will be present as undissolved particles. The concentration of drug in solution will depend upon its solubility. If the drug degrades in solution it will be replaced by drug from the suspended particles so that the drug concentration in solution remains constant, despite the degradation. This gives rise to apparent or pseudo zero-order reaction kinetics.

Figure 17.8 Graphs of first-order kinetics

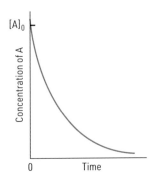

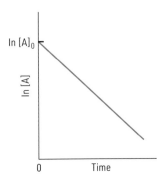

The units for a first-order rate constant are time^{-1}. The equation which can be used to determine the half-life of a first-order reaction is,

$$t_{0.5} = \ln 2/k$$

ln 2 has a value of 0.693 and so equation

$$t_{0.5} = 0.693/k$$

is often used. Note that half-life of a first-order reaction is independent of the initial concentration of the reactant (see Integration Box 17.3 Example calculation of half-life).

 In first-order reactions the reaction rate is dependent upon the concentration of only one of the reactants.

17.3.3 Second-order reactions

These are reactions where the rate is dependent on the concentration of two reactants. This may be two identical species reacting (i.e. 2A → products) or when two different species react (A + B → products). The relevant rate equations are thus,

$$-d[A]/dt = k[A]^2 \quad or -d[A]/dt = k[A][B]$$

Integration of the first of these equations yields

$$1/[A] = 1/[A]_0 + kt$$

A plot of this equation will be linear and the half-life of such a reaction can be determined using the expression

$$t_{0.5} = 1/k[A]_0$$

INTEGRATION BOX 17.3	EXAMPLE CALCULATION OF HALF-LIFE

The graph (Figure 17.8) shows a first-order (linear) relationship between ln % drug remaining and time in a degradation reaction. The slope of the line is 5×10^{-2} h^{-1}. Thus, for first-order kinetics, the slope of the straight line $-k/2.303 = 5 \times 10^{-2}$. Therefore, $k = 0.115$ h. Thus, from equation $t_{0.5} = \ln(2)/k = 0{,}693/0.115 = 6.02$ hours.

A reaction of the type (A + B → products) is very complex to investigate. However, if the reaction involves a reactant which can be kept in a large excess (such as the hydrolysis of a drug substance where the water will be in a large excess), then effectively this becomes a pseudo first-order reaction. The half-life can be calculated using the previous equation. Note the difference from a truly first-order reaction in that the rate of reaction is proportional to the initial concentration of the reactant.

 In second-order reactions the reaction rate is dependent on the concentration of two reactants.

17.4 **FACTORS AFFECTING DRUG DEGRADATION**

Collision theory states that reaction between molecules will only take place when molecules collide with the correct orientation, and if their combined energies exceed the activation energy, i.e. the minimum energy requirement for the reaction to take place. This can be represented diagrammatically by an energy diagram (see Figure 17.9). The factors affecting drug degradation reaction rates can be considered in terms of their influence within collision theory.

17.4.1 **The presence of moisture**

If a drug substance is susceptible to hydrolysis, the rate of this type of degradation reaction will be increased by the presence of moisture simply because there will be more water molecules available to collide with the drug substance. It is important, therefore, if hydrolysis is identified as a degradation reaction, to control the presence of water during processing, formulation and storage.

17.4.2 **The presence of oxygen**

Another common degradation reaction is that of oxidation, where the drug substance reacts with oxygen. Possible means of reducing the amount of oxygen would be packaging in an inert atmosphere (e.g. nitrogen), adding an antioxidant such as sodium metabisulphite or ascorbic acid, or adding a metal chelator such as EDTA as autoxidation is often catalysed by metal ions.

Figure 17.9 Energy profile for a reaction

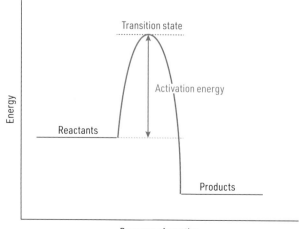

17.4.3 The presence of light

The irradiation of molecules can cause them to be converted to a higher energy form thereby increasing the number of molecules in a collision with sufficient energy content to exceed the activation energy. Photolytic degradation is relatively easy to reduce, by protecting from light, usually by storage in amber glass bottles which block light of wavelengths below 470nm (thus including protection against ultraviolet irradiation).

 Degradation reaction rates can be increased by an increase in the presence of water, oxygen and light for hydrolysis, oxidation and photolysis respectively.

17.4.4 The influence of pH

Because hydrolysis is often catalysed by acid or base or both, it is important to monitor the stability of a drug substance over a range of pHs. However, the pH-stability profile may be complex and there may not be a linear relationship between rate of hydrolysis and pH and different pH-stability profiles may be obtained (see Figure 17.10). A U-shaped profile indicates acid catalysis at low pH and base catalysis at high pH (see Figure 17.10a). Much more complex profiles can be obtained if the hydrolysis reaction exhibits a variety of pH-dependent behaviours (see Figure 17.10b).

 Degradation by hydrolysis is particularly susceptible to pH changes.

17.4.5 The influence of temperature

The factor influencing reaction rate, which is usually studied in greatest detail, is that of temperature, as an increase in temperature will increase both the frequency of collisions and the energy content of the species which are colliding. As temperature increases, the fraction of molecules possessing the requisite energy for reaction will increase. The influence of temperature on reaction rate was first investigated by Arrhenius. It was in 1889 that Arrhenius conceived the concept of activation energy. He made the empirical observation that reaction rates generally doubled with every 10K increase in temperature. Subsequently, this observation led to the development of the Arrhenius equation,

$$k = Ae^{-(E_a/RT)}$$

where k is the reaction rate constant, A is a constant related to the number of molecules which possess the energy to react, E_a is the activation energy, R is the universal gas constant, and T is the absolute temperature. Again the logarithmic form of this equation,

$$\log k = \log A - E_a/2.303 \times 1/RT$$

produces a linear expression. When log k is plotted against 1/T it yields a straight line with a gradient of $E_a/2.303R$. This allows the activation energy to be calculated. The most useful aspect of a so-called Arrhenius plot is the ability to extrapolate the results obtained at higher temperatures to room temperature in order to determine the shelf-life of a drug (**> XR Section 17.6**).

 Generally the rate of a degradation reaction is increased by an increase in temperature.

Figure 17.10 Hydrolysis pH-stability profiles

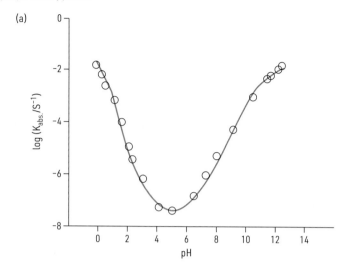

(a)

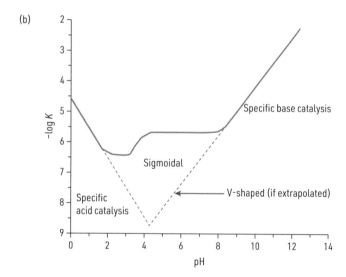

(b)

17.5 **STRESS TESTING**

During preformulation studies it is important to determine any potential degradation as quickly as possible. This is achieved by what is known as stress testing, i.e. subjecting the potential drug substance to reaction conditions which are more extreme than those likely to be encountered normally. Because at this stage of drug development only a small amount of material will be available, the effect of temperature (>40°C) and humidity (>75 per cent) is usually carried out on a single sample. The conditions to be used are contained in the ICH guidelines Q1A(R2)(2003). Hydrolytic degradation can be investigated by heating in 5M HCl and 5M NaOH. Samples will also be stored in the presence and absence of oxygen and in the presence and absence of light. The testing of photostability is subject to an ICH guideline (ICH Q1B 1996).

Stress testing, i.e. subjecting a drug substance to extreme storage conditions, is useful in identifying degradation reactions quickly and allows the calculation of the shelf-life of a drug.

17.6 ACCELERATED STABILITY TESTING AND SHELF-LIFE

Regulatory submissions for new drugs require accelerated stability testing to be carried out at least
at 40°C and 75 per cent relative humidity. It is also a requirement to provide 6 months of stability
data. At this stage in drug development, some indication of the nature of any degradation will be
available (from stress testing). Usually accelerated stability testing is carried out at a series of higher
temperatures and the degradation rate constants for each temperature determined. When this data
is plotted, extrapolation to lower temperatures provides an indication of the degradation rate at, say,
room temperature much more rapidly than would be obtained by a study at room temperature (hence,
accelerated).

Having obtained the degradation rate constant for a temperature at which the drug is likely to be
stored, this information can be used to calculate the shelf-life for the product. The shelf-life of a drug
product is defined as the total period of time from manufacture during which a product can be safely
used. It reflects the time taken for the concentration of the active substance(s) to fall to a value which
is still regarded as acceptable. Often this value is 90 per cent of the original concentration.

It must always be remembered that in using an Arrhenius plot for generating this data there are
some assumptions made. One assumption is that the mechanism of degradation at the higher temperatures is the same as at lower temperatures. The second assumption is that the Arrhenius plot is
legitimately a straight line, but, in reality, this may not be correct, although data is usually obtained
over a narrow range so that this is likely to be so. In determining an accelerated shelf-life from storage
data, climatic variation must always be taken into account. For regulatory submission the ICH defines
the required long-term storage conditions (at least 12 months) according to four climatic zones (see
Table 17.1).

 Accelerated stability studies are required as part of a regulatory submission and must include climatic
variations.

Table 17.1 Climatic zones and associated ICH storage conditions

Zone	Climate	Example countries	Temp.°C	Relative humidity %
I	Temperate	UK, US, Russia, N. Europe	21	45
II	Mediterranean/ Subtropical	S. Europe, Japan	25	60
III	Hot and dry	India, Iraq	30	35
IVA	Hot and humid	Egypt, Iran	30	65
IVB	Hot and very humid/ Tropical	Brazil, Malaysia	30	75

? Questions

1. What would you expect to be the major degradation reactions for the following drugs: procaine, paracetamol, enalapril, fentanyl, diazepam?

2. Why is it not possible for reactions taking place in the solid state to be described in terms of molecularity?

3. Compound A degrades according to first-order kinetics. 10g of A degrades to 2g in 30 minutes. What is the half-life of the reaction?

4. How do sodium metabisulphite, ascorbic acid and EDTA act as antioxidants?

5. The reaction rate constants for a reaction at 25°C and 30°C were found to be 9×10^{-3} L/mol and 3×10^{-2} respectively. What is the activation energy for the reaction?

↻ Chapter summary

- Physical instability is usually associated with dosage forms, although drug substances can pose problems if a metastable polymorph is used.

- Chemical instability is often a problem and the main degradation reactions are hydrolysis, oxidation, and photo-degradation.

- Chemical degradation can lead to a loss of therapeutic activity and/or toxic effects.

- Knowledge of the reaction kinetics of any degradation is useful in understanding the nature of the reaction and being able to prevent that reaction.

- Degradation reactions may follow zero-, first- or second-order reaction kinetics with first-order being most common in pharmaceutical circumstances.

- Because of the types of degradation reaction which are most common, the presence of moisture, air and light tend to increase drug degradation.

- Hydrolytic degradation is often significantly influenced by pH.

- An increase in temperature usually increases the rate of degradation.

- The Arrhenius equation can be used to determine the activation energy of a degradation reaction and, hence, the shelf-life of a drug.

- Stress testing involves subjecting a drug to more extreme conditions than normal in order to investigate any potential degradation reactions more rapidly.

- Regulatory submissions require accelerated stability studies to have been carried out including climatic variations.

▥ Further reading

Florence, A.T. and Attwood, D. (2015) *Physicochemical Principles of Pharmacy*. 6th edn, London: Pharmaceutical Press, ISBN 978-0-85711-174-6.

This book contains a chapter on drug stability.

Loftsson, T. (2014) *Drug Stability for Pharmaceutical Scientists*. Oxford: Elsevier, ISBN 978-0-12-411548-4.

A book which covers all aspects of drug stability, including numerous examples.

WHO (1997) Guidelines for stability testing of pharmaceutical products containing well established drug substances in conventional dosage forms, in *Quality Assurance of Pharmaceuticals* Volume 1, Geneva: WHO.

A comprehensive guide to regulatory requirements regarding stability testing of pharmaceuticals.

Baertschi, S.W., Alsante, K.M., and Reed, R.A. (eds) (2011) *Pharmaceutical Stress Testing: Predicting Drug Degradation*. Chichester, UK: Taylor and Francis, ISBN 9781439801796.

A guide to designing, executing and interpreting stress testing studies for drugs and their products.

Frokjaer, S. and Otzan, D.E. (2005) Protein drug stability: A formulation challenge, *Nature Reviews Drug Discovery* 4: 298–306.

An account of the problems posed to conventional drug stability knowledge by newer drug substances.

PART 5

Clinical Research

Clinical research is comprised of investigations into human disease and involves human subjects. It is a very broad subject and encompasses research into the origins and causes of disease, the prevention of disease, the diagnosis of disease, the outcomes of disease, and the treatment of disease. In order to ensure the safety and efficacy of a new drug, preclinical testing is first carried out. Preclinical research involves, mainly, investigations carried out in the laboratory both *in vitro* and *in vivo* and, increasingly, *in silico* (i.e. by computer) during which the pharmacology, pharmacokinetics and toxicology of the drug is investigated. These aspects have been referred to in previous chapters in this volume (XR Chapters 9, 12, and 14) and will not be dealt with further in this Part. Following preclinical testing, clinical testing, if appropriate, is carried out in humans. Clinical research carries out these investigations in volunteers and patients, eventually involving investigations in the entire human population. Clinical research in humans (clinical trials), in particular, are a vital part of the investigation of a new drug candidate (XR Chapter 18). Clinical trials are highly regulated and must be subject to very careful management and require a series of evidenced documents in order for authorization for clinical trials to begin—indeed, an entire industry has been established which undertakes and manages clinical trials. The design of clinical trials and their management (XR Chapter 19) are very important in order to ensure the safety, efficacy, and validity of any new drug product.

18

Clinical Research and Its Regulation

Clinical trials have a very long history (▶ **XR Section 18.1**) but it is only since the 1940s that the ethical considerations of such trials began to become important. Even so it wasn't until 1990 that the current integrated regulatory framework was developed, known as the International Conference on Harmonisation (ICH) (▶ **XR Section 18.2**). This framework is administered by various bodies worldwide (▶ **XR Section 18.3**) with the aim of harmonizing the application of guidelines and requirements for new product registration. Clinical trials are required to take place in a number of steps, referred to as the phases of clinical trials (▶ **XR Section 18.4**), all of which should be conducted according to the principles of good clinical practice (GCP) (▶ **XR Section 18.5**).

18.1 HISTORY OF CLINICAL TRIALS

It is generally acknowledged that the 'father' of clinical trials was the Scottish physician James Lind (see, however, Box 18.1 Bezoar stones).

In 1747 Lind, as a naval surgeon, performed the first recorded controlled clinical trial on twelve sailors suffering from scurvy. Lind was testing his theory that eating citrus fruits cured scurvy. The twelve sailors were divided into six pairs, each pair receiving a different treatment, in addition to their normal diet. The treatments were cider, seawater, vinegar, a mixture of garlic, mustard and horseradish, elixir of vitriol (sulphuric acid), and citrus fruits (oranges and lemons). The two sailors receiving the citrus fruits were the only ones who showed improvement in their condition. Having retired from the Navy Lind became a physician and published his work on scurvy which, however, was not acted upon by the Navy until 1795.

The use of **placebos** was first introduced into clinical trials in 1863 by an American physician, Austin Flint, who compared a placebo preparation with an active remedy for rheumatism. The first randomized clinical trials were introduced in 1923, thus removing possible bias, as doctors did not know which patients had received the active drug and which the placebo. The first multicentre clinical trial was in 1948, investigating the use of streptomycin in pulmonary tuberculosis, and was organized by the Medical Research Council (MRC).

> **BOX 18.1   BEZOAR STONES**
>
> A bezoar stone is a mass which grows in the gastro-intestinal tract of animals and humans and is composed of material that cannot be digested by the body. The first bezoar stone was isolated from the stomach of a Middle Eastern goat. The stones were, for many years, thought to be an antidote to poison (in Persian bezoar means counter-poison). This antidote theory was disproved in an experiment by the French surgeon Paré in 1575. A poison was administered to a man condemned to be hanged, followed by a bezoar stone. The condemned man agreed to this trial as, if he survived the poisoning, he would escape the hanging. He died in great pain, proving that bezoar stones were no antidote to the poison used which was sublimate of mercury. Oddly though, bezoar stones can be bought on Ebay—do not try this at home!

Because of unethical practices which took place in World War Two (medical experiments were conducted on concentration camp prisoners without their consent), ethical considerations with respect to clinical trials became increasingly important. This led to the introduction of the Nuremberg Code in 1947 and the Declaration of Helsinki, developed by the World Medical Association and amended at regular intervals to the current date.

 Although the first generally acknowledged clinical trial took place in 1747, the clinical trial system, as it is today, only began after World War Two.

18.2 INTERNATIONAL CONFERENCE ON HARMONISATION (ICH)

Founded in 1990, the ICH was formed because of a recognized need to 'achieve greater harmonization worldwide to ensure safe and effective and high-quality medicines are developed and registered in the most resource-efficient manner'. Initially this involved the bringing together of the regulatory authorities of Europe, the United States and Japan. The primary aim of ICH was to achieve greater harmonization in the interpretation and application of guidelines and requirements for drug product registration. In doing so, it was intended to minimize duplication of experiments and monitoring of drugs worldwide and to minimize any delay in delivering new treatments to the target population. The founder members from the three regions were from Europe, the European Commission, and the European Federation of Pharmaceutical Industries and Associations; from Japan, the Ministry of Health, Labour and Welfare, and the Japanese Pharmaceutical Manufacturers Association; and from the United States, the Food and Drug Administration, and the Pharmaceutical Research and Manufacturers of America. In addition to these founding members, there are now members from Canada, Switzerland, Brazil, and Korea. There are also a number of observers which act as links to non-ICH countries and regions, the most significant of which are the World Health Organization (WHO) and the European Free Trade Association (EFTA). The aspects involved in the ICH guidelines are divided into four categories—quality, safety, efficacy, and multidisciplinary. All guidelines are given a unique code (e.g. Q1A) and if they are revised, which many are on a regular basis, the revision is coded Q1AR (date of revision).

 The International Conference on Harmonisation was founded in 1990 to ensure the development of safe and effective medicines worldwide.

18.2.1 Quality guidelines

This aspect relates to the chemical and pharmaceutical quality assurance. It includes aspects such as the conduct of stability studies (❯ XR Section 17.5), impurity testing, harmonization of pharmacopoeial standards and good manufacturing practice (GMP) for active pharmaceutical ingredients. Each of these items is the subject of specific coded guidelines, e.g. Q1A–Q1F for stability studies, Q3A–Q3D for impurities, Q4A–Q4B for pharmaceutical harmonization, and Q7 for good manufacturing practice. There are a total of twelve guidelines within this aspect of the ICH.

18.2.2 Safety guidelines

These guidelines relate largely to *in vitro* and *in vivo* preclinical studies and deal with potential toxicological risks such as carcinogenicity, genotoxicity and reproductive toxicity (❯ XR Chapter 14). There are also guidelines which relate to pharmacokinetic studies, immunotoxicity studies and the safety of biopharmaceuticals. In total, there are eleven guidelines within this part of the ICH.

18.2.3 Efficacy guidelines

This is the aspect concerned with the design, conduct, safety, and reporting of clinical trials. There are eighteen items in these guidelines including aspects of clinical trials such as Good Clinical Practice (GCP) (❯ XR Section 17.5) and aspects such as the content and structure of clinical trial reports, statistical principles and guidelines for clinical trials in geriatrics and paediatrics which will be covered in detail in the following chapter (❯ XR Chapter 19). More recently guidelines have been introduced for biotechnologically-derived products (❯ XR Chapter 11) and the use of pharmacogenetics and pharmacogenomics (❯ XR Chapter 13).

18.2.4 Multidisciplinary guidelines

Essentially these are guidelines which do not fit uniquely into one of the previous aspects. They include medical terminology (MedDRA), the Common Technical Document (CTD), and the Electronic Standard for Transfer of Regulatory Information (ESTRI) Guidelines for gene therapy.

 The ICH produces guidelines on, amongst others, quality, safety, and efficacy.

18.3 REGULATORY BODIES

Most countries have a drug regulatory body which governs new drug approval. We shall only consider those which are most likely to be encountered—the MHRA in the UK, the EMA in the European Union, and the FDA in the United States.

18.3.1 Medicines and Healthcare products Regulatory Agency (MHRA)

This agency was established in 2003 by the merger of the Medicines Control Agency (MCA) and the Medical Devices Agency (MDA). It regulates medicines, medical devices and blood components for transfusion within the UK and is an executive agency of the Department of Health. This regulatory role is to ensure the safety, quality and effectiveness of medicines and medical devices. In terms of drug development this is the body to which applications need to be made in order to license a medicine for sale within the UK and Europe.

18.3.2 European Medicines Agency (EMA)

The EMA is a scientific agency (as opposed to a regulatory authority) and provides guidance and support to companies developing human medicines, including scientific and regulatory information. Topics covered include quality guidelines, non-clinical guidelines, clinical trials guidelines, ICH guidelines and the manufacture, characterization, and control of biologicals. The EMA is also responsible for the evaluation of marketing authorization applications within the European member states. It was formed in 1995 and is located in Amsterdam.

18.3.3 Food and Drug Administration (FDA)

The FDA is an agency of the US Department of Health and Human Services and is responsible for protecting and promoting public health, amongst many responsibilities, by the control and supervision of prescription and OTC drugs, vaccines, and biopharmaceuticals. The FDA, in its current form, arose as a result of pressure brought about by the sulfonamide tragedy (➤ **XR Integration Box 14.1**). The refusal of the FDA to authorize the marketing of thalidomide protected the USA from the tragedy that took place by the release of this drug in Europe. The branch of the FDA that deals with drugs is known as the Center for Drug Evaluation and Research. New drugs are subject to scrutiny in a process called a new drug application (NDA). Biologically-derived therapeutic agents are subject to approval by the Biologics License Application (BLA), which is overseen by a separate branch of the FDA, the Center for Biologics Evaluation and Research.

 The authorities that control new drug approval processes are the MHRA, the EMA and the FDA in the UK, Europe and the United States respectively.

18.4 CLINICAL TRIALS

Once preclinical trials have been successfully completed, the next steps in the development of a new drug are to determine the effectiveness of the medication in the target population—clinical trials. Clinical trials are carried out in a number of phases, 0 and 1 to 4 (often written I to IV). Each clinical trial phase has a particular aim, including safety, efficacy, and dose determination (see Table 18.1).

 There are five phases of clinical trial, each with its specific purpose in terms of safety and efficacy.

Table 18.1 Details of phases of clinical trials

	Phase 0	Phase 1	Phase 2	Phase 3	Phase 4
Outcome	Confirmation of preclinical studies	Safety in humans	Efficacy	Efficacy	Efficacy/long-term safety
Specific endpoints	Confirmation of preclinical studies	Side effects/dosage	Effectiveness side effects	Effectiveness side effects	Long-term safety
Types of study	Sub-clinical doses	Single or multiple doses	Dose escalation Placebo controlled	Comparative to existing treatment Randomized	Post-marketing studies
Participants	Healthy volunteers	Healthy volunteers	Patients with condition	Patients with condition	Various populations
Numbers	~10	Small <100	Larger >100	1000s	Possibly millions

18.4.1 Phase 0 clinical trials

These trials aim to find out if a drug behaves in humans as expected from laboratory studies in animals. They usually involve a small number of subjects (~10) and utilize what is regarded as a sub-therapeutic dose of the drug. Because of the low dose involved, phase 0 studies provide no safety or efficacy information. What are examined are pharmacokinetic parameters, especially the oral bioavailability and half-life of the drug. Phase 0 studies are often used by pharmaceutical companies to make decisions about which drug candidates are worth taking forward for further development.

18.4.2 Phase 1 clinical trials

Phase 1 clinical trials utilize relatively small numbers of healthy volunteers (~100) and their time scale is around 6 months. They have three categories—single ascending dose studies (SAD), multiple ascending dose studies (MAD) and food effect studies. The volunteers in the trial are monitored closely in order to obtain information about the safety, tolerance, pharmacokinetics and pharmacodynamics of the drug. The ascending dose studies are intended to provide initial information regarding what might be the correct clinical dosage. Also at this stage, the **maximum tolerated dose (MTD)** can be determined. The food effect studies involve administration of the drug in the fasted state and after food, thus allowing the recommendation 'to be taken before, with or after food'. Occasionally, in special circumstances, Phase 1 clinical trials can be carried out on volunteers who are not healthy (such as cancer patients). Usually these individuals have not responded to any currently available treatments.

 Phase 1 clinical trials utilize small numbers of healthy volunteers and are primarily used to establish the safety and the dosage of the drug in humans.

18.4.3 Phase 2 clinical trials

Once a drug has been shown to be safe for use in humans in Phase 1 trials, Phase 2 trials are instigated although at this stage the drug is still not presumed to have any therapeutic effect. In this phase slightly larger numbers (100–300) are involved, but this time the subjects are patients who have the target disease. Once again data is collected on pharmacological activity, dose requirement, safety and efficacy. In many ways Phase 2 trials are a scaled-up version of Phase 1 trials and are carried out over a longer time scale, usually 1–2 years. Because these trials involve patients the regulatory requirements become more stringent in terms of ethics approval and the investigatory personnel. This is the stage at which placebo control is introduced.

 Phase 2 clinical trials use larger numbers of subjects and are conducted on patients with the condition for which the drug is intended.

18.4.4 Phase 3 clinical trials

This phase of clinical trials is the most complex. Whereas in Phase 2 trials placebo treatments have been included, in Phase 3 trials large numbers of subjects with the target disease (up to 3,000) are investigated in multiple centres using randomized control groups (❯ XR Chapter 19). The new drug is usually compared for efficacy with an existing treatment and any adverse effects monitored. However, if the drug target is new, there may not be an existing treatment. The time scale for Phase 3 clinical trials is usually at least 3 years and often continues after marketing approval is sought. Once sufficient satisfactory evidence of efficacy and safety has been obtained, this evidence, together with all other relevant information, is submitted to the appropriate regulatory authority as a new drug application (NDA).

 Phase 3 trials involve much larger numbers of patients with the condition for which the drug is intended to be used, involve multiple centres, and comparison with an existing treatment for the condition.

18.4.5 Phase 4 clinical trials

This phase of clinical trials takes place after the drug has been marketed and it is also known as post-marketing surveillance. The subjects in this phase are, probably, very large numbers—in fact all the patients taking the medication. During Phase 4 clinical trials the efficacy of the drug will continue to be monitored. The main aim of Phase 4 trials is to provide any additional information about the long-term safety of the drug, a process known as pharmacovigilance (Section 18.4.6). As women of child-bearing age are normally excluded from Phase 3 clinical trials, there is now an opportunity in Phase 4 trials to monitor any effects on pregnant women and the unborn child.

 Phase 4 clinical trials are effectively an ongoing monitoring of the drug once it has been marketed, looking for any long-term safety issues.

18.4.6 Pharmacovigilance

Pharmacovigilance is a term which refers to the ongoing monitoring of the safety of a medicine once it has reached the market. It includes an assessment of risk involved in its use and also provides information about a medicine's safety both for health professionals and patients. Pharmacovigilance rules are necessary for the protection of public health in order to prevent, detect and assess adverse reactions to medicinal products. Adverse drug reactions (ADR) reporting can arise from a variety of sources. These include Individual Case Safety Reports (ICSRs) from a number of potential sources such as pharmaceutical companies, clinical research organizations, regulatory agencies, and literature reports. Healthcare professionals and patients are also encouraged to submit reports of suspected ADRs. In the UK, this is achieved by the use of the yellow card system. This involves the reporting of suspected adverse drug reactions and applies to all medicines including over the counter and herbal medicines. For newly released medicines, all adverse drug reactions should be reported. For established medicines, only serious adverse drug reactions need to be reported, e.g. those that are life-threatening or result in prolonged hospitalization or death of a patient. All the data arising from these sources is monitored and reviewed in the European Union via the Eurovigilance programme of the EMA (see Integration Box 18.1 Eurovigilance in action).

INTEGRATION BOX 18.1   EUROVIGILANCE IN ACTION

The increase in obesity in the general population has led to an increased search for an effective weight loss medicine. Rimonabant is a cannabinoid receptor antagonist that, amongst other properties, modulates the intake of highly palatable sweet or fatty foods. It was introduced as an anti-obesity drug in 2006. Subsequent data, however, reported an increased risk of psychiatric ADRs (depression, anxiety, aggression, sleep disorders, suicide) vs a placebo. Because options to minimize these risks were limited, the marketing authorization was suspended, and the drug was withdrawn in 2009.

Pharmacovigilance is a set of procedures which ensure the safety of a drug after it has been marketed.

18.5 GOOD CLINICAL PRACTICE (GCP)

The definition of GCP, contained in the EU directive from 2001, is 'a set of internationally recognised ethical and scientific quality requirements which must be observed for designing, conducting, recording and reporting clinical trials that involve the participation of human subjects'. GCP provides assurance that the rights, safety and wellbeing of trial subjects are protected and that the results of the trials are credible and accurate. GCP is based in a set of principles that originated from the Declaration of Helsinki (1964) and has had numerous revisions in subsequent years (see Integration Box 18.2 Reasons for the introduction of GCP).

INTEGRATION BOX 18.2   **REASONS FOR THE INTRODUCTION OF GCP**

The advent of the guidelines for GCP arose as a result of a number of uncontrolled clinical trials which have taken place over the years. During World War Two, experiments were conducted on concentration camp prisoners. These experiments resulted in disfigurement, disability and death. The 'medical experiments' included injection with gasoline and live viruses, forcing people to ingest poisons, and deliberately causing wounds and infecting them with live bacteria. A number of the doctors who performed these experiments were brought to trial, sixteen were found guilty and seven were sentenced to death. This situation led to the development of the Nuremburg Code of Medical Ethics and, ultimately, to the Declaration of Helsinki. Despite the introduction of these guidelines, there still continued to be examples of trials carried out, the nature of which caused great concern. Starting in the 1930s but continuing until 1970, the Tuskegee syphilis study recruited African-American men with syphilis. No informed consent was obtained and some of the procedures carried out were termed 'special free treatment'. Even after the advent of penicillin in the 1940s, which treats syphilis effectively, the men were not treated with penicillin. In 1963, a study was conducted at the Jewish Chronic Disease hospital in New York, looking into the body's ability to reject cancer cells by injecting cancer cells into debilitated patients. Again, there was no informed consent and the medical staff at the hospital had not been informed of the nature of the research. Also in the 1960s and again in New York, at an institution for 'mentally defective' children, newly admitted children were deliberately injected with a hepatitis virus in order to gain insight into the natural history of infectious hepatitis. All of these cases, and the disgust that they caused, finally led to the production of the ICH guidelines on Good Clinical Practice.

A summary of the principles is as follows:
1. Conduct trials according to GCP.
2. Weigh risks vs benefits.
3. Wellbeing of subjects has priority over science.
4. There should be adequate information to justify the trial.
5. There should be a clear, defined protocol.
6. The protocol should be approved by the relevant institutional review board/independent ethics committee.
7. The trial must use qualified physicians.
8. There must be trained and qualified support staff.
9. Informed consent must be obtained.

10. Information must be recorded appropriately.
11. Records must respect privacy and confidentiality.
12. The product under investigation must comply with good manufacturing practice (GMP).
13. The entire system must be quality assured.

 Good clinical practice ensures that clinical trials are conducted in a safe and effective manner, with particular emphasis on the rights and wellbeing of trials subjects.

? Questions

1. What are the essential differences between preclinical and clinical trials?

2. What are the essential differences between Phase 1 and Phase 2 clinical trials?

3. The thalidomide tragedy was avoided in the United States because the FDA did not approve the use of the drug. Why was approval not given?

4. Statins have an established role in prevention of cardiovascular disease. They also have a known risk of myopathy, namely myalgia. It has been suggested that all males over 65 and all females over 75 should be prescribed statins. However, there have been recent studies which do not support this view. After reviewing the evidence what is your view—and does it agree with the EMA?

⟳ Chapter summary

- The first controlled clinical trial took place in 1747 and involved treatments for scurvy.

- Placebos in clinical trials were first used in 1863 and the first randomized trials took place in 1923.

- The International Conference on Harmonisation (ICH) was founded in 1990 with a view to bring together worldwide regulatory authorities and the pharmaceutical industry to ensure the development of safe, effective, and high-quality medicines.

- The ICH has been responsible for producing guidelines on safety, efficacy, and quality of medicines.

- The authorities that control new drug approval processes are the MHRA, the EMA and the FDA in the UK, Europe, and the United States respectively.

- Clinical trials are carried out after preclinical trials have established that a new drug is likely to be safe for use in humans.

- Phase 0 clinical trials are used to ascertain if a drug behaves in humans as expected from laboratory studies.

- Phase 1 clinical trials which take place with healthy volunteers are mainly involved with establishing the safety and dosage levels of a new drug.

- Phase 2 clinical trials, which take place with patients who have the condition for which the drug is intended, are concerned both with safety and efficacy of the new drug.

- Phase 3 clinical trials also involve patients with the condition and involve comparison of the new drug with an existing treatment for the condition.

- Phase 4 clinical trials, also known as post-marketing surveillance, involve ongoing monitoring of a marketed drug for safety.

- Pharmacovigilance ensures the continued monitoring and evaluation of adverse drug reactions.

- Good Clinical Practice (GCP) is based on a set of principles designed to ensure ethical and scientifically conducted clinical trials.

Further reading

ICH Publications, www.ich.org

This is the website for the ICH, which contains material about its development, role, and guidelines.

Hackshaw, A. (2009) *A Concise Guide to Clinical Trials*, UK: Wiley-Blackwell, ISBN 978-1-4051-6774-1.

A comprehensive overview of the design, conduct and analysis of clinical trials.

Waller, P. and Harrison-Woodrych, M. (2017) *An Introduction to Pharmacovigilance* 2nd ed., Wiley, ISBN 9781119289746.

An introduction to the key principles of pharmacovigilance

HMSO publications. MHRA (2012) Good clinical practice guide, HMSO, ISBN 978-0-11-708107-9.

Provides practical advice for implementing the principles of good clinical practice within the EU.

19

Design and Management of Clinical Trials

There are many aspects which need to be taken into consideration when designing a clinical trial. The design of a clinical trial requires a plan of each element of the trial that is to be carried out, with the overall aim of ensuring that the results of the trial are valid. To quote the ICH, 'the scientific integrity of the trial and the credibility of the data from the trial depend substantially on the trial design'. The design of the trial requires regulatory authority approval before commencing. The objective of the trial should be clearly set out, as this will influence all aspects of the trial, such as target population, and patient selection (▶ XR Section 19.1), and the nature of the disorder and treatment duration (▶ XR Section 19.2). In clinical trials the choice of treatment is strictly controlled (▶ XR Section 19.3). In order to ensure comparability between test and control groups of subjects a process of randomization is utilized (▶ XR Section 19.4). It is also important that the endpoints to be measured are clearly defined (▶ XR Section 19.5). In order to eliminate any bias in the conduct of the clinical trial a process of blinding is utilized (▶ XR Section 19.6). There are a number of standard designs for clinical trials (▶ XR Section 19.7), each of which may be utilized in order to address the objective of the trial. Because clinical trials involve volunteers or patients there are ethical issues that must be addressed (▶ XR Section 19.8). The final aspect, which can have a significant effect on the credibility of the data from the trial, is that of data management, known as clinical data management (▶ XR Section 19.9), which utilizes good data management practice (GDMP), which like GMP and GCP is based upon ICH guidelines.

19.1 TARGET POPULATION AND SUBJECT SELECTION

The protocol for a clinical trial needs to define the subject population and must avoid selection bias by avoiding a population choice by the investigator. A set of eligibility criteria will be established by which the target population is defined, from which eligible subjects can be recruited. Eligibility criteria will typically consist of a set of inclusion criteria and a set of exclusion criteria. The inclusion criteria will outline the target subject population and the exclusion criteria will be used to fine tune the target subject population by removing unwanted sources of variability (see Integration Box 19.1 Examples of inclusion and exclusion criteria). The subject population may change according to the phase of the trial, with Phase 1 using healthy volunteers, Phase 2 will be restricted according to the criteria specified in the protocol, and Phase 3 will sample the entire patient population who may receive the drug under test. As noted previously (**➤ XR Section 18.4**), the numbers will vary between phases. It is important that both test and control groups (**➤ XR Section 19.3**) match all the criteria. The overall recruitment criteria will typically include such aspects as the nature of the disorder, the stage of the disorder in the subjects, any other disorders suffered by the subjects including medication for such disorders, age and sex.

INTEGRATION BOX 19.1 | **EXAMPLES OF INCLUSION AND EXCLUSION CRITERIA FOR A CLINICAL TRIAL**

Factors that allow an individual to participate in a clinical trial are inclusion criteria. Factors that do not allow participation are exclusion criteria. In general these factors are based on age, gender, type and stage of condition, previous treatment history and other medical conditions. Examples of these criteria are best considered by looking at a particular clinical trial. For a clinical trial of apixaban vs warfarin in patients with atrial fibrillation (AF), the criteria can be seen in Table 19.1 taken from *the New England Journal of Medicine*, 2011, 365, 981–2.

Table 19.1 Example of inclusion and exclusion criteria

Inclusion criteria	Exclusion criteria
Atrial fibrillation (AF) at time of enrolment	AF due to a reversible cause
2 episodes of AF at least 2 months apart in the last year	Moderate to severe mitral stenosis
Presence of at least one of the following risk factors	Other conditions requiring anticoagulant therapy
At least 75 years old	Stroke within past 7 days
Previous stroke	A requirement of aspirin >165mg daily or a requirement for both aspirin and clopidogrel
Transient ischemic attack	Severe renal insufficiency
Systemic embolism	
Symptomatic heart failure within past 3 months	
Left ventricular ejection fraction of no more than 40 per cent	
Diabetes	
Hypertension requiring drug treatment	

 The protocol for a clinical trial needs to establish clear eligibility criteria, both for inclusion and exclusion of subjects.

19.2 THE NATURE AND STAGE OF THE DISORDER

The design of a clinical trial should take into account the type of disorder and the nature of the the treatment. Disorders can be broadly classified into acute (has a rapid onset and/or a short duration, e.g. a cut or a broken bone, flu, an asthma attack) and chronic (is a long-lasting condition, usually longer than three months, e.g. heart disease, diabetes, osteoporosis) and this classification will determine the duration of the trial, the subject population, and the overall design of the trial. It should also be recognized that some disorders are cyclical (a condition that occurs at regular intervals, e.g. cyclic **neutropenia**, migraine) whilst others may be seasonal (e.g. hay fever) and the design of the trial will have to take this into account to rule out inappropriately biased results.

 Disorders may be acute, chronic, cyclical, or seasonal and clinical trials need to be designed to account for this.

19.3 CONTROLS IN CLINICAL TRIALS

The regulatory authorities such as the Medicines and Healthcare products Regulatory Agency (MHRA) and the Food and Drug Administration (FDA) require clinical trials to be well-controlled in order to eliminate bias, to minimize variability, and to enhance the accuracy and reliability of the outcome of the study. There are three types of control—the treatment under investigation is compared with no treatment, the treatment is compared with a placebo, and the treatment is compared with an active comparator, although the first of these is rarely used except in Phase 1 trials. In comparison with a placebo, the placebo contains no active ingredient and must be identical in appearance, taste, etc. to the treatment under investigation in order to prevent bias. This type of controlled trial is used to determine the efficacy and safety of the treatment under investigation. What are being looked for are efficacious results and an absence of adverse events. There are, of course, ethical issues (**❯ XR Section 19.8**) with this type of control because a proportion of the subjects (who have the disease) are receiving no treatment. Of more value is where the control is an active comparator, then both test and control contains an active drug, although again they must be identical in appearance, taste etc. In this type of trial, the efficacy and safety of the new treatment is directly compared with a drug already on the market, usually a market leader. The active comparator should be one which is widely used with established efficacy under identical conditions of usage. There may be some practical issues, e.g. different drugs may be used in different countries at different doses.

 There are three types of control used in clinical trials—comparison with no treatment, comparison with a placebo, and comparison with an active comparator.

19.4 RANDOMIZATION

The process of randomization takes place after the subjects for a trial have been recruited but before the trial actually commences. Randomization is carried out because it eliminates selection bias, with the aim of ensuring that the test and control groups are comparable. In this process subjects are allocated to treatment or control groups in a pre-determined random manner. A variety of different randomization procedures can be used and the choice of procedure depends on a number of factors. In reality, a combination of the various randomization types tends to be used. Examples of the types of randomization that are used can be seen in Figure 19.1.

Figure 19.1 Examples of types of randomization: **a)** Restricted simple randomization: **b)** Unrestricted simple randomization: **c)** Alternative randomization

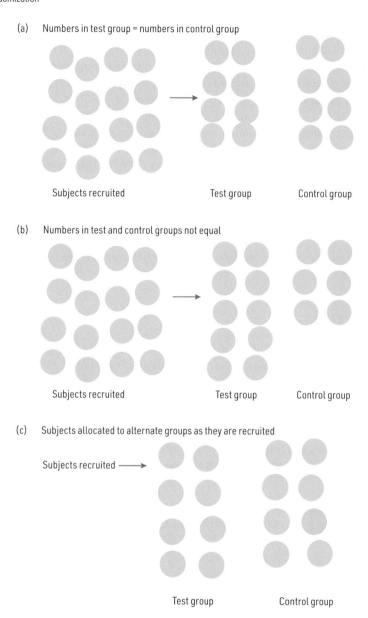

(a)   Numbers in test group = numbers in control group

Subjects recruited   Test group   Control group

(b)   Numbers in test and control groups not equal

Subjects recruited   Test group   Control group

(c)   Subjects allocated to alternate groups as they are recruited

Subjects recruited ⟶

Test group   Control group

 The process of randomization in clinical trials eliminates selection bias and ensures that test and control groups are comparable.

In restricted simple randomization, the number of subjects in the test group and the control group are the same and subjects are randomly allocated to the groups in equal numbers. In unrestricted simple randomization, the numbers of subjects in the test group and the control group are not equal. Usually there will be more subjects in the test group than the control group. This provides more information about the treatment under test. This type of randomization works best with larger population numbers (generally >1,000). Alternative randomization is where the subjects are allocated into alternate groups as they are enrolled onto the study. The disadvantage of this method is that the groups may not be comparable and there is no blinding (**XR Section 19.6**), leading to possible bias. Stratified randomization is quite a complex process and can be used to identify such aspects as age or sex differences. The subjects are divided into sub-groups (strata), and then each stratum is randomized separately. Each stratum should contain equal numbers of subjects. In adaptive randomization, as the term suggests, subjects are randomized according to an analysis of the results already obtained. In this way, if a group has a 'better' response, a higher proportion of subjects can be allocated to that group, thus obtaining more useful information, although the data analysis for this method can prove difficult. Finally, in the random permutated block method, subjects are randomized in blocks as they continue to be enrolled onto the trial. This method is primarily for use in trials that are likely to last for prolonged periods (e.g. 5 years) where it can be difficult to retain subjects for the whole period of the trial due to dropouts for a variety of reasons, e.g. change in circumstances, other illnesses, cure, death.

 There is a variety of randomization strategies, each of which is appropriate to clinical trials with different circumstances.

19.5 OBJECTIVES

It is important that the objectives of the trial are clearly set out in the trial protocol, along with the measurements and endpoints to be used. Trials usually have primary and secondary objectives and the measurements and endpoints may be quite different between them (see Integration Box 19.2 Cancer drug trial objectives). The protocol should also be quite clear whether the measurements and endpoints are likely to be influenced by factors other than the treatment itself, such as time of day taken, with or without food. The measurements may be subjective or objective and, usually, the latter is preferred. If subjective judgements are involved in the measurements, there is always the possibility of bias, which can be eliminated by the use of blinding (**XR Section 19.6**).

INTEGRATION BOX 19.2 **CANCER DRUG TRIAL OBJECTIVES**

In the example of a clinical trial of a new anti-cancer drug in the treatment of lung cancer, the objectives can be divided into primary and secondary objectives. The primary objectives of the trial (which is a randomized parallel-group trial) is to demonstrate that the one-year survival rate of patients with pre-treated advanced non-small-cell lung cancer receiving the investigational drug orally is not inferior to those receiving intravenous docetaxel. The secondary objectives of the trial are to evaluate overall survival rate, time to progression, time to response, improvement in quality of life, and qualitative and quantitative toxicities.

 The objectives of a clinical trial, and how they will be evaluated, must be clearly defined and set out in the trial protocol.

19.6 **BLINDING**

The purpose of blinding is to eliminate bias in some or all of the participants in the trial, both investigators and subjects. Blinding is defined as an experimental condition in which the knowledge of the treatments assigned to subjects is withheld from investigators and/or subjects, depending on the type of blinding utilized. There are three types of blinding used in clinical trials—open-label, single-blinded and double-blinded (see Table 19.2). Occasionally triple-blinding is used, where in addition to the investigators and subjects, the data analysts do not know which group received a particular treatment.

In an open-label study everyone knows who is receiving which treatment, i.e. there is no blinding. Such a study may only be used where knowledge of treatment cannot influence the endpoint of the study. Examples of where open-label trials are inevitable are where psychotherapy or physiotherapy is being compared with a drug treatment. A single-blinded study is one in which only one party to the investigation (either investigator or subject) knows the nature of the treatment received, although more usually it is the subject who is blinded. Once again, there is a potential for bias in this method of investigation. A double-blinded clinical trial is one where neither the investigator nor the subjects are aware of the identity of the treatments given. In this case, it is necessary to have contingency plans if something goes wrong with the trial and these must be included in the protocol, as well as how the overall blinded nature of the trial is to be maintained. If the test and comparator have different characteristics (e.g. different dosage regimes), then a system known as double dummy blinding can be used (see Figure 19.2).

Table 19.2 Types of blinding used in clinical trials

Type of blinding	Description
Open-label	All parties are aware of the treatment the patient is receiving
Single-blinded	Only one party (usually the patient) is unaware of the treatment the participant is receiving
Double-blinded	Both participants and investigators are unaware of the treatment the participant is receiving
Triple-blinded	Participants, investigators and data analysts are all unaware of the treatment the participant is receiving

Figure 19.2 Double dummy blinding

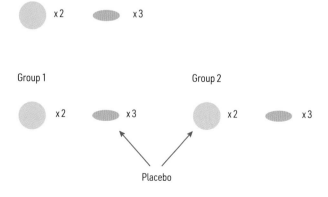

Blinding is a process by which bias can be eliminated from a clinical trial.

19.7 TRIAL DESIGNS

Clinical trials can use a number of different designs depending on the reason for conducting the trial, the phase of the trial, and the primary endpoint measurements. Broadly speaking, there are two types of design—comparative and non-comparative, with the former being the type most often employed.

The parallel group design is a completely randomized trial in which each subject receives either only the test material or only the control treatment. In this way, there is a direct comparison between the treatment groups and there is no possibility of drug interaction. Because of the shorter duration of this type of trial, the stability (or otherwise) of the disorder is not an issue.

The crossover design type of trial involves each subject receiving the test treatment and the control treatment at different times during the trial. This design has the advantage that smaller numbers of subjects can be used, but, conversely, the timescale of the trial will be longer. Additional potential drawbacks to this design are that data obtained may be affected by the timeframe of the disorder, and side effects may cause a double-blinded trial to become un-blinded.

Whichever design of clinical trial is used, a washout, or lead-in, period will be used. A washout period acts to remove effects of any previous drug therapy. It can also be used to establish baseline data for the disorder, to identify any placebo responses, and to assist in assessing subject compliance. Often this period is used as a training period for subjects, investigators, and other staff involved in the trial. In crossover studies a washout period is essential to ensure that there is no carry-over of the first treatment in the subjects. There may be, of course, clinical issues posed by having subjects free of treatment for any period of time.

An important aspect of trial design is a decision regarding the number of patients to involve. If the number is too small it may not be able to address the objective of the trial and, thus, would be a waste of resources. It could also be thought unethical because patients may be put at risk with no apparent benefit. Conversely, too large numbers of patients may also be a waste of resources if fewer patients would be sufficient.

One further type of design is the cross-sectional study. This is an observational study that collects data from a population and usually examines the relationship between a disease or condition and observable variables related to them. They examine the chosen population at a particular point in time and can include questionnaires, surveys, and laboratory tests. They are often used to assess the health needs of a population with a view to planning and allocation of health resources.

 The main type of clinical trial design is comparative, which includes parallel group and crossover designs.

19.8 ETHICAL ASPECTS OF CLINICAL TRIALS

Because of the operation of a number of uncontrolled clinical trials carried out in a variety of circumstances (❯ XR Integration Box 18.1), the ICH guidelines on Good Clinical Practice (GCP) were introduced, incorporating ethical principles (❯ XR Section 18.5). These principles protect the rights, safety and well-being of clinical trial subjects. Randomized controlled trials are generally regarded as the gold standard of intervention studies. There are, however, some ethical issues associated with them, in terms of informed consent, placebo usage, randomization, and participant protection.

Informed consent is considered to refer to the understanding of the risks and benefits of the treatment that may be received, an understanding of the procedures involved (including randomization and blinding), an understanding that participation is voluntary, and an understanding of the purpose of the trial.

The use of a placebo treatment in a trial gives rise to the problem of deception. The patients receiving the placebo treatment must believe they are receiving an active treatment. More seriously, there is a possibility that patients may be harmed by receiving a placebo instead of active treatment (e.g. by increased pain, aggravation of their condition). This situation can be alleviated by the use of a crossover trial.

Randomization and blinding are necessary to eliminate any bias from the trial and this may conflict with the individual interest of the participants (e.g. those in the placebo group not receiving active treatment of their condition).

There is a considerable emphasis on protecting participants from the risks of research and this is enshrined in the Helsinki Declaration. A potential issue here is that, because of the strict regulations in place in developed countries, there has been a tendency to outsource clinical trials to countries where the regulations are less strict.

 Because the ICH guidelines on GCP place considerable emphasis on ethical principles, there are some key issues that need to be addressed in designing a clinical trial.

19.9 CLINICAL DATA MANAGEMENT (CDM)

The aspect of clinical trials that ensures the validity, quality and integrity of the data collected is known as clinical data management (CDM). It involves the use of computer-based data systems. During the trial the investigators collect data of various types which is then pooled and statistically analysed, usually by the sponsor of the clinical trial (e.g. a pharmaceutical company). In order for regulatory authorities to be assured that any clinical trials data presented to them is valid, CDM is a regulatory requirement.

The process of CDM initially involves the development of a case report form (CRF) and this will take place at an early stage in the protocol development. The CRF is designed to capture all data recorded in the trial in a standardized format and in such a way as to allow scanning and analysis. The CRF may be traditional paper-based or an e-CRF, where the study data is entered directly into a computer (see Figure 19.3).

Whatever form is used will be required to contain several standard sections:

- Inclusion/exclusion criteria
- Baseline data and demography data
- Data specifically required by the protocol
- Any dose and/or therapy (including non-trial therapy) taken and/or modified
- Adverse events, concomitant medications and inter-current illnesses
- Visits that participants fail to make, tests that are not conducted, and examinations that are not performed
- All withdrawals and dropouts of enrolled participants from the trial reported and explained

Following on from design of the CRF will be the development of a database which, although based on standard formats, will be specific to the requirements of the particular clinical trial. Prior to use the database will be tested and reviewed in a test environment (i.e. a non-study environment), and then made available for use in the clinical trial.

Despite all these precautions it is possible for CDM to encounter problems such as a failure to collect the necessary useful information, the collection of irrelevant information, or the data collection may be of poor quality due to missing values or discrepancies. To deal with issues such as these, by what is

Figure 19.3 Example case report form

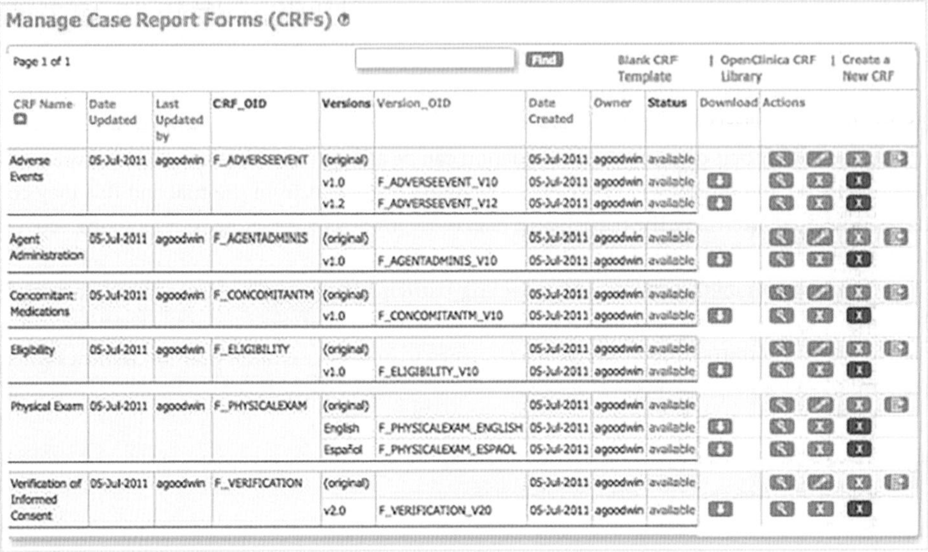

Manage Case Report Forms (CRFs) ⊕

Page 1 of 1   [Find]   Blank CRF Template | OpenClinica CRF Library | Create a New CRF

CRF Name	Date Updated	Last Updated by	CRF_OID	Versions	Version_OID	Date Created	Owner	Status	Download	Actions
Adverse Events	05-Jul-2011	agoodwin	F_ADVERSEEVENT	(original)		05-Jul-2011	agoodwin	available		icons
				v1.0	F_ADVERSEEVENT_V10	05-Jul-2011	agoodwin	available	download	icons
				v1.2	F_ADVERSEEVENT_V12	05-Jul-2011	agoodwin	available	download	icons
Agent Administration	05-Jul-2011	agoodwin	F_AGENTADMINIS	(original)		05-Jul-2011	agoodwin	available		icons
				v1.0	F_AGENTADMINIS_V10	05-Jul-2011	agoodwin	available	download	icons
Concomitant Medications	05-Jul-2011	agoodwin	F_CONCOMITANTM	(original)		05-Jul-2011	agoodwin	available		icons
				v1.0	F_CONCOMITANTM_V10	05-Jul-2011	agoodwin	available	download	icons
Eligibility	05-Jul-2011	agoodwin	F_ELIGIBILITY	(original)		05-Jul-2011	agoodwin	available		icons
				v1.0	F_ELIGIBILITY_V10	05-Jul-2011	agoodwin	available	download	icons
Physical Exam	05-Jul-2011	agoodwin	F_PHYSICALEXAM	(original)		05-Jul-2011	agoodwin	available		icons
				English	F_PHYSICALEXAM_ENGLISH	05-Jul-2011	agoodwin	available	download	icons
				Español	F_PHYSICALEXAM_ESPAOL	05-Jul-2011	agoodwin	available	download	icons
Verification of Informed Consent	05-Jul-2011	agoodwin	F_VERIFICATION	(original)		05-Jul-2011	agoodwin	available		icons
				v2.0	F_VERIFICATION_V20	05-Jul-2011	agoodwin	available	download	icons

referred to as discrepancy management, involves the use of a good clinical data management practice (GCDMP), which is a set of procedures which assesses the validity, quality, and integrity of the collected clinical data within the database.

At the end of the clinical trial the database will be locked to ensure that there can be no further manipulation of the data during its analysis. The data is now ready to be extracted from the database and subjected to detailed statistical analysis (the methods used are beyond the scope of this text). However, there are some key principles which should be adhered to. All outcome measures included in the trial protocol must form part of the analysis. There should be methods for handling missing data and multiplicity of data and justification for utilization of non-standard statistical techniques. Finally, there should be documentation to ensure that any statistical manipulations performed on the original data can be repeated and is all filed at the completion of the trial. All of this analysis will, ultimately, lead to the creation of a clinical study report (CSR) which is then submitted to the appropriate regulatory authority.

 Clinical data management is the process which ensures the quality, integrity and validity of the data collected and analysed during a clinical trial.

? Questions

1. What would you consider to be the potential sources of bias within a clinical trial and how would you design a trial to minimize bias?

2. What is meant by randomization and why is it used in clinical trials?

3. What problems might arise when subject compliance is poor in an intervention study?

4. In a clinical trial of a new statin therapy, what would be used as a primary endpoint—its ability to lower blood cholesterol levels or its ability to prevent heart attacks and ischaemic strokes? What type of trial design would be used?

Chapter summary

- The subjects for a clinical trial will be selected on the basis of predefined inclusion and exclusion criteria.
- The design of a clinical trial needs to take into account the nature and stage of a disorder, which may be acute, chronic, cyclical, or seasonal.
- Clinical trials must be controlled to eliminate bias, reduce variability, and enhance reliability of the outcome.
- The main types of controls used in clinical trials are comparison with no treatment, comparison with a placebo, and comparison with an active comparator.
- In order to eliminate selection bias in clinical trials, a process of randomization is used.
- There are a number of different processes of randomization each of which is applicable to a particular set of circumstances.
- The objectives (both primary and secondary), measurements and endpoints of a clinical trial need to be clearly defined in the trial protocol.
- Blinding is a process designed to eliminate bias in the participants of a clinical trial.
- Clinical trials may be open-label, single-blinded, double-blinded, or triple-blinded.
- A consideration of ethical issues is of great significance in the operation of clinical trials.
- Clinical data management is the process which ensures the quality, integrity, and validity of the data collected and analysed during a clinical trial.

Further reading

Hackshaw, A. (2009) *A Concise Guide to Clinical Trials*. Chichester, UK: Wiley-Blackwell, ISBN 978-1-4051-6774-1.

> A comprehensive overview of the design, conduct, and analysis of clinical trials.

David Brown (2016), see www.ema.europa.eu/docs/en_GB/document_library/.../2016/.../WC500202535.pdf

> This is a pdf of a presentation by David Brown of the MRHA which covers all aspects of clinical trials design, including analytical methods.

Pfeiffer, J. and Wells, C. (2017) *A Practical Guide to Managing Clinical Trials*. CRC Press, Abingdon, Oxfordshire: Taylor & Francis. ISBN 9781138196506.

> A basic, comprehensive guide to managing clinical trials.

(T) CASE STUDY 19.1   CLINICAL TRIALS—IS IT TIME FOR A CHANGE?

The current regulatory system with respect to marketing a new drug involves testing of the drug candidate *in vitro* and in animals followed by at least three lengthy clinical trials in humans. Only at this stage does the pharmaceutical company request a marketing authorization. However, because of the enormous costs in bringing a drug to market, the clinical trials system is increasingly under scrutiny as maybe not being entirely fit for purpose. There are a number of challenges being encountered by the current system, namely recruitment and retention of participants, regulatory constraints, unmet need medical conditions, personalized medicines, and the targets of more complex disease mechanisms.

Recruitment of participants to clinical trials is currently proving problematical. A clinical trial will only be effective if the appropriate patients can be recruited in sufficient numbers. It is not clear whether the problem lies with

→

the unwillingness of patients to participate or a lack of information about how to get involved in a clinical trial. To date, clinical trials have concentrated on measurable outcomes, with little concentration on the patient experience. With the dramatic increase in on-line fora and chatrooms, patients now feel that they should have greater input to a clinical trial rather than simply acting as human 'guinea pigs'.

Safety concerns are the reason why clinical trials are so highly regulated (and rightly so). However this makes it more difficult for pharmaceutical companies to bring a much-needed new product to market. Often different regulatory authorities across the world require different clinical data, requiring companies to undertake multiple clinical trials in order to get world-wide approval. The current clinical trial system was developed for the approval of small molecule drugs but an increasing number of new therapies are being brought forward and this poses different issues (what are these issues?), with the type of information from preclinical studies and clinical trials being more complex.

Related to the problems posed by new therapies are the issues of unmet need conditions and the development of personalized medicines. These could be regarded as 'niche' markets which do not fit within the established clinical trials regulatory framework. However both the FDA and the EMA have introduced alternative pathways for such situations. The FDA, in 2012, introduced a breakthrough therapy design which can speed up the authorization of drugs for patients with serious or life-threatening conditions. However this is largely restricted to a commitment to a fast-track review of an application (60 days compared with the standard of 10 months). The EMA has also introduced a similar approval process for drugs treating conditions with unmet needs. Additionally, the EMA is looking at the introduction of so-called adaptive pathways. These enable a drug to be approved rapidly for a specific patient subgroup, allowing the provision of more detailed clinical data once the drug has been put into clinical usage. Depending on the results, the approval can be widened to other patient groups. Personalized medicine will actively require a movement away from the standard clinical trial format. This type of therapeutic approach will render large-scale clinical trials redundant and they would be required to be replaced by many much smaller trials.

The move towards more complex targets does mean that preclinical studies will become even more important before clinical trials (of whatever format) are carried out. We have already referred to one such instance, where preclinical animal testing did not produce the same outcome as happened in the first human trial (**⟩ XR Integration Box 14.4**). This was where a therapy was targeting a receptor in the immune system but the animals used in the preclinical studies did not express the receptor, and so the human outcome was not predicted in the animal studies. Such differences are maybe to be expected when targeting the immune system as immune systems of all species are not identical. More recently (2016), another clinical trial resulted in a similar outcome—one death, and serious neurological damage, even though preclinical animal studies had not shown any adverse effects. The drug candidate in this instance was an enzyme inhibitor, the enzyme in this case being fatty acid amide hydrolase (FAAH). The inhibition mechanism was by covalent binding—a mechanism used in other established drugs such as aspirin and penicillin antibiotics. Once again, no such toxic effects were observed in rodent toxicity studies and, indeed, another FAAH inhibitor had not shown such toxicity in humans. The answer to this anomaly is likely to involve interactions with enzymes other than the target. There are other hydrolases which are present in the brain and, perhaps equally significantly, are much less active in mice. It is vital, therefore, that any changes to the clinical trials regulatory framework must be based upon detailed, and appropriate, preclinical studies.

GLOSSARY

agonist a molecule that activates a particular receptor to produce a specific response

aminoglycoside a compound with two or more amino sugars joined by a glycoside link to a hexose unit

anaesthesia artificially induced loss of ability to feel pain or other sensations

antagonist a molecule that binds to a receptor but does not trigger the usual response and can block the binding of, and activation by, an agonist at the same receptor

antiarrhythmic a drug used to regulate disturbances of the electrical impulses which control the beating of the heart

anticodon a triplicate tRNA nucleotide sequence that is complementary to the codon in an mRNA sequence

antidepressant a drug used to treat depressive disorders

antimetabolite a substance that competes with, replaces or antagonizes an endogenous metabolite

atrial fibrillation an irregular and usually abnormally fast heartbeat

aziridinium ion the protonated form of a three-membered ring containing an amine group

bacteriophage a virus that infects a bacterium and reproduces inside it

bioavailability the proportion of an administered drug which reaches the systemic circulation unchanged

bioisosteres groups with similar physical or chemical properties which produce broadly similar biological effects

biomarker an objective indication of a medical state observed outside the patient which can be measured accurately and reproducibly

β-blocker an antagonist at β-adrenergic receptors

blood dyscrasia a pathological condition of the blood, usually relating to the cellular components of the blood

bone marrow micronucleus test a test in which erythrocytes sampled from the bone marrow are examined for the presence of the formation of micronuclei which is indicative of induced chromosomal damage

broad spectrum effective against a wide range of diseases or organisms

capillary electrophoresis an analytical technique that separates analytes based on their mobility under the influence of an electric field

capture group functional group within a molecule to which a radiolabelled substrate can be linked

chelate a compound formed by ligand bonds to a central metal atom at two or more points

chelator a compound which combines with metal ions to form stable complexes involving coordinate bonds

chimeric relating to a monoclonal antibody produced from the cells of an organism in which the constant region has been replaced by a sequence of human DNA

chiral a chiral molecule is non-superimposable with its mirror image. A chiral carbon has four different groups bonded to it

chiral auxiliaries a group incorporated into an organic compound in order to control the stereochemical outcome of a synthesis by favouring the production of one stereoisomer in preference to the others

chiral environment an environment that can distinguish one enantiomer from another

clastogenicity disruption or breakages of chromosomes

cloning replication of a fragment of DNA and placing it in an organism to analyse genes or manufacture protein

codon a sequence of base triplets which represents a single amino acid

comet assay an assay which detects DNA strand breaks in eukaryotic cells

compact a compact is formed by the process of compression and consolidation of a powder, e.g. a tablet. Compression involves particle rearrangement under relatively low pressure and consolidation involves formation of a compact mass at relatively high pressure

compaction the conversion of a loose powder into a solid object

compressibility the extent to which a powder is reduced in volume when subjected to an applied pressure

configuration the three-dimensional arrangement of atoms in space

conformation the spatial arrangement or shape of a molecule

depolarization when an excitable cell goes from having a negative resting potential to having a positive internal charge

diastereoisomer stereoisomers not related as object to mirror image

discriminant analysis a statistical analysis used to predict the value of a dependent variable by one or more independent variables

electronic configuration the distribution of electrons of an atom or molecule

electrostatic potential the potential energy due to a positive charge

enantiomeric pertaining to an enantiomer

enantiomers a pair of chiral molecules that are non-superimposable mirror images of each other

endocrine messenger a substance that is secreted directly into the bloodstream

endocytosis process of entering the cell without passing through the cell membrane

endofacial facing towards the interior of a cell

endogenous originating from or produced by an organism

endoplasmic reticulum a series of folded membranes within the cytoplasm of the cell which are associated with protein synthesis and storage

entropy measure of the disorder within a system

exofacial facing away from the interior of a cell

filgrastim a granulocyte colony-stimulating factor (G-CSF) analogue used to treat neutropenia caused by chemotherapy or bone marrow transplantation

formulation the science of converting a drug into a form that is suitable for presentation to a patient

fractional crystallization method of separating substances based on differential solubilities in a particular solvent

freeze-drying a drying process in which the solvent (usually water) is sublimed from the solid (frozen) state

genome `the complete set of genes present in an organism

genomics the study of genes, their function and related techniques

genotype the entire set of genes in an individual

geometrical isomers occur when groups of atoms are arranged asymmetrically about an element of rigidity such as a double bond or a ring

glucuronidation the addition of glucuronic acid to a substrate

glycolipid a lipid containing carbohydrate groups

glycoprotein a protein molecule with carbohydrate groups attached

good manufacturing practice a system for ensuring that products are consistently produced and controlled according to quality standards

gout a type of arthritis in which crystals of sodium urate form in and around the joints

haematocrit the percentage of whole blood that is made up of red blood cells

haemopoiesis the formation of blood cellular components

heteroaromatic an aromatic ring that contains one or more atoms other than carbon

HOMO/LUMO acronyms for highest occupied molecular orbital and lowest unoccupied molecular orbital. The energy difference between these two molecular orbitals relates to **chemical reactivity** the higher the difference the more reactive

homologous series a series of compounds, having similar structures and properties, which differ by a single parameter, usually the length of a carbon chain

hybridoma a hybrid cell used for the production of antibodies in large amounts

hygroscopicity the property of absorbing water from the atmosphere

hyperpolarization when the internal negative charge of an excitable cell becomes more negative

hypersensitivity a set of undesirable reactions produced by the immune system

IC$_{50}$ the concentration at which an antagonist displaces half of the endogenous ligand from a receptor

immortal cells a population of cells which do not undergo natural senescence and can continue to divide allowing them to be grown for prolonged periods *in vitro*

immunoconjugate a complex of an antibody and a toxic agent used to destroy a targeted antigen

immunosuppressant a drug which can suppress or prevent the immune response

immunosuppression suppression of the immune response which may result from certain diseases, certain drugs or may be deliberately induced to prevent rejection of a transplant

inductive effect arises as a result of a difference in electronegativity between two atoms and is transmitted through sigma bonds

intercalator a planar molecule capable of interacting with DNA by insertion between the base pairs of the DNA helix

isoelectric point the pH at which a molecule carries no electrical charge

isosterism groups that exhibit similarities in their chemical and/or physical properties.

isozymes (isoenzymes) enzymes which differ in amino acid sequence but catalyse the same reaction

kinase an enzyme that catalyses the transfer of a phosphate group from one substrate to another

leukaemia production of abnormal white blood cells

leukopenia reduction in the number of white blood cells

linear regression analysis a technique for modelling the relationship between one dependent variable and one or more independent variables

maximum tolerated dose the dose that produces an acceptable level of toxicity or, if exceeded, would put patients at unacceptable risk of toxicity

melting endotherm the peak in DSC caused by absorption of heat due to the transition of a crystalline solid to a liquid

mesomeric effect the transmission of electronic charge by delocalized electrons through the overlapping p orbitals of a molecule such as those within conjugated π bonds

micromass test a test which is based upon the ability to detect the inhibition of the formation of cell foci in the mid-brain of mammalian origin

microtubule hollow cylindrical protein found in the cytoplasm of eukaryotic cells

milling process for reducing the size of particles

mitosis a type of eukaryotic cell division where two identical daughter cells are produced

modified and sustained release formulations these are products which alter the timing and/or the rate of release of a drug, as opposed to immediate release (conventional) products. They include controlled-release and sustained- release as well as delayed-release products (e.g. enteric coated tablets)

molecularity the number of species (molecules or ions) that participate in the rate limiting step of a reaction

monoclonal antibodies antibodies that are produced by identical immune cells which are all clones of a unique parent cell

mucopeptide a peptide found in combination with polysaccharides containing muramic or sialic acids

multiple ascending dose study patients receive multiple low doses of the drug in order to examine the pharmacokinetics and pharmacodynamics of multiple doses. The dose is subsequently escalated to a predetermined level

muscarine an alkaloid found in certain mushrooms which mimics some of the actions of acetylcholine

mutagenic capable of inducing or increasing the frequency of mutation

myelogenous refers to the non-lymphocytic white blood cells

myelotoxic toxic to the bone marrow

myopathy a condition in which muscle fibres do not function correctly, leading to muscle weakness

nephrotoxicity toxicity towards the kidneys

neuropathic pain pain caused by damage or injury to the nerves that transfer information between the central nervous system and the muscles, skin and other parts of the body

neurotransmitter a chemical that transmits a nerve impulse from one nerve cell to another or to a muscle fibre

neutropenia abnormally low number of neutrophils in the blood

NHEJ non-homologous end-joining

nicotine an alkaloid found in plants of the family Solanaceae which mimics some of the actions of acetylcholine

oestrogens are the primary female sex hormones

oligomeric containing a small number of monomeric units

oligonucleotide short sequence of nucleotides forming part of DNA or RNA molecules

optical isomers isomers which rotate plane polarized light in opposite directions (also called enantiomers)

organogenesis the origin or development of organs

paracrine messenger a substance which is released by cells affecting only those cells in close proximity to the site of release

Parkinsonism a progressive disease of the nervous system marked by tremor and muscular rigidity

pattern recognition the identification of patterns in large data sets, using appropriate mathematical methodologies

peptidoglycan a polymer of amino acids and sugars which forms the cell wall of bacteria

p-glycoprotein a protein which pumps many foreign substances out of cells

pharmacodynamic relating to the biochemical and physiological effects drugs have on the body

pharmacogenomics the study of the role of the genome in drug response

pharmacokinetic relating to the absorption, distribution, metabolism and excretion of drugs administered to the body

pharmacophore the structural aspects of a molecule responsible for its biological activity

phenotype physical and biochemical characteristics of an organism as determined by its genetic constitution

phosphoramidase an enzyme that breaks down phosphoramide groups

pili hair-like structures on the cell capsule of prokaryotic cells which allow attachment to other cells and the sharing of genetic material

placebo a treatment that has no therapeutic effect, used as a control when testing new drugs

plasmid a circular double-stranded unit of DNA that replicates within a cell independently of chromosomal DNA most commonly found in bacteria

polyene macrolide molecules which are characterized by a large macrocyclic lactone ring also containing a large number of alkene groups

polymerase chain reaction (PCR) a technique used to make multiple copies of a segment of DNA

polymorphism a discontinuous genetic variation resulting in the occurrence of different types of individuals among the members of a single species

potentiometric titration a volumetric method in which the potential between two electrodes (reference and indicator electrodes) is measured as a function of the added reagent volume

powder density the mass of a powder per unit volume

preformulation the characterization of the physicochemical properties of a drug substance

proteomics that branch of biotechnology relating to the analysis of proteins produced by the genes of a particular cell, tissue or organism

pseudocholinesterase (plasma cholinesterase) an enzyme present in the blood and other organs which hydrolyses acetylcholine more slowly than acetylcholinesterase

quench-cooling the rapid cooling of a molten substance

racemic mixture an equimolar mixture of enantiomers

recessive gene a gene that produces its characteristic phenotype only when its allele is identical

resolving agent an enantiomerically pure compound which when reacted with a racemic mixture forms two diastereoisomers, which can be separated, because they have different physical properties

retrosynthesis the process of designing the chemical synthesis of a target molecule by starting at the target and working backwards to readily available compounds

reverse transcriptase an enzyme that permits DNA to be made using RNA as the template

scintillation fluid a fluid containing molecule(s) which absorbs the energy emitted by radioisotopes and re-emits that energy as light, usually fluorescence

single ascending dose study patients receive a single dose of the drug and if the pharmacokinetics are as expected the dose is escalated to a predetermined level

sink conditions normally requires use of a volume of dissolution medium that is at least five to ten times the volume required to produce a saturated solution of the drug under test

spray-drying method of producing a powder by atomizing a liquid within a hot drying gas

square planar complex a central metal atom is surrounded by constituent atoms which form the four corners of a square in the same plane

statins a group of drugs that act to reduce blood levels of cholesterol

stereoisomers molecules with the same molecular formula and arrangement of atoms that differ from one another in three-dimensional space

supercooled liquid a liquid which has been lowered below its freezing temperature without it becoming a solid

supersaturated solution a solution with more dissolved solute than the solvent would normally dissolve

synthons structural units within a target molecule which is related to a possible synthetic procedure

tautomerism isomers that are in rapid equilibrium with each other

tertiary structure the three-dimensional shape of a protein

T_g glass transition temperature

thrombocytopenia a disorder in which there is an abnormally low amount of platelets in the blood

transesterification the changing of one ester group into a different one

transgenic relating to an organism where genetic material has been altered by the transfer of one or more genes from another species

transgenic animal an animal whose genetic code has been altered

transpeptidation the process of transferring an amino acid from one peptide chain to another

transposon a small piece of DNA which inserts itself into a different place in the genome

xenobiotic a substance that is not normally found in the body

x-ray crystallography used to determine the atomic and molecular structure within a crystal by analysing the diffraction pattern of incident X-rays

zwitterion a molecule that contains both positive and negative charges

INDEX

tables, figures, and boxes are indicated by an italic *t*, *f*, and *b* following the page number